Totally Accessible MRI

Totally Accessible MRI

A User's Guide to Principles, Technology, and Applications

Michael L. Lipton, MD, PhD

With a Foreword by Emanuel Kanal, MD, FACR, FISMRM, AANG

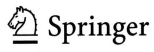 Springer

Michael L. Lipton, MD, PhD
Associate Professor of Clinical Radiology, Psychiatry and Behavioral Sciences
Medical Director, MRI Services
Director of Radiology Research
Albert Einstein College of Medicine and Montefiore Medical Center
Bronx, NY
USA
and
Senior Research Scientist
The Center for Advanced Brain Imaging
The Nathan S. Kline Institute for Psychiatric Research
Orangeburg, NY
USA

ISBN: 978-0-387-48895-0   e-ISBN: 978-0-387-48896-7
DOI: 10.1007/978-0-387-48896-7

Library of Congress Control Number: 2007932970

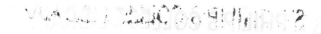

Dedicated to the memory of my grandfathers:

Samuel Parelman
Samuel B. Lipton
Meyer Light
Herman Blitz
Siegfried Rosenthal

Stature of character and ethic,
Unqualified love and support
Justifiable pride in their enduring legacy
Stand as an example for us all.

May their memory be a blessing.

Foreword

BS"D

All magnetic resonance technologists and all radiologists who work with magnetic resonance (MR) technology can be divided into two subgroups: (1) those who understand the underlying physics principles and how to apply them; and (2) those who do not.

For so many patients and for so many diagnostic considerations, the difference between membership in these two groups is minimal. One can easily diagnose a vestibular schwannoma and accurately differentiate it from a cerebellopontine angle meningioma without being that well versed with many of the concepts underlying the creation of the MR images on which these tumors are depicted. One by rote can generate images of the pelvis that are quite diagnostic and aesthetically pleasing without really understanding the intricate interrelationships between the varying imaging parameters used in the generation of the obtained image contrast.

There are certain situations, however, for which a more in-depth understanding is required. For example: Seeing tissue signal disappear on a short T1 inversion-recovery sequence yet recognizing that it does not have to originate from fat but may come from methemoglobin or some other short T1 tissue may prove clinically vital for arriving at the correct diagnosis. For such circumstances, understanding the underlying principles that govern the creation of the image and the contrast contained therein is critical and sets one apart—and distinctly ahead—of the competition, who cannot make this claim.

In the two-plus decades during which I have taught my courses on MR physics entitled, "Clinical MR Physics: Understanding and Applying," I have had the good fortune to teach literally thousands of eager students. Among the most eager and most persistent was Dr. Michael Lipton. Never satisfied with a superficial understanding, he always asked for more and continually sought a deeper level of understanding of the underlying concepts in a never-ending effort to build upon and improve upon that which we already know.

vii

With this text, Dr. Lipton attempts to impart some of his vast knowledge to one just starting out on a journey toward understanding this fascinating technology. In a clearly written and disarmingly informal style more reminiscent of conversational tone than formal lecture, Dr. Lipton breaks down many of the concepts involved in the clinical magnetic resonance imaging process into bite-sized pieces that are easy to swallow and digest. Steering clear of most mathematics and quantum mechanics and remaining firmly grounded in classical physics and explanations, Dr. Lipton sheds light on many topics that can be so difficult to so many. By so doing, he is attempting to modify the ratio of "understanders" to "rote performers" we find in our MR society today. I hold this to be quite a commendable objective, and I applaud Dr. Lipton for his efforts. You, too, are to be commended, because reading this book is clear evidence that you have taken your first steps in trying to switch camps to the "understanders" group.

With G-d's Help and through the assistance of Michael's pen, may you be granted the wisdom to attain your objectives and, more importantly, apply them to the benefit of the patients entrusted to your care.

Emanuel Kanal, MD, FACR, FISMRM, AANG
Pittsburgh, Pennsylvania

Why This Book?

Nam et ipsa scientia potestas est [Knowledge itself is power].
—Sir Francis Bacon (*Of Heresies*, 1597)

The pages that follow are, in a very large part, an outgrowth of an intensive but accessible course in the physical basis and practical use of magnetic resonance imaging (MRI) technology that I have had the privilege and pleasure to present semiannually at Montefiore Medical Center/Albert Einstein College of Medicine since 1997. It is at the urging of numerous current and former students that I finally undertook to transform the contents of the course and its syllabus into a cohesive written work. My approach in preparing this book has been to mirror the experience of the course, to the extent that is possible given the restrictions of a one-sided conversation.

The course remains oriented toward and open to anyone who wishes to understand MRI, from the ground up, as used in clinical medicine; it is not merely a crash course to review for the radiology physics examinations. When the study of physics and technology is broached among clinical radiologists, a common refrain is "why, beyond passing our exams, do we need to know it." The fact is that most clinical radiologists, simply because of its seemingly overwhelming complexity and their heavy clinical workloads, remain largely in the dark with regard to the physical basis of the technology they wield. However, as we will see, a large part of the diagnostic power of MRI lies in understanding the physical basis of the images you examine. Further, when, inevitably, images do not turn out as they should, a modest awareness of the "inner workings" of MRI leaves the user poised to understand and perhaps remedy the problem. I maintain that everything contained in these pages has direct importance and utility in clinical imaging. Nonetheless, as a part-time scientist, I believe the material is equally useful and important for nonclinicians. The responses of several graduate students and faculty scientists who have attended the course looking for a rigorous but very approachable introduction have borne this out.

In the interest of making the material as accessible as possible to as wide an audience as possible, I assume no specific background whatsoever on the part of my students. (Attendees range from undergraduates to full professors but are predominately radiology residents.) Although it is certainly true that mathematics is exquisitely well-suited for expression of the concepts underlying MRI, I choose to take an entirely nonmathematical approach; only one equation need be learned and recalled in order to fully absorb the information. Where I do include equations, it is for the benefit of those who find it a useful way to consolidate their understanding of concepts.

Above all, this book is intended for users of MRI; it is not an exhaustive reference work and not a pulse sequence developer's handbook. The book is designed to be read. Most importantly, however, I implore you to take the concepts detailed in the following pages with you as you review clinical images, assess abnormalities, and confront artifacts and otherwise suboptimal images. One thing I can virtually guarantee: when it comes to MRI, it is use it or lose it. Come join the users; the alternative doesn't sound very good!

Michael L. Lipton, MD, PhD

A User's Guide

The scientists of today think deeply instead of clearly. One must be sane to think clearly, but one can think deeply and be quite insane.
—Nikola Tesla (*Modern Mechanics and Inventions*, 1934)

We are forced to live with [scientific advances] whether we want or not and try to make the best out of it.
—Richard R. Ernst (Nobel Banquet Speech, 1991)

This book was written to be read. It is not a reference book but rather a conversation of sorts that you are invited to join. Our common goal will be a clear understanding of MRI. I begin at the beginning: the only prior knowledge required is of the most basic concepts of vectors—their addition and decomposition. A concise exposition of this essential foundation topic is provided in Appendix 1. With this small bit of background in hand, the book can be approached as a self-contained narrative, in sequence, providing a comprehensive understanding of nuclear magnetic resonance (NMR) and basic and advanced MRI techniques.

Always keep clearly in view that our goal is to understand essential principles to the extent that they facilitate our understanding and enhance our application of clinically relevant imaging techniques. In order to maintain a readable narrative format, I have deliberately avoided specific literature references for the myriad concepts and applications described in these pages. It goes without saying, however, that I come as an expositor and not an originator of these concepts. As Dr. Emanuel Kanal once remarked to me (I paraphrase): As we struggle to understand this stuff, remember that someone figured it out the first time around! Those readers interested in more in-depth, specialized, or mathematical approaches may wish to consult one of the sources listed in Appendix 4 and the original research cited in those references.

I have divided the book into three parts. Part I covers the concepts of NMR, *without creating an image*, just an NMR signal. This part is important because it develops all of the concepts underlying image contrast that are central to clinical imaging. In discussing the basics of the NMR phenomenon, I have not, as is customary in introductory texts, shied away from the quantum mechanical nature of this phenomenon. My rationale is simple: using analogies of classical mechanics and electromagnetism is misleading, wrong, and ultimately proves more confusing than helpful. To keep this section open and accessible, however, I have taken a qualitative approach and not delved into the mathematics. I believe the presentation is, nonetheless, a truthful description of NMR and provides a more satisfying and complete explanation than one forced using classical physics analogies.

The concepts of excitation and relaxation and the parameters T1, T2, and T2* are essential principles developed in Part I that will be referred to over and over again in subsequent chapters. Additionally, be advised that without understanding the concepts underlying the spin echo, you cannot understand spin echo or turbo spin echo imaging or magnetic susceptibility–related contrast (Parts II and III).

Part I ends with an overview of the hardware elements of the MRI scanner system. Some overall understanding of the components is extremely useful when we delve into imaging in Part II. A thorough understanding of the concept of the gradient magnetic field, however, should be considered an absolute prerequisite to understanding imaging in Parts II and III.

A word of caution: It is quite common for students who attend my course to inquire about skipping the first day and a half when basic NMR and image reconstruction concepts (Parts I and II in this book) are covered. These individuals, busy as they are, are understandably interested in attending only those sessions that address clinical imaging applications such as pulse sequences, artifacts, magnetic resonance angiography (MRA), and diffusion imaging. I always balk at these requests, generally refusing them outright. On the rare occasion when I accede to a persistent plea, it inevitably backfires. Simply put, if you are not equipped with a basic understanding of NMR, you will certainly be lost and frustrated trying to understand, say, turbo spin echo imaging. I implore you to strongly consider reading the chapters in order.

Part II encompasses the basics of *imaging*. In the first portion of this part, we cover the building of an MRI image from a spatially encoded NMR signal. Be advised that this part (Chapter 6) is, hands down, the most difficult material in the entire book. Keep in mind that our goal in covering this material is not to become experts in the raw physics or the design of MRI pulse sequences but rather to understand the components of an image and a pulse sequence and how choices made when selecting these elements impact image quality, imaging time, and other outcomes. Take heart! From this point on, the material will begin to "jell" as we unify our background knowledge to begin *imaging*. The remainder of Part II introduces our basic pulse sequence types: spin echo and gradient echo. A clear understanding of the basics of these imaging methods forms a solid foundation for our discussion of more advanced techniques in Part III. Safety and image quality are also included in Part II precisely because they are *basics*.

Whereas Parts I and II form a continuous narrative that is best studied in sequence, Part III allows, perhaps, more room for discretion and selection. Each chapter explores an advanced topic in MRI. Although each chapter builds on the material presented in Parts I and II, the chapters of Part III do not specifically depend one on the other. Bear in mind that each of the topics in Part III could be the subject of an entire textbook. I have aimed to distill the essential elements of each technique and point out its practical application. Sources for further study are listed in Appendix 4.

The language of MRI is almost a field unto itself. Abbreviations and acronyms seem to propagate endlessly. Although the abundance of jargon and catchy but cryptic abbreviations presents a challenge to the newcomer, it is simply a fact of life that is not likely to change. To bridge the language barrier somewhat, Appendix 2 contains a glossary of essential MRI terms used in the book. Although each term is defined when it is introduced in the text, this one-stop reference will prove useful when reading later chapters that do not redefine each and every term. Appendix 3 contains a rather long list of MRI symbols, abbreviations, and acronyms. I have endeavored to include those items that surface throughout the book but have also listed many that are not mentioned at all. Consider this a ready reference when an unintelligible string of letters confronts you in a journal or rolls off your physicist's tongue.

It is my fervent hope, and I dare say my expectation, that anyone who reads through as outlined above will find themselves better equipped to not merely understand but also to *use* MRI in their day-to-day practice. Then, recalling (or looking up) the principles discussed can truly open your eyes to important nuances of your images that went unnoticed before. Constantly holding your images to this higher level of scrutiny will enhance your understanding and, as far as physics is concerned, how you will use it, not lose it!

Michael L. Lipton, MD, PhD

Acknowledgments

I have learned much from my teachers, even more from my colleagues, but I have learned the most from my students.

—Babylonian Talmud—Taanit

The Talmudic dictum is apt in considering the major forces that drove the development of this book. It is more than 10 years of teaching radiology residents and others about MRI that has honed my approach and presentation. To all of my former and current students, I owe tremendous recognition for their interest, patience, and perseverance. Their many insightful questions and demands for clarification and substantiation have been perhaps the single most important influence on my understanding of MRI and its presentation in this book. Thankfully, they have never let me get away with anything! Although the list of individual students is too long to include here, I do wish to specifically acknowledge the first small group who was willing to sit around a conference table in the original Harold G. Jacobson Library at Montefiore Medical Center and bear with my first iterations: Ginny Bakshi, Bruce Berkowitz, and Janet Spector.

My continuous tenure at Albert Einstein College of Medicine and Montefiore Medical Center is somewhat unusual by academic standards. In no small part, it has evolved this way because of the exceptional support I have received from our chairman, Steve Amis, and the exceptional and collegial faculty and staff with whom I have had the pleasure to work. The many facets of my career that have developed over the past years benefited greatly from the support, guidance, and mentoring I have been fortunate to receive from Jacqueline A. Bello, director of neuroradiology. Without her support and sacrifice, the circumstances that led to this publication would not have transpired.

I have been fortunate to tap two wellsprings in developing an understanding of MRI. Manny Kanal was my first actual teacher of MRI physics. By welcoming me not only to Pittsburgh but into their home, he and his wonderful wife, Judy, set the stage for an ongoing correspondence that has been an invaluable resource. I am further certain that Manny's rigorous yet accessible teaching style has influenced me as well.

My position in the Center for Advanced Brain Imaging (CABI) at the Nathan S. Kline Institute for Psychiatric Research provided me immersion in MRI as well as an ongoing interaction with MR scientists and developers. To the founding director of CABI, Joe Helpern, and its current director, my mentor Craig Branch, I express my appreciation for the opportunity to benefit from the CABI and their interest and expertise. My colleagues at the CABI—David Guilfoyle, Honza Hrabe, David Lewis, Gaby Pell, Jody Tanabe, and Bob Bilder—have been a welcome influence as well.

The manuscript was read in part by Tamar Gold and Bill Gomes and has benefited from their insightful suggestions. David Lewis and David Guilfoyle each helped me with image reconstruction techniques used to generate selected figures. I am indebted to my photographic assistants Gittel, Miriam, Shmuel, and Chava and my reliable model Tamar.

My editor at Springer, Rob Albano, as well as Sadie Forrester have been extremely gracious—and patient—in allowing this project to come to fruition. Liz Corra, developmental editor for Springer, has been an absolute pleasure to work with and has provided organizational suggestions that truly enhance the user-friendliness of the book. Liz patiently waited for and promptly processed each component of the manuscript I sent her way, no matter how stale my promise may have been. I thank my dedicated assistant, Jessica Delvalle, for her prompt attention to detail.

My dear father, Dr. Arthur Lipton, spent many hours reading the entire manuscript in detail, providing numerous suggestions that have enhanced it considerably. I further owe any writing ability I wield to my father. He, more than any professional teacher of English, taught me to express myself using the written word. It is my hope that this book is in some way a testament to his efforts.

To my parents, Arthur and Judith Lipton, I, of course, owe everything. A special belated note of appreciation is due for their unending and unconditional support. In the same vein, my parents-in-law, Gary and Rose Ann Rosenthal, have been a cornerstone of support since I merited to join their family almost 19 years ago.

Gittel, Miriam, Tamar, Shmuel, Chava, Aaron, and Rafael graciously indulged the time their father devoted to the writing of this volume. Although this endeavor only added to many other time-intensive professional commitments, they nonetheless allowed me the quiet to finish the job, interrupting only to express encouragement and offer suggestions.

To my precious wife, Leah, I owe more than everything. These pages would be empty were it not for her support, encouragement, and perseverance.

Michael L. Lipton, MD, PhD

Contents

Part I
In the Beginning: Generating, Detecting, and Manipulating the MR (NMR) Signal

1
Laying the Foundation: Nuclear Magnetism, Spin, and the NMR Phenomenon

The Overall Aim

If we bring together a group of people involved in magnetic resonance imaging (MRI) and present them with a magnetic resonance (MR) image, each will see something different in that image. Radiologists will hone in on subtle pathology, psychiatry researchers will notice minute asymmetries in cortical sulci, technologists may pick up on poor positioning, and physicists will evaluate signal-to-noise and detect artifacts. What are we all trying to achieve at the end of the day? Regardless of the type of image acquired or the purpose for which it was acquired, our single common goal in MRI is this:

> Differentiate the tissue in two adjacent locations based on the way that tissue behaves in the MRI environment.

If the signal extracted from those two locations is identical, we cannot differentiate the two tissues from each other. This could be because each location does in fact contain the same tissue (e.g., two locations within the cortex of the kidney) or because the MR image was not made sensitive to the difference between the two tissues. In this latter case, a tumor could be virtually indistinguishable from the normal tissue within which it is growing.

To accomplish our goal of differentiating adjacent tissues of different composition, two tasks must be accomplished in properly designing the MRI examination: (1) resolving the tissues to unique locations in the image and (2) detecting different signal amplitude (intensity) from the two tissues.

Spatial Resolution

The image must be physically capable of resolving the two locations of interest in the tissue to distinct locations within the image; that is, the image must have sufficient *spatial resolution*. An MR image represents a slice of tissue with a defined thickness. This slice is then divided into a two-dimensional array of prism-shaped pieces that we call voxels (for "volume elements"). If we are trying, for example, to differentiate a 5-mm nodule in the liver of a cancer patient from the surrounding normal liver tissue, the voxel must be close to or, preferably, smaller than 5 mm. This is because each voxel is sampled as a single MRI signal that is an average of signal arising from *all* of the tissue within the voxel. In our example liver nodule, if the voxel is so large, say 10 mm, that it contains more normal tissue than abnormal, the average signal we sample will be dominated by normal tissue. Because this signal is no different than that arising from adjacent voxels containing normal liver, the nodule may go undetected.

Contrast Resolution

The MRI acquisition must also elicit a different signal from each of the tissues we wish to separate. That is, the image must have sufficient *contrast resolution*. Even if the image has exceptional spatial resolution (i.e., very small voxels much smaller than the lesion of interest), if both the nodule and normal liver yield the same signal, we will be unable to differentiate the nodule from normal liver tissue. In an effort to maximize the difference in signal between tissues, we modulate the measured signal by adjusting the parameters of the MR acquisition.

As we progress in our understanding of MRI, do not lose sight of the fact that all we are ever trying to do is to differentiate two adjacent tissues based on their different MR signal. The same is true for any and all MRI images whether spin echo, diffusion weighted, or even functional MRI.

Where Does the MRI Signal Come From?

Before we venture into the realm of imaging, we must first understand how the MR signal is generated and measured. To keep things manageable, the following disclaimer should be kept in mind: *Until further notice*, we will limit our discussion to the measurement of signal from a homogeneous sample (maybe a bowl of Jell-O?). *No* attempt will be made, at this point, to determine where in the sample the signal comes from; the signal comes from everywhere in the entire sample.

Nuclear Magnetic Resonance

Nuclear magnetic resonance (NMR) is a physical phenomenon that occurs when *certain* elements interact with a magnetic field. NMR is the process by which the signal detected in MRI is generated; it is the foundation on which MRI is built. Some common elements that demonstrate NMR are

TABLE 1-1. Some elements that undergo NMR.

^{1}H	^{31}P
^{13}C	^{19}F
^{15}N	^{129}Xe

listed in Table 1-1. In order to qualify for this list (and other elements and isotopes do qualify), the element must have a nonzero magnetic moment. It is not necessary for us to delve into what a nonzero magnetic moment is, but it will be present when either the number of protons *or* neutrons in an atom is odd. Thus, helium can never undergo NMR because its nucleus is composed of two protons and two neutrons. So why is it so important that the atom have an odd number of protons or neutrons? A truthful answer requires a discussion involving quantum mechanics. We will touch on this a bit in the following sections. The bottom line, however, is only those nuclei with nonzero magnetic moments demonstrate a property called *spin angular momentum*. The essential role of spin angular momentum in NMR will be introduced shortly.

Spin Semantics

Although many nuclei can undergo NMR, we will confine our discussion to the hydrogen nucleus (^{1}H). The type of sample we will be imaging and the question that we wish to answer directs the choice of nucleus to be examined. In human tissue, which is composed largely of hydrogen-containing water (H_2O), hydrogen is the most abundant of all the NMR-capable nuclei. For this reason, human MRI is focused almost exclusively on hydrogen. However, if we wished to look at energy metabolism and ATP, ^{31}P would be the nucleus of choice. If we were interested in glucose metabolism, ^{13}C would be best.

Because the hydrogen nucleus contains a single proton and nothing more, hydrogen nuclei are also referred to merely as

What about the electrons?

As small charged subatomic particles, electrons also demonstrate magnetism and spin. Thus, they demonstrate both magnetism and spin angular momentum. Why, then, are we ignoring them in our discussion of NMR? Because of their much smaller mass, electrons have a much higher gyromagnetic ratio and precess at frequencies in the gigahertz range; signals in this frequency range will not be detected by our detection hardware (see Chapter 5). Additionally, their resonance signal—called electron spin resonance, or ESR—is comparatively weak relative to the NMR signal. The magnetic fields expressed by electrons, however, are quite important, as they induce variability in the static magnetic field of the MRI scanner (B_0), causing the chemical shift effects so important in spectroscopy and imaging.

protons. As we will see shortly, the nucleus must have a quantum mechanical property termed *nuclear spin*. For this reason, nuclei are also commonly referred to merely as spins. Note that

> For human MRI, the terms *nucleus, proton,* and *spin* are interchangeable.

in the case of NMR of nuclei other than ^{1}H, the term *proton* would be incorrect, whereas the term *spin* would be appropriate.

Prerequisites to NMR: Nuclear Magnetism

NMR is based on the presence of two properties of the atom: (1) magnetism and (2) spin angular momentum. The protons within the nucleus of any atom contain electric charge and generate a magnetic field. Whereas it is tempting to think of such nuclear magnetism in terms of classic electromagnetic phenomena with spinning charges generating a magnetic field based on Faraday's law of induction, nuclear magnetism is in fact a quantum mechanical phenomenon, and nuclear particles do not, as currently understood, actually spin in the physical sense.

Nuclear magnetism does, nonetheless, result in a very real magnetic field that is local to the nucleus and behaves just like the magnetic field of a permanent magnet or compass needle. Magnetic field lines describe this nuclear magnetic field and are identical to those generated by a common bar-shaped permanent magnet (Fig. 1-1).

Basic Electricity and Magnetism: *Faraday's Law of Induction*

Moving charge (i.e., electricity) will induce (generate) a magnetic field. It really is that simple. The key to understanding NMR, however, is that *Faraday's law also works in reverse! Moving magnetic fields induce electricity—voltage and/or current in a conductor.*

A real-life example: In a hydroelectric dam, the rushing water pushes turbines that spin large magnets nestled within huge coils of wire. The moving magnets induce voltage in these wires, ultimately sending electric current through the power lines that provide the electricity that runs your toaster. *Remember: We require magnets in motion. In the case of the hydroelectric dam, the magnets are permanent; in MRI, they are water protons.*

Field lines are not something magical. They are very real and a useful way to describe the strength, orientation, and homogeneity of a magnetic field (see Chapter 5). For our descriptions of nuclear magnetism, however, it will suffice to describe the magnetic field of the nucleus using a single vector. The orientation of this magnetic field vector will indicate the orientation of the nuclear magnetic field, and the length of the vector will indicate the strength of the field. In the absence of any magnetic field external to the nucleus, orientation of the nuclear magnetic field will be random. In

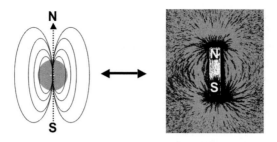

FIGURE 1-1. The proton's magnetic field. The magnetic field lines of a common bar magnet (right) are shown by the distribution of iron filings. The magnetic field of a proton (left) behaves in the same manner, exhibiting field lines and polarity identical to those produced by the bar magnet.

the presence of an externally applied magnetic field, however, the nuclear magnetic field will align with the externally applied magnetic field, much as a compass needle aligns with the earth's magnetic field.

At this point, we have described the magnetism of the ^{1}H nucleus and can see that our proton essentially behaves as a tiny magnet, aligning with an external applied magnetic field. To demonstrate NMR and be useful for MRI, however, the proton must also have *spin angular momentum*.

Prerequisites to NMR: Nuclear Spin Angular Momentum

Spin angular momentum is a property of certain nuclei (those that exhibit NMR). Its existence becomes apparent when we observe the interaction of such a nucleus with an externally applied magnetic field. Though not precisely applicable to the world of small particles like atomic nuclei, a real-world example can at least give us a feeling for what angular momentum is. When a figure skater crouches into a high-velocity spin, the skater may wobble. If we ask the skater what he or she felt during that spin, they will describe a centrifugal force pushing his or her body away from its vertical alignment. In fact, any Olympic hopeful skater will tell us that it takes substantial energy to resist this force and maintain the spin. Similarly, if we take a small weight, tie it to the end of a string, and whirl the string and weight overhead like a lasso, what happens? The string remains taut. Again, this centrifugal force is at work. The physical phenomenon that produces this centrifugal force is called *angular momentum*. The same force causes the wobble of a spinning top.

Spin angular momentum is an analogous force that is applicable to small particles such as atomic nuclei. Consider another macroscopic example. Tie a permanent magnet to a string and suspend it a few centimeters above a tabletop; the entire system will lie at rest with the string plumb to gravity. Next, place a second permanent magnet on the tabletop and slide it under the suspended magnet. What happens? The suspended magnet will begin to swing from side to side over the magnet placed below it on the tabletop (Fig. 1-2A). The magnet below attracts the suspended magnet, causing it to move closer. Momentum of the suspended magnet causes it to overshoot the location of the magnet below. Next, the suspended magnet is drawn back toward the magnet on the tabletop. Ultimately, the suspended magnet swings back and forth in a straight line until it eventually slows and comes to rest over the magnet that was placed on the tabletop. Why does the suspended magnet stop swinging? The system comes to rest only because of friction within the suspensory mechanism. If a completely frictionless system could be developed to suspend the magnet, it would swing back and forth forever! By the way, although the direction in which the magnet swings is completely unrestricted, it will swing back and forth in a straight line.

Let's complicate the system slightly. Install a small motor at the point where the string is suspended and rotate the string at this point. Note that the string is still free to swing back and forth. What happens now? Instead of swinging back and forth in a straight line, the spinning magnet moves in a circular trajectory around the magnet lying on the table below (Fig. 1-2B). If we would map the path of the suspending string, it would delineate a cone. This change from a linear to a circular path is due only to the pres-

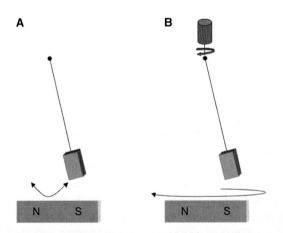

FIGURE 1-2. Spin angular momentum. (A) The magnet suspended from a universal joint is free to swing in any direction. (N and S refer to the poles of the magnet.) When a second magnet is placed underneath it, the suspended magnet will swing back and forth through a plane parallel to the magnetic field of the stationary magnet. Only because of friction at its point of attachment will the suspended magnet eventually come to rest. (B) When the point of attachment is connected to the shaft of a small motor, angular momentum is added to the system. When the second magnet is positioned underneath, the suspended magnet circles so that the string to which it is attached traces the surface of a cone.

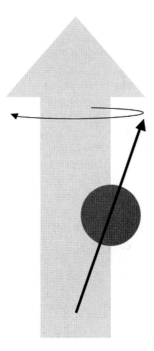

FIGURE 1-3. Precession. Interaction of the magnetic field of the proton with an applied magnetic field leads to precession. The vector describing the proton's magnetic field circles that describing the static magnetic field. Its path traces the surface of a cone.

ence of angular momentum. This same phenomenon is responsible for the wobbling of a gyroscope, top, or *dreidel.* Because such devices have "spin," when they interact with the earth's gravitational field, they pursue the same conical trajectory.

Now let's look at the same phenomenon as it pertains to nuclei. Nuclei have charge that confers nuclear magnetism. When placed in an externally applied magnetic field, they will interact with that field in much the same way as a compass needle interacts with the earth's magnetic field: they will oscillate. If the nucleus also has spin angular momentum, it will not oscillate but will *precess* around the externally applied magnetic field, pursuing the same type of conical trajectory described above (Fig. 1-3).

What Is Spin?

The preceding description of spin angular momentum drew on examples from classical mechanics. These examples are useful but are ultimately inadequate for accurately describing the behavior of very small particles such as nuclei. Quantum mechanics is required to fully explain the effects of spin angular momentum at the nuclear level. Although a full quantum mechanical description is beyond our scope and is *not* necessary for an understanding of MRI, it is worthwhile to be aware of the quantum definition of "spin" described in the box in this section. Note that nuclear spin does not imply that the nuclei actually spin in the physical sense; in the world of quantum mechanics, small particles such as nuclei exhibit angular momentum, *but do not actually spin.*

Based on the background we have developed thus far, the "requirements" for the NMR effect can be succinctly stated as follows:

1. Nonzero charge provides nuclear magnetism.
2. Nonzero spin provides spin angular momentum.

Both of these characteristics are central in determining the nature of the interactions of nuclei with an externally applied magnetic field, and both must be present before an MRI signal or image can be obtained.

Nuclear Spin

Is a quantum mechanical phenomenon describing the behavior of very small particles;

Is proportional to spin angular momentum:

○ More spin = greater spin angular momentum;

Is described by the spin number: either 0, a whole integer, or a noninteger multiple of ½:

○ Spin = 0, if there are an even number of *both* protons and neutrons. Such nuclei (like He) do not exhibit NMR;
○ Spin is an integer if there is an odd number of *both* protons and neutrons;
○ Spin is a noninteger multiple of ½ for all other nuclei;
○ Spin ranges from 0 to 7; *higher spin number = greater spin angular momentum.*

Spin determines the *gyromagnetic ratio.* This constant value is unique for each element and independent of magnetic field strength. It describes the strength of the NMR response (the frequency of precession ω) of a nucleus, and, thus, we will see it directs how we will be able to detect that nucleus using NMR.

Interaction of Protons with a Static Magnetic Field (B)

In the absence of a magnetic field external to the one exhibited by the spins, the orientation of the spins' magnetization will be completely random such that the vector sum of their magnetization will be zero. We must consider two consequences of the spins' interaction with B. First, just as a compass needle will align with the earth's magnetic field, the proton's magnetic field will align with B. Spins tend to align parallel *or* antiparallel (parallel, but pointing in the opposite direction) to B. After the spins' magnetizations align with B, the vector sum will be nonzero, yielding a net magnetic field. In this state, we say that the sample has become magnetized. The alignment of spin magnetization is in some way analogous to the preferred alignment of two permanent magnets. The "antiparallel" orientation is in fact the most likely to occur. When you press two small bar magnets together, the north pole of each will tend to align with the south pole of the other. Whereas two bar magnets will *always* assume this "antiparallel" alignment, the magnetization of our spins will align both antiparallel and parallel. This is because of the quantum mechanical nature of nuclear magnetism. The majority of the magnetization will yield a vector sum of zero with only a small excess vector sum detectable in the antiparallel orientation. This small excess is approximately equivalent to the magnetization of six nuclei in a sample of 10,000. That tiny net magnetization is the signal we must detect in order to make an MR image. However, we will soon see that this tiny component of magnetization cannot be detected unless we manipulate its orientation using the NMR effect. Second, because the spins precess about B they never fully assume a truly parallel orientation with respect to B. The influence of spin angular momentum leads to the proton's magnetization vector describing a cone (Fig. 1-3). This pattern of motion is termed *precession*. The gyromagnetic ratio—indicated by the Greek letter γ and expressed in units of MHz/T—is the unique value for each nucleus that allows us to determine the frequency (think of it as rate or speed) at which the nucleus will precess around a static magnetic field B. The gyromagnetic ratio in combination with the strength of B tells us the frequency of precession (i.e., the rate or "speed" at which each proton precesses around the axis of B), indicated by the Greek letter ω: $\omega = \gamma B$. This is the famous Larmor equation.

In the ensuing discussions, we will, until further notice, assume a constant and perfectly homogeneous externally applied magnetic field (B), referred to from now on as B_0. This means that the strength and orientation of B_0 is exactly the same in every location, so that each and every spin "sees" the same B_0. Because we will be dealing with a homogeneous magnetic field B_0, we will speak in terms of the Larmor frequency of the nucleus at that field strength. It is termed ω_0. Thus,

$$\omega_0 = \gamma B_0$$

You *must* know this equation, but this is the *only* equation that you will have to know.

Describing a Real-Life Sample: Dealing with Many Spins

In reality, whether our sample is a solution in a test tube or the human body, we never observe a single proton. Rather, billions of protons are observed *as a group*. The signal that we measure is the aggregate signal generated by *all* spins in the sample. Just as we measure the aggregate signal, in our discussions of NMR and MRI we will deal with this composite signal rather than discuss the behavior of individual spins. Although each proton is an individual, so to speak, we can describe this entire group of spins without misrepresenting the contribution of even one individual spin. The net magnetization vector (NMV), also called M_0, gives us this "bird's-eye view" of the whole sample of spins. Here we will put vector addition into practice.

In order to find the NMV, we first decompose the vector of each spin into components parallel and perpendicular to B_0. Adding the component vectors parallel to B_0, which we call longitudinal component vectors, yields a single vector that is also parallel to B_0. This vector will be called M_z. Next we will deal with the component vectors perpendicular to B_0, calling them transverse component vectors, or M_t. Although all spins precess at the same rate (ω_0)—remember, they all "feel" the same B_0, and $\omega = \gamma B_0$—they are not all at the same point in their precession about B_0. That is, the transverse components do not all point in the same direction at any one point in time. In fact, the arrangement of the spins along the path of precession is completely random. We call this *random phase*. Given a large sample of spins— remember that we are dealing with millions, billions, or trillions of spins—we will find a transverse component vector with orientation exactly opposite each and every component vector. These transverse component vectors yield a vector sum of zero. In other words, for each transverse component vector, there is another one pointing in the opposite direction to cancel it. Recall that the magnitude of each of these component vectors is identical because each derives from a single proton experiencing an identical B_0. Random phase means that all transverse components cancel each other.

The *net* magnetization is now *correctly* represented as a single vector parallel to B_0 with a magnitude equal to the sum of the longitudinal component vectors. Note that whereas each protons' vector demonstrates precession, the NMV is stationary because the "precessing component" of magnetization has summed to zero.

The Energy Configuration Approach: A Painless (Really!) Bit of Quantum Mechanics

Overview

Explanations of the NMR phenomenon that employ principles of classical mechanics and electromagnetism abound in introductory texts on NMR and

MRI. This approach, however, inevitably runs aground, unable to really explain what is going on. This is because classical physics is not capable of explaining the behavior of very small particles such as nuclei undergoing NMR. In order to understand what is going on during NMR, we must view the events through the lens of quantum mechanics. The problem is that a full understanding of quantum mechanics is well beyond the scope of this book

> **A note to the faint-hearted:** This is a nonmathematical explanation of a nonetheless complex topic. It is, I believe, a more satisfying explanation than the forced classical physics descriptions. Once we understand this approach to NMR, the inconsistencies inherent in the prevalent classical explanations will be glaring. You *do not*, however, need to do the math in order to grasp the key concepts presented here.

and beyond what most MRI users (even MRI scientists) want and need to know. So, on the one hand we have relatively easy to understand phenomena (classical approach) that do not accurately explain NMR. On the other hand, esoteric and more difficult to understand phenomena (quantum mechanics) can elegantly explain the physical basis of NMR. It is indeed tempting to take the easy path and use the classical explanations, hoping that some hand waving will suffice where the approach fails.

Another approach for those who reject the simpler but inadequate classical physics explanations is to simply accept various tenets of the NMR phenomena as postulates or articles of faith.

Our approach, on the other hand, will be to take the "high road" and invoke quantum mechanical explanations to expose the truth of MRI. The catch is that we propose to do so without delving into the more esoteric details of quantum mechanics and certainly not into the mathematics. Although the mathematics provides the clearest and most complete delineation of these concepts, it is not necessary in order to gain adequate insight to support a very good working knowledge of MRI. Our rationale for this approach is that it affords "an explanation that actually makes sense" and allows the student of MRI to see a logic behind the apparent NMR voodoo. This understanding of basic mechanisms is not an end in itself but in turn enhances understanding of concepts such as spin relaxation and facilitates retention of important concepts and their application to other aspects of NMR and MRI.

Probability and Certainty

The world of quantum mechanics is very different from the world that we are accustomed to. First, we perceive a continuous spectrum of possibilities. Human vision, for example, does not generate images composed of individual pixels but a continuous spectrum of color and objects. Second, we are accustomed to having "certain" knowledge of the state of affairs at any moment in time. In the quantum mechanical world, things cannot be "anywhere" but only in specific discrete ("quantized") states—hence the name *quantum*. Perhaps most curiously, items subject to the rules of quantum mechanics can exist in a combination of two or more different states at once. One example of this curiosity is wave-particle duality; small discrete particles can exist and behave simultaneously as continuous waves—yes, this has been shown to be true by experiment. Finally, we can never know the exact state of individual components of the system (e.g., spins), only the likely state of the system as a whole at a specific point in time. Although the quantum mechanical approach may seem unusual, it is very well-suited to describe the behavior of very small particles like hydrogen nuclei. In fact, quantum mechanics is the only truthful and satisfying means through which to understand MRI. The contrived classical explanations simply do not cut it.

Like any system, quantum mechanics operates by a set of rules. However, these rules are unlike others, such as the rules of English grammar or etiquette, in that the rules of quantum mechanics are true and absolute; there are *no* exceptions. In the world of quantum mechanics, we can describe particles (such as nuclei or protons) in terms of their location, velocity, energy, and so forth, but there are limits set on how much we can know about any one particle at any one time.

Energy Levels

Quantum mechanics identifies a discrete number of states for a given nucleus. These states are known as energy levels, and the number of energy levels varies with the type of nucleus. In the case of ^1H, there are only two energy levels, making it a relatively simple system to discuss. Rather than thinking of the energy levels as places where the spins physically reside, think of energy level "filling" and the relative predominance of one energy level or the other as a means to describe the overall "energy configuration" of the system.

Note that, based on the foregoing, it is *not* strictly correct to say that spins exist within or "occupy" one energy level or the other, because the energy levels describe the energy of spins, *not* their physical location. As discussed above, items subject to the rules of quantum mechanics, such as our hydrogen nuclei, can, in fact, exist in more than one state at once, termed *superposition*. The only restriction on our hydrogen protons is that they show a linear combination of the available energy levels. It is, therefore, inaccurate to describe the spins as moving between energy states. Although spins can exist with a combination of energy levels, however, there is a catch. The nature of quantum mechanics only permits us to observe spins within one energy level at a single point in time. As strange as it seems, it is actually our observation of the system that "forces" it to "choose" a single energy level. This is just another peculiar aspect of the quantized nature of the world according to quantum mechanics.

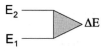

FIGURE 1-4. Energy states. Protons exist in a system of two energy states, where a shift from the lower energy state E_1 to the higher energy state E_2 requires input of an amount of energy ΔE. Conversely, a shift from E_2 to E_1 results in the release (emission) of an equal amount of energy.

Minimizing the Energy Configuration

The example shown in Figure 1-4 depicts a system with two energy states— E_1 and E_2—which is the actual number of states available to ^1H nuclei. As described above, spins must exist with energy corresponding to some linear combination of the available energy levels. When spins change their energy distribution among the available energy levels, we will observe a change in the overall energy configuration of the system. Because energy must always be conserved, in order for such a change in the energy configuration to occur, the spins must either absorb or emit energy (ΔE in Fig. 1-4), depending on the direction of shift in the energy state balance. When the lower energy level E_2 is dominant, we describe the system as being in a low-energy configuration. This is in comparison with a situation where the higher energy level E_1 predominates, yielding a high-energy configuration. The second law of thermodynamics tells us that any system will always tend toward the lowest possible energy configuration. At this lowest energy configuration, entropy (randomness) is maximal. In our case, this means an energy configuration where the lower energy state E_2 predominates. The lowest net energy configuration is called the state of maximum entropy. The corollary to this law is that maintaining a low-entropy/high-energy state requires input of energy.

These quantum mechanical laws of energy levels and distribution are ubiquitous and also govern the behavior of many things well within our daily experience. To put this into perspective, I like to think of the "household definition of entropy": Your home is a system, and, if it is to function according to the second law of thermodynamics, there must be a distribution among energy states. Organization, where each of your possessions is in its place, represents a high-energy configuration, and complete disarray is a low-energy configuration. The second law of thermodynamics tells us that things will tend to become disorganized; to maintain order at home, we must put energy into the system (home) in the form of cleaning effort.

If any system will move to maximize entropy by shifting to the lowest energy configuration possible, why is the higher energy level E_1 not vacated entirely? This is because of thermal energy within the spin system. At absolute zero, where molecular motion stops because of the complete absence of thermal energy, spins will in fact only exist at the lowest energy level.

The Uncertainty Principle

At all temperatures exceeding absolute zero (see earlier discussion), the distribution of spins among the available energy levels is not static but constantly in flux. The Heisenberg uncertainty principle dictates that we cannot know the state of an individual spin at a discrete point in time. Nonetheless, we can know the probability of finding a certain distribution of spins among the available energy states, given a specific set of ambient conditions. We can demonstrate this by making experimental measurements of the system. We will always be able to confirm our predictions about the energy configuration *as a* whole by making a large number of measurements.

The corollary of the description above follows: by measuring the energy configuration of the system (something that we will measure as the MRI signal intensity), we will be able to infer the distribution of spins among energy states. Once again, these statements apply *only* to the system as a whole, not to the specific state of individual spins. In the following section, we will see how the MRI signal intensity can be most completely described in terms of these energy distributions.

Summary

These, then, are the ground rules for our quantum mechanical approach:

- We can never know the energy state or location of any individual spin, only the *probability* of finding spins in a certain distribution among energy states under given conditions. We are only permitted to talk about the configuration of the whole system.

  What any one spin is doing is none of your business.

- Energy levels describe the nature of the system but do not imply physical location of the spins in one level or another. Spins' energy can exist with a combination of energy levels.
- The predominance of specific energy levels can be described as the energy configuration of the whole system.
- The system energy configuration cannot change without input or emission of energy.

Making the Quantum Mechanical Approach Specific to MRI

First, let us identify the energy configurations we will be dealing with. As we have already established, all of our discussions here will concern the NMV and its longitudinal and transverse components. Earlier when we introduced the NMV, it had *no* transverse component because all of the individual spins that contribute to the NMV have random phase. As a result, their transverse components cancel out. This is true if we place our sample in the B_0 field and observe it at rest. However, we will see shortly that, in order to measure the MRI signal, we must disturb this resting state and create a net transverse component to the NMV.

In a low-energy configuration where population of the lower energy level (E_1) predominates, we will observe the longitudinal component of magnetization—we will call this M_z from now on—parallel to B_0. In addition, in this low-energy configuration, we will observe that random phase predominates. This means that there will be no net transverse magnetization (referred to as M_t from now on); all the randomly oriented transverse components will add to 0. Note that this is the resting state where we observe the NMV as originally described: a stationary vector parallel to B_0.

A higher-energy configuration, where population of the higher energy level (E_2) is greater than at rest, can only be observed if energy is added to the system. The details of how we add energy to disturb the resting NMV and what happens when we disturb it are the subject of the next chapter. When we do observe this higher-energy configuration, net longitudinal magnetization (M_z) will be lower than at rest. Simultaneously, phase coherence of the spins contributing to the NMV will increase, yielding net transverse magnetization (M_t). The degree to which we observe these phenomena—decreasing M_z and increasing M_t—depends on the extent to which we shift toward a higher-energy configuration. This, of course, is a function of the amount of energy that we add to the system.

At this point it should be very clear how essential vector addition is to understanding the behavior of spins in a magnetic field. (See Appendix 1 if vectors and their addition and decomposition are not completely clear.) As M_z declines and M_t increases, the vector sum (i.e., the NMV—originally parallel to B_0) does not change in magnitude but becomes oriented at an angle to B_0. If enough energy is deposited, the NMV will form a 90° angle with respect to B_0 (Fig. 1-5), and, if even more energy is deposited, the orientation with respect to B_0 will exceed 90°. How we achieve this "flip" in the orientation of the NMV with respect to B_0 is, believe it or not, *best* understood through the distribution of spins among energy states and how that distribution is altered by the input of energy. Attempts at classical (mechanical/electromagnetism) explanations of this phenomenon simply fall flat on their face.

Remember that energy must always be conserved. Just as adding energy to the system will cause a shift of spins toward a higher-energy configuration, redistribution of spins back to the lower-energy state requires loss of energy from the spin system. In a subsequent chapter, we will discuss how energy can be transferred to the environment or to other spins to accomplish this return to a lower (resting) configuration. Finally, notice that the longitudinal and transverse components are in balance:

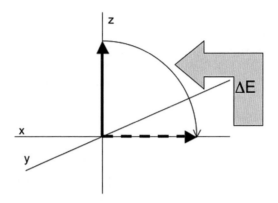

FIGURE 1-5. Excitation. In this example, B_0 is parallel to the z axis. The consequence of addition of energy and the resultant shift to a higher-energy configuration is the rotation of the NMV from its alignment parallel to B_0 (thick arrow) toward one perpendicular to it (broken arrow).

- Adding energy yields: $\Downarrow M_z$ *and* $\Uparrow M_t$ = flip of NMV of 90°, or more or less depending on the amount of energy added;
- Loss of energy yields: $\Uparrow M_z$ *and* $\Downarrow M_t$ = return of NMV to rest (M_0) parallel to B_0.

The following chapters will address how we cause these shifts in the energy state of the system and will examine in much greater detail what happens when we sit back and watch things move back to "normal": maximum entropy/lowest energy configuration, that is, of course!

One More Thing . . . What Exactly Is the MRI Signal That We Measure?

As we will see in the next chapter, MR signal intensity is the measured magnitude of M_t. If we are measuring magnetization, why not just measure M_z? The short answer is that the MRI signal from tissue is so small relative to B_0 that *we would be looking for a needle in the proverbial haystack.* If we chose to use a gaussmeter (a device used to measure magnetic field strength) to measure the magnetization of tissue, our instrument would be swamped by the huge amount of B_0 magnetization. The tiny amount of tissue magnetization would be undetectable. In the next chapter, we will learn that, because M_t is in a different *orientation* than B_0, we can detect it independently and with great sensitivity.

2
Rocking the Boat: Resonance, Excitation, and Relaxation

Introduction: How Can We Find a Signal to Measure?

As we concluded the previous section, a sample of protons was described by its energy configuration, the distribution among energy levels. The magnetization of the sample was shown as the NMV. Nonetheless, we could not measure the NMV because it was so small relative to the static magnetic field B_0. This chapter answers the question: How then can we measure the magnitude of magnetization in the sample?

At Rest, Signal Is Not Detectable

Faraday's law of induction tells us that moving charge will induce a magnetic field. It is conversely true that a moving magnet will induce an electric field. In the presence of a conductor (a loop of wire—AKA antenna—that we will call a receiver coil), a voltage will be induced by the moving magnet. This is exactly how we measure the signal in NMR and MRI; the magnetization of the sample induces voltage in a receiver coil. In our case, however, what voltage will be induced in a receiver coil placed adjacent to our sample of protons that has been placed into a static magnetic field B_0? Surprisingly, perhaps, we will measure absolutely nothing! This is because the net magnetization of our sample (the NMV) is stationary. Remember that, although each individual spin is precessing about B_0 with a frequency of ω_0, because the spins precess with random phase, all transverse magnetization cancels. If the net magnetic field of our sample (i.e., NMV) does not move, no signal (voltage) will be induced in the coil (wire).

Net Transverse Magnetization Is Detectable

If the sample of protons can be altered so that there is nonrandom phase of precession of the individual spins that comprise the NMV, there will be a net transverse component to the NMV. The NMV will no longer be parallel to B_0 but rather will be oriented at an angle with respect to B_0. We call this the *flip angle* or *angle of nutation*. Most importantly, because there is now net M_t, the NMV itself will now precess about B_0. The NMR signal that we measure is induced by the transverse component of the NMV (the portion that is perpendicular to B_0). Notice again that the NMV is *no longer stationary*; it precesses around the axis of B_0. The frequency of precession, of course, is ω_0.

Generating Net Transverse Magnetization

How then do we get the NMV to flip and generate net transverse magnetization?

The short answer is that flip of the NMV results when energy is added to the spin system, shifting it into a higher-energy configuration. The new orientation of the NMV (flipped) is the observable manifestation of this higher-energy configuration. To efficiently transfer energy onto the spins in our sample, we exploit the concept of resonance.

Resonance

The basis of resonance—a major scientific contribution of Nikola Tesla—is that everything has a unique "natural frequency" at which it will oscillate under a given set of ambient conditions. Think, for example, of a "C" tuning fork. When we add energy to the tuning fork by striking it against a desktop, it oscillates at a unique frequency, a C note. If we place a second C tuning fork adjacent to the ringing C fork without making contact, the second fork will also begin to ring. This is due to resonance; sound energy from the ringing fork is so efficiently transferred through the air that contact is unnecessary. If we next place an "A" tuning fork in proximity to the ringing C fork, it will not ring. This is because the energy source (the C fork) and the receiver (the A fork) do not have the same natural frequency. Without a precise match of frequencies, resonance is absent and efficient transfer of energy cannot occur.

One of my favorite examples of resonance was featured in a famous commercial for Memorex cassette tapes. When Ella Fitzgerald, a professional vocalist, sings a high note that happens to match the natural frequency of a nearby crystal glass, sound energy from her voice is deposited with such great efficiency that the glass shatters. Of course, energy not matching the natural frequency of the crystal—such as a blow from a hammer—can also shatter the glass; it makes up for the mismatch in natural frequencies with amplitude. Consider the difference in amplitude between the sound wave and the hammer blow.

Another example of resonance had more dramatic consequences. In 1940, the Tacoma Narrows Bridge opened for travel across Puget Sound, Washington. The suspension design was state of the art and designed to withstand winds up to 120 miles per hour. The bridge earned the nickname "Galloping Gertie" because of the way it would undulate in the wind. Four months after opening, the bridge collapsed into the sound during only a 45 mile per hour wind. Although there is some debate about the cause of the collapse, it has largely been attributed to the phenomenon of resonance. In even gentle breezes, the bridge would undulate and sway at its natural frequency.

For our purposes, resonance is a process by which energy is transferred with great efficiency from one system to another. This requires a source of energy and a subject that receives the energy. In our case, the subject is the spin sample. Its natural frequency, ω_0, is determined by the Larmor equation we discussed previously. The energy source will be a second magnetic field that, while weaker than B_0, will change its orientation over time at a frequency that matches ω_0. This time-varying magnetic field is called B_1, and it is described as a "rotating magnetic field." Because B_1 must rotate at ω_0, which is in the same range as the frequencies used in FM radio, it is also called the radiofrequency (RF) field and is said to deliver a radiofrequency (RF) pulse.

What Is a Rotating Magnetic Field (Radiofrequency Field)?

Consider a magnetic field B_1 that is oriented perpendicular to the static magnetic field of the MRI scanner, B_0. B_1 is described by a vector representing field strength and orientation. If we turn the magnetic field B_1 on and leave it on at a constant strength and direction, graphing the strength of the magnetic field B_1 versus time yields a horizontal line as shown in Figure 2-1. Now, let us turn the magnetic field B_1 on only for an instant at strength of B and then immediately turn it off. After a delay, we will turn the field on for another instant, but will change its orientation by 180°. This is the

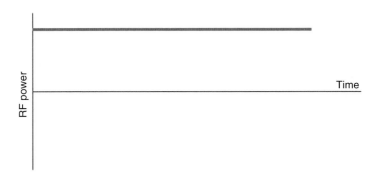

FIGURE 2-1. A constant magnetic field. Graphical representation of B_1 turned on at a constant strength for an extended period of time.

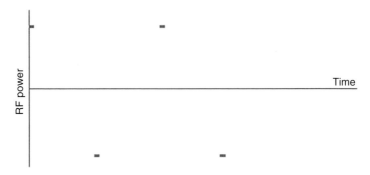

FIGURE 2-2. Intermittent application of a magnetic field. Graphical representation of B_1 turned on for brief periods with alternating polarity but equal magnitude.

same as applying it with strength of −B within a plane perpendicular to B_0. Assuming that it is in fact possible to turn B_1 on at maximum strength for only an instant and then turn it off instantaneously, we will have the pattern shown in Figure 2-2. In reality, of course, the pattern will continue, with the vector describing B_1 oscillating back and forth through a plane perpendicular to B_0. In this scheme, described in Figure 2-3, we see that the magnitude of B_1 is described as a sine function and that its magnitude is less than maximum for much of the cycle. This approach can be used for MRI if we oscillate B_1 at ω_0, but it is inefficient because little magnitude is transmitted during much of the cycle.

In almost all modern implementations of MRI, RF is not transmitted in such a simple manner. Consider a case where B_0 is oriented along the z dimension. We create two magnetic fields (B_{1x} and B_{1y}) within the xy plane orthogonal to B_0, so that the vectors representing B_{1x} and B_{1y} are oriented at 90° to each other within this plane. Both B_{1x} and B_{1y} oscillate at the same

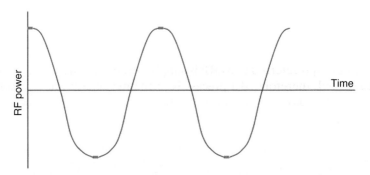

FIGURE 2-3. The oscillating magnetic field. Connecting the dots in Figure 2-2 reveals a sinusoidal oscillation. This is the real time course of B_1 that includes ramp-up and ramp-down periods.

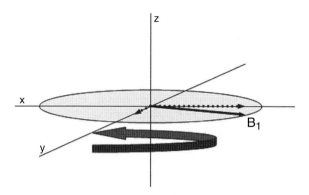

FIGURE 2-4. The rotating magnetic field B_1. Dotted arrows represent the two components of B_1. Each oscillates at the same frequency but 90° out of phase with the other. The vector sum of these two components is represented by the solid arrow. This net B_1 *rotates* through a plane (xy in this example) that is orthogonal to B_0 (parallel to the z axis in this example).

frequency, but the two components are out of phase by 90°. What is the appearance of the vector sum of B_{1x} and B_{1y} (B_1) over time? As the two components B_{1x} and B_{1y} oscillate out of phase, one component declines toward zero whereas the other rises toward its maximum and vice versa. B_1 will have constant magnitude while its orientation *rotates* through the xy plane, orthogonal to B_0 (Fig. 2-4). The hardware that transmits B_1 in this manner is called a quadrature RF coil. It will be discussed in more detail in Chapter 5.

We will be invoking such a rotating field in the next sections. This rotating field will be referred to as B_1 or the RF. It is described by two properties:

- Strength: What is its maximum field strength?
- Frequency(ω): What is the rate of rotation? This must match ω_0 of water protons in order to achieve resonance.

The reason B_1 is referred to as RF is simply because the frequency at which protons (and, therefore, B_1) precess is in the megahertz range commonly used in FM radio. At 1.5 Tesla, the frequency or precession/rotation is about 64 MHz.

What Happens When the Radiofrequency (B_1) Is Turned On?

The short answer is that we observe rotation of the NMV away from its parallel orientation with respect to B_0. We previously learned that we can resolve the vector representing the NMV into component vectors parallel and perpendicular to B_0. By definition, if the NMV is not parallel to B_0, a component of the NMV must be present that is perpendicular to B_0. This *transverse component magnetization* (M_t) precesses about B_0. According to Faraday's law of induction, the precessing M_t—because we are only considering transverse component magnetization, rotating would be more accurate—can induce voltage in a conductor (i.e., a receiver coil). Thus, the voltage induced in the receiver coil by M_t is the MR signal intensity.

As we indicated previously, classical physics is not adequate for a full explanation of the behavior of small particles such as nuclei. Only quantum mechanics will suffice. This is certainly true for the generation of the MR signal where classical electromagnetism cannot explain the flip of the NMV due to interaction with the RF field. Using quantum mechanical concepts, on the other hand, nicely and completely explains the phenomenon.

Let us view the RF as a means for adding energy to the spin system. When we add energy to the system, it must shift to a higher-energy configuration in order to conserve energy. In this state, we describe the sample of spins as "excited." As energy is added to the system, M_z will decline and M_t will increase with resultant rotation of the NMV. It is tempting to identify phase coherence of M_t as "a manifestation of the higher-energy state." However, continuing to add energy to the system will actually flip the magnetization further to 180° and beyond. Beyond 90° of rotation, the spins are in a higher-energy configuration (more RF energy has been introduced), but phase coherence and, consequently, net M_t will actually decline. If phase coherence is the manifestation of the higher-energy state, how does further addition of energy lead to this decrease in phase coherence that is present as the NMV moves beyond 90°? The answer is that the higher-energy state does not correspond directly with a specific physical configuration of the spins such as phase coherence. Rather, each increment of increase in energy will alter the configuration resulting in an effect on the NMV that defies the simplistic logic of assigning each energy level to a specific spatial state of the spins. In this scheme, the following is the case:

- At rest the NMV has a 0° orientation with respect to B_0.
  - This is the lowest energy state.
- Until 90°, incremental excitation is characterized by:
  - *Increase* in phase coherence and net M_t
  - *Decrease* in net M_z
- From 90° to 180°, incremental excitation is characterized by:
  - *Decrease* in phase coherence and net M_t
  - *Increase* in magnitude of M_z with orientation opposite the resting M_z
- From 180° to 270°, incremental excitation is characterized by:
  - *Increase* in phase coherence and net M_t
  - *Decrease* in the magnitude of net M_z

- From 270° to 360°, incremental excitation is characterized by:
  - *Decrease* in phase coherence and net M_t
  - *Increase* in magnitude of M_z with orientation opposite the resting M_z

These changes in orientation of the NMV are the result of quantum mechanical phenomena (altering the energy configuration of the system). Although the orientation of the NMV is a manifestation of a given energy configuration, it is not true that a specific orientation of the NMV can tell us what the energy configuration is. For example, although the orientation of the NMV is the *same* at 0° and 360°, the energy configuration is not! 360° is a higher energy configuration than 0°.

After we have added an appropriate amount of energy, the NMV will flip 90°, generating an amount of net M_t equal in magnitude to that of M_z at rest. In the following sections and chapter, we will discuss how this leads to a detectable MR signal and what happens next.

Generating MR Signal

What is the MR signal and at what point do we have it? As described at the beginning of this chapter, net transverse magnetization is detectable. This net M_t is a moving magnetic field, and when we place a conductor (antenna, coil) in close proximity to M_t, a voltage will be

> Transverse Magnetization (M_t) = Signal Intensity (SI)

induced in the coil. The magnitude of the induced voltage is proportional to the magnitude of M_t. Thus, net transverse magnetization is signal intensity. As we will see in the following chapter, signal is present as soon as we begin to flip the NMV toward the transverse plane, and it is entirely up to you when you choose to measure that signal.

Points of View: The Laboratory and Rotating Frames of Reference

The laboratory frame of reference refers to the real-world phenomenon where, after excitation, we observe precession of the NMV about B_0 in the transverse plane. It is easier, however, to view the behavior of the NMV from a different vantage point termed *the rotating frame of reference*. Because the concept of this alternative vantage point was developed by scientists to better understand NMR phenomena they were investigating in the laboratory, they came to call the real-life viewpoint *the laboratory frame of reference*. We will see shortly why the alternative viewpoint is termed *the rotating frame of reference*.

Think of someone sitting at the center of a carousel in the dark with a lantern in hand. Their arm represents the NMV, which is flipping (nutating,

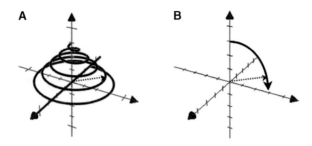

FIGURE 2-5. The laboratory and rotating frames of reference. (A) Reality (the laboratory frame of reference. The NMV follows a spiral trajectory due to precession of the transverse component magnetization about B_0. (B) The rotating frame of reference accurately depicts the same process by having the observer rotate at ω_0.

rotating, etc.) 90° from vertical (parallel to B_0) to horizontal (perpendicular to B_0). That is, they are lowering their hand up to down in a continuous arc. The rotation of the carousel represents precession about B_0. When we make and examine a time exposure of the lantern light in motion, it shows an expanding spiral as the path of the precessing NMV (Fig. 2-5A). This is what we observe in the *laboratory frame of reference*.

Now mount the camera onto the carousel and make the same time-exposure photograph. The light merely moves in an up to down arc. Precession is not perceived (Fig. 2-5B). This is the *rotating frame of reference*. It is a 100% accurate and a much more convenient means for visualization of the behavior of the NMV. Do not forget, however, that precession is still occurring; we just cannot see it in the rotating frame of reference.

We *correctly* represent the behavior of the magnetization as a vector moving in two dimensions, even though the reality is a three-dimensional motion.

3
Relaxation: What Happens Next?

What Happens When the Radiofrequency Is Shut Off?

We saw in the previous chapter that the power deposition provided by the RF (B_1) leads to a higher-energy configuration for the sample of spins. To keep our discussion manageable, we will restrict ourselves to the case in which just the right amount of energy is added to generate a 90° flip of M_0 (the NMV at rest). The manifestations of this higher-energy configuration can be described in two ways. First, longitudinal magnetization (M_z) has declined. Second, phase coherence of the precessing spins has developed, leading to net transverse magnetization (M_t). At the exact moment at which the NMV reaches 90°, $M_z = 0$ and $M_t = M_0$.

Because this energy configuration is higher than at baseline, it cannot be maintained without the input of energy. As a result, when the energy source (RF) is shut off, we will observe the system return to a lower-energy configuration with the emission of energy equal to the amount of energy added by the RF during excitation. This return to the resting state is called *relaxation*. To keep things relatively straightforward, we will first describe what we observe as the energy configuration returns to the resting state, and only then will we delve into the mechanisms. Keep in mind, however, that these shifts in the energy configuration of the spin sample represent quantum mechanical phenomena. Thus, we can know what the entire system (sample of spins) is doing but not what individual spins are up to.

Separate, but Equal (Sort of): Two Components of Relaxation

Though relaxation is a unified process, we can describe what happens to the two orthogonal components of M_0 in order to more completely understand the whole. The behavior of the longitudinal component of magnetization (M_z) and the transverse component of magnetization (M_t) can be

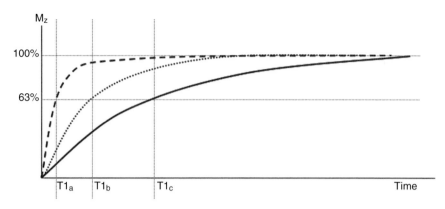

FIGURE 3-1. Longitudinal relaxation. At t = 0, a 90° RF pulse has just been delivered, and all magnetization is in the transverse plane. T1, the time at which 63% of M_z has recovered, describes the rate of recovery. In this example, each line represents a different tissue: The dashed line represents fat, which has a short $T1(T1_a)$, the solid line represents CSF, which has a long $T1(T1_c)$, and the dotted line represents brain, which has an intermediate $T1(T1_b)$.

viewed as two separate, but related, processes. Keep in mind, however, that these two processes describe the same sample and occur simultaneously. One does not occur without the other.

Recovery of Longitudinal Magnetization

During the course of relaxation, M_z "grows back" to reach M_0, its magnitude prior to the RF. The rate of recovery of longitudinal magnetization is defined by the time constant T1. Rather than looking at the equation describing longitudinal relaxation, it will suffice for us to know that the time T1 is the time required to recover 63% of M_z. No matter how much of the M_z has been recovered, T1 will always tell us the time required to recover 63% of what is left.

Figure 3-1 shows a graph of the recovery of M_z versus time. t = 0 represents the instant at which a 90° flip is achieved and the moment at which the RF is turned off. Full recovery of M_z to the point where $M_z = M_0$ requires a time interval of approximately 5 times T1. However, there is actually never full recovery of M_0; the longitudinal magnetization approaches M_0 asymptotically but never fully reaches M_0. Note that the shorter T1, the greater the shift in the longitudinal magnetization recovery curve to the left.

Loss of Transverse Magnetization

Simultaneous with the recovery of M_z, net M_t must diminish in order to comply with the principle of conservation of energy. Net M_t is lost as spins

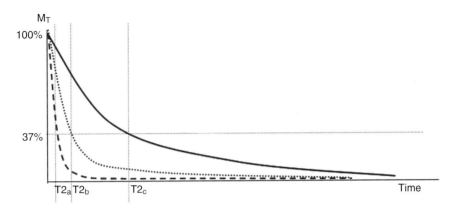

FIGURE 3-2. Transverse relaxation. At t = 0, a 90° RF pulse has just been delivered, and all magnetization is in the transverse plane. T2, the time at which 63% of M_t has dissipated and 37% remains, describes the exponential rate of signal loss. In this example, each line represents a different tissue as described in Figure 3-1. Note that tissues with long T1 also have long T2 and vice versa.

assume increasingly random phase such that the vector sum of the transverse component of magnetization approaches zero. As with relaxation of the longitudinal component magnetization, M_t never fully relaxes to reach a vector sum of zero but approaches it asymptotically. The process of transverse relaxation is depicted by an exponential decay (Fig. 3-2). As in the case of longitudinal component relaxation, it is not necessary to remember the equation that describes the process. It is useful, however, to remember the time constant that governs transverse component relaxation: T2. Because of the nature of the exponential decay, the time constant T2 is the time required for 63% of M_t to be lost. Regardless of the amount of M_t remaining at a specific point in time, T2 will always be the time required to lose 63% of the M_t that remains.

Relaxation Mechanisms

It is tempting to think that the recovery of M_z and M_t is simply due to alignment of spins with B_0. If this was so, the trajectory of recovery would mirror that of excitation with rotation of the NMV back to its resting state (Fig. 3-3A). The reality is that the NMV traces a very different route (Fig. 3-3B). This is because longitudinal and transverse relaxation occurs at very different rates, with transverse relaxation much more rapid than longitudinal relaxation. This phenomenon is reflected in the physical requirement that T2 be shorter than T1.

In order to fully explain the process of relaxation, we must refer back to our understanding of the quantum mechanical nature of the behavior

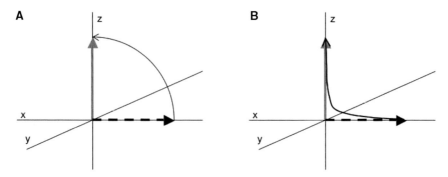

FIGURE 3-3. The trajectory of excitation versus relaxation. (A) Excitation entails rotation of the NMV along the course of the curved arrow through 90° to generate an amount of M_t (broken arrow) equal to M_0 (gray arrow). During excitation, the longitudinal and transverse components of magnetization change at the same rate. (B) During relaxation, however, the transverse component changes much more rapidly than the longitudinal. This follows the physical requirement that T2 always be shorter than T1, generally much shorter.

of spins. Because our spin sample is in a higher-energy configuration after the 90° flip, the spins must emit energy in order to assume the lower-energy configuration that is the resting state of the NMV. In compliance with the principle of conservation of energy, there must be some source to receive the energy emitted by the spins in our sample. Two different means for transfer of energy out of the spin sample exist: transfer to the surrounding environment and transfer to other spins. As we will see, each of these mechanisms is specific to one component of relaxation. This difference confers the difference in the rate of relaxation for each component.

Spin-Lattice (Longitudinal) Relaxation

The slower component—longitudinal relaxation—occurs when spins transfer energy to the environment, principally as heat. Longitudinal relaxation does not describe energy transfer to other spins. The environment is termed the *lattice* as a carryover from the earliest days of NMR applications in chemistry. It follows—remembering our quantum mechanical world in which exact knowledge is limited at any one point in time—that T1 describes the probability that spins will be able to transfer energy to the lattice. This probability increases with the complexity of the lattice and decreases as the lattice becomes increasingly sparse. Thus, in cerebrospinal fluid (CSF) where there is limited lattice, T1 is very long. In tissue, where a rich lattice is present, T1 is much shorter because energy is readily transferred onto the lattice.

Spin-Spin (Transverse) Relaxation

This faster component of relaxation occurs when spins transfer energy to other spins, causing energy to flow through the sample. Analogous to T1 in spin lattice relaxation, T2 is a time constant that describes the likelihood that two spins will interact and exchange energy. When this likelihood is high, T2 will be short and vice versa. In CSF, where diffusion of spins is relatively unrestricted, the probability that two spins will interact for a long-enough time to exchange energy is relatively low compared with the probability of such an interaction between spins in tissue where the structure of the tissue impedes movement of spins, in turn increasing the likelihood of a spin-spin interaction. Consequently, the T2 of CSF is much longer than the T2 of tissue.

The Effects of Variation in B_0: T2′

We said earlier that, for the purposes of our discussion, we would assume that B_0 is absolutely homogeneous such that all spins experience exactly the same B_0 and precess at exactly the same ω_0. In this idealized case, T1 and T2 will accurately and completely describe spin relaxation. In reality, however, there is no such thing as perfect homogeneity of B_0. Even if the MRI scanner generated a perfectly homogeneous magnetic field, as soon as we place the patient in the scanner, the field strength will vary depending on the type of tissue present at each location in the scanner. This interaction of tissue with the magnetic field that causes these effects is a result of differences in the magnetic susceptibility of tissue and will be discussed further in Chapter 18.

The consequence of this spatial variation in B_0 is that adjacent spins will not experience the same field strength and, consequently, will not precess at the same frequency. With time, spins precessing at different frequencies will lose phase coherence. The longer we observe a sample of spins exposed to a heterogeneous B_0, the greater the loss of phase coherence and, of course, the greater the resultant decline in the net M_t of our sample. Because M_t *is* signal intensity, we can see that variability in B_0 causes a loss of M_t over time. Sound familiar? The observed phenomenon is the same as that described earlier by T2: loss of M_t over time due to loss of phase coherence. The mechanism is entirely different, however.

It turns out that there are two different mechanisms that lead to loss of M_t over time. First is the quantum mechanical energy transfer among spins described by T2. Second is the *additional* loss of M_t caused by variability of B_0. This second process leads to an exponential decay of M_t just like the first process, but it is described by a different time constant, T2′. Note that, for either mechanism, we can only observe the net effect on the sample (loss of M_t), not the actual mechanism (energy exchange or loss of phase coherence): the effects of T2 and T2′ look the same. We will see shortly that

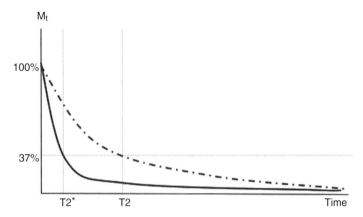

FIGURE 3-4. T2 and T2*. The shapes of the T2 and T2* curves are similar, but their time constants differ. T2* is essentially the T2 curve shifted to the left due to the addition of relaxation due to T2′.

there is a method that can recover the signal lost due to T2′ relaxation. However, because the T2 mechanism is a quantum mechanical phenomenon, it will always be present and we can never observe T2′ in the absence of T2. The time constant that describes the net rate of signal loss due to T2 *and* T2′ is termed T2*. T2* is a composite of T2 and T2′, described by the relationship:

$$1/T2* = 1/T2 + 1/T2′$$

It is *not* important to remember the equation, but it is essential to understand that T2* represents a composite of T2 and T2′ effects.

Figure 3-4 shows the loss of M_t over time due to T2* and T2. Notice that, because T2* is the composite of T2 + T2′, the time constant T2* is shorter and the relaxation curve is steeper for this composite effect. As discussed above, T2′ cannot be measured directly, but the difference between the T2 and T2* curves, of course, represents T2′; T2′ can be calculated.

The Spin Echo

The spin echo is a method for "recovering" M_t lost due to heterogeneity of the magnetic field, essentially neutralizing T2′ effects. The background principle underlying the spin echo (also called a Hahn echo after its discoverer, Erwin L. Hahn) is that, when spins experience different B_0, they lose phase coherence with time. If we consider adjacent spins precessing at different rates, one will be accelerating ahead of the other. If we can instantaneously invert the phase of the spins so that the one precessing faster is now "behind" the one precessing slower, the spins will come back into phase as the faster spin "catches up" with the slower one. Just as there is a continuous loss of phase coherence before we invert the phase of the spins, there will be a continuous gain of phase coherence after we do so. If we allow an amount of time x to elapse before we invert phase, the spins will have maximal phase coherence after an equivalent time x has elapsed after the inversion of phase. Simply said, to achieve maximal recovery of lost phase coherence due to T2′ effects, we must invert the phase of the spins exactly midway between the initial RF excitation and TE, the time at which we sample the signal. Another way to put this is to say that the phase inversion *must* occur precisely at the time TE/2 after the initial RF excitation.

What is an echo? The term *echo* can be a cause of confusion, but its usage is strictly descriptive. An ordinary echo occurs when you walk into a tunnel and yell "hello." The vocalization trails off as the sound waves travel away from you. Because of the reflection of sound waves off of the sides of the tunnel, after the word *hello* trails off, it will be heard with increasing volume as the reflected sound comes closer. In NMR, we will encounter situations where the MR signal declines, but then, after a time delay, increases again. Because the pattern is similar to that of an echo, it was once named accordingly and the name stuck. The term *echo* is ultimately kind of ordinary nonetheless. We could call it Jim, spook, or Wonko just as well. You will be hearing about two types of echoes: spin echoes and gradient echoes.

An RF pulse that flips the magnetization 180° accomplishes inversion of phase of the spins. The RF pulse must deposit twice the amount of energy as the 90° pulse in order to achieve a flip of exactly 180°. After the 180° RF pulse, the spins do *not* change physical location and, therefore, continue to precess with the same difference in frequency (due to variability in B_0: T2′ effects). However, the 180° RF pulse reverses their "order." The "faster" spin accelerated relative to the slower one during the time between the 90° and 180° RF pulses, leading to a phase difference, after the 180° RF pulse. Although the "faster" spin is still out of phase relative to the "slower" spin by the same amount, it is now positioned "behind" the "slower" spin. Thus, during the interval between the 180° RF pulse and TE, the phase difference decreases. Maximal rephasing occurs at TE.

Figure 3-5 shows the transverse component magnetization of two example spins during the process of generating a spin echo. To keep the demonstration simple, we will only show the T2′ effects. In reality, of course, this is not possible, as T2 effects are always present. Initially, spins have random phase such that net $M_t = 0$. Immediately after the 90° RF pulse (Fig. 3-5A), all spins are in phase yielding net M_t. Over a time of length, TE/2 spins lose phase coherence due to T2′ (Fig. 3-5B). An 180° RF pulse is applied that inverts the phase of the spins by rotating them through a 180° arc out of

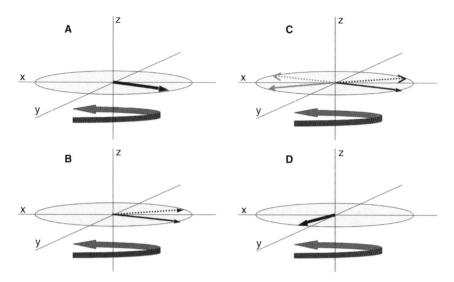

FIGURE 3-5. The spin echo. (A) Immediately after the 90° RF pulse has been applied, spins are all phase coherent, represented by one large vector in the transverse plane. (B) After a period of time, spins will dephase due to T2′ effects. Note that the dotted arrow is "ahead" of the solid arrow with respect to the direction of precession (curved arrow). (C) The 180° RF pulse rotates, spins out of and then back into the transverse plane, effectively inverting their phase. Now, the dotted arrow is "behind" the solid arrow. (D) After an additional period of time equal to that between (A) and (B), the spins are back in phase, creating a spin echo.

and back into the transverse plane (Fig. 3-5C). Because the spins still precess at the same frequency, but the "faster" now lags behind the slower," after a second period of time also of duration TE/2, phase coherence recurs with no net loss of M_t due to T2′ effects (Fig. 3-5D).

Figure 3-6 shows the relaxation of M_t during a spin echo. M_t initially declines with the T2* curve. The 180° RF pulse initiates recovery of phase lost due to T2′ effects. We observe the consequence of this recovery of phase: increase in signal. The phase recovery is maximal at TE where the 180° RF pulse is placed exactly midway between the 90° RF pulse (t = 0) and TE. Notice that, at the point where maximum signal recovery occurs, the measured signal intersects the T2 relaxation curve. This, of course, is because all T2′ effects have been eliminated and the signal, at that moment, represents only the effects of T2 relaxation.

Notice that, when structured with requisite symmetry, signal loss due to T2′ effects is minimized at TE. Before *or after TE*, however, signal will be lower due to T2′ effects. As soon as the echo occurs, signal will again begin to decline due to T2′.

Often, students ask what happens to M_z that has recovered by the time the 180° RF pulse is applied. The implication of this question is certainly

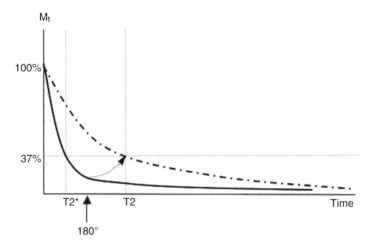

FIGURE 3-6. The spin echo corrects T2' effects. Initially, signal decays along the T2* curve for a time x. After the 180° pulse, signal begins to increase until at time $2x$ it intersects the T2 curve. It is at this point that T2' effects have been fully recovered, producing a spin echo.

true: the M_z is also flipped 180°. However, because TE is generally much shorter than T1, very little M_z has recovered by the time we apply the 180° RF pulse, and the effect on contrast—essentially resetting recovery of M_z—is not significant.

A Different Case of the Spin Echo

It turns out that any time we apply two RF pulses in a row, a spin echo is generated, regardless of the nature of the RF pulses. Two 90° RF pulses generate a spin echo just like a 90° followed by an 180°. As shown in Figure 3-7c, this is because, when we apply the second 90° RF pulse, some of the M_t is rotated from the transverse plane into a plane orthogonal to the transverse plane. Still, a component of this rotated M_t will be detectable in the transverse plane and will form a spin echo after a time elapses equal to the time between the two 90° RF pulses. However, because only a portion of the magnetization exists in the transverse plane, the magnitude of M_t is

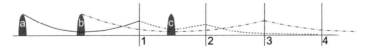

FIGURE 3-7. Echoes after a string of RF pulses. Each pair of RF pulses a, b, and c produces a spin echo; a and b produce a spin echo at TE = 1, b and c at TE = 3, and a and c at TE = 4. A stimulated echo is induced by the combination of a, b, and c and occurs at TE = 2.

smaller than in the case in which we apply an 180° RF pulse. In that classic case, of course, *all* of M_t is rotated out of *and back into the transverse plan* to generate signal at TE.

The Stimulated Echo

As we have seen, a spin echo will occur whenever we have two successive RF pulses. In fact, if we apply three RF pulses in a row, we will generate *three* separate spin echoes (Fig. 3-8). This is because each unique pairing of RF pulses will generate a spin echo after a time elapses equal to the time between the two RF pulses. This is true for any pairing of RF pulses *even if another RF pulse intervenes between the two.*

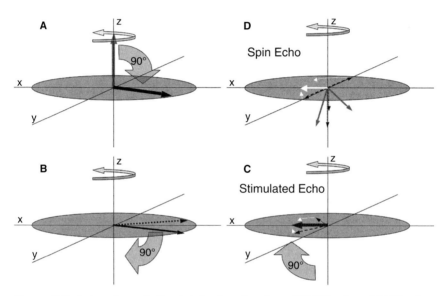

FIGURE 3-8. Spin echo and stimulated echo after three 90° RF pulses. (A) The first 90° RF pulse (large, curved gray arrow) rotates M_z into the transverse plane, creating phase coherent M_t (thick black arrow). (B) A second 90° RF pulse (large, curved gray arrow) is applied after a time interval has passed, and, consequently, some dephasing of M_t has occurred. When this RF pulse is applied, M_t is represented by two component vectors that are out of phase with each other (solid and broken arrows). (C) The components of M_t in (B) have been rotated into the yz plane (gray arrows). This magnetization can be described as two components: M_t (dashed black arrows) along the y dimension and M_z (dotted black arrows) along the z dimension. With time, the M_t components rephase to form a second spin (white arrow). The curved white arrows show the trajectory of rephasing. M_z components remain in the yz plane. (D) The third RF pulse (large, curved gray arrow) rotates the M_z components into the xy plane generating M_t (broken arrows), but not phase coherence. With time, this M_t rephases (white arrows) to form a stimulated echo (thick black arrow).

Another perhaps unexpected phenomenon occurs whenever we have a series of three RF pulses. In addition to the three spin echoes described above, an additional echo will be generated called a stimulated echo. To understand the stimulated echo, consider the example in Figure 3-7 in which we have three 90° RF pulses in a row. Recall that in addition to the effect on M_t, any M_z present at the time of the second 90° RF pulse will be inverted. This results in retention of M_z, which is then present when the third 90° RF pulse is applied and forms an additional echo termed a *stimulated echo*. We saw that the magnitude of a spin echo created using two successive 90° RF pulses is lower than when an 180° RF pulse is used for refocusing. It turns out that the sum of the first (spin) echo and the stimulated echo created by the third RF pulse approximates the magnitude of a spin echo created using an 180° RF pulse. In essence, the component of M_t that was not rotated into the transverse plane but remained parallel to M_z is ultimately refocused when the final RF pulse rotates this component into the transverse plane and the stimulated echo is formed.

Measuring the MR Signal

As soon as we excite the spins in our sample by applying an RF pulse, we have generated net M_t and therefore have NMR signal. Simultaneous with the cessation of the RF, M_t begins to diminish with the time constant $T2^*$. This inexorable decline in signal is called a *free induction decay*, or FID. As mentioned above, the time at which we sample the signal is called TE for time to echo. This terminology is used because we almost always sample an echo (a spin echo, a gradient echo, or a hybrid combination of the two).

The signal is always there; we choose when during relaxation to record it.

It is most important to recognize that the time at which we sample the signal (TE) can be whenever the operator of the MR scanner chooses. From the T2 and $T2^*$ relaxation curves (Fig. 3-4), we can see that a shorter TE (earlier sampling) will yield more signal and a very long TE (late sampling) will detect very little signal. In the next chapter, we will explore the way in which our choice of the NMR parameters TE and TR modulate the degree to which differences between T1 and T2 of different tissues contribute to the contrast present in the MR image.

4
Image Contrast: T1, T2, T2*, and Proton Density

We began our discussion in Chapter 1 with the concept of contrast resolution:

> The MRI acquisition must elicit a different signal from each of the tissues we wish to separate.

If we do not meet this requirement, our images will be incapable of demonstrating a difference between normal and abnormal and will be essentially useless. We generate image contrast by exploiting differences between tissues in their behavior within the magnetic field. Specifically, differences in proton density, T1, T2, and T2* can be enhanced or minimized by our choice of the parameters used in generating and sampling the signal. In this chapter, we will examine the contrast modulation by the parameters TE and TR. Other means for modulating contrast include (but are certainly not limited to) flip angle and TI. These will be presented later in Chapters 8 and 12.

First, let's review the concept that longitudinal (T1) and transverse (T2 or T2*) relaxation occur *simultaneously* but *independently*. Neither one can be suppressed, turned off, tuned out, or ignored. As we will see, this means that every NMR measurement and, therefore, every MRI image contains contrast dependent on *both* longitudinal (T1) and transverse (T2) relaxation.

T2/T2* Contrast

Looking at Figure 4-1, we see that the two tissues whose transverse relaxation curves are shown lose net M_t at different rates. The tissue with the shorter T2 (or T2*) will lose M_t faster. If we set TE to occur immediately after the RF is turned off (making TE as close to 0 as possible), we will detect very little difference in the M_t (read signal intensity) from the two tissues. As a result, we will be unable to distinguish the tissue in our image.

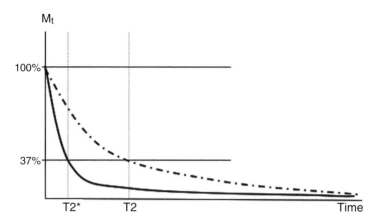

FIGURE 4-1. Transverse relaxation. The two lines represent different relaxation processes for the same tissue. The broken line describes loss of net M_t due to quantum spin-spin energy exchange and is described by the time constant T2. At the time T2, 63% of M_t has been lost (37% remains). The solid line describes loss of net M_t due to quantum spin-spin energy exchange *plus* that due to variability in B_0. This process is described by the time constant T2*. Analogous to the time T2, at the time T2*, 63% of Mt has been lost.

A longer TE, however, will reveal a large difference in signal from these tissues. That signal difference (read image contrast) is entirely dependent on differences in T2 (or T2* if we do not employ a spin echo). Thus, T2 and T2* contrast is modulated by TE. To put it simply:

Maximal T2 contrast: Long TE
Minimal T2 contrast: Short TE

Figure 4-2 shows a series of MR images of the same subject all obtained during one scanning session. Each image represents the same slice of tissue and was acquired using exactly the same parameters except for TE. As indicated in the figure, TE varies from very short to very long. These happen to be gradient echo images. We will learn in Chapter 8 that this means no spin echo is employed. As a result, varying TE varies the T2* contrast in the image. Notice how, as we progress from short to long TE, the image contrast completely changes. In fact, it inverts with CSF, changing from dark to bright and gray matter lower signal relative to white matter at low TE but higher signal than white matter at longer TE. Modifying TE can have dramatic effects on image contrast through modification of the degree to which T2* (or T2 in the case of a spin echo image) affects image contrast.

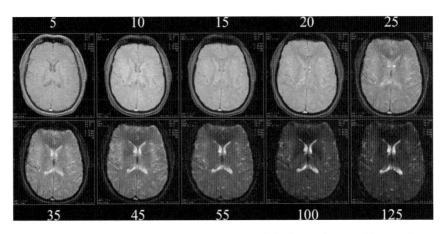

FIGURE 4-2. T2* contrast is determined by TE. TE is indicated by the white numbers. As TE is varied (all other parameters are unchanged), tissue contrast changes dramatically from one reflecting T1 differences to one reflecting T2* differences. When using a short TE, signal is sampled before signal differences because of disparate T2* manifest. When using a long TE, however, such differences in signal manifest substantially by the time we sample the signal at TE. Notice also that signal to noise declines with TE because less net M_t remains.

T1 Contrast

The manipulation of T1 contrast is a bit (but only a bit!) more complicated and requires that we lay down an additional background concept.

Multiple Repetitions Required

By recording the signal induced by M_t after a single RF excitation, we will detect such a small amount of signal that it, by itself, will be virtually useless. In order to obtain usable amounts of signal, we must repeat the RF excitation multiple times. This signal will then be combined through an involved process to generate an image. We will explore this process in detail in Chapter 6. However, the simple concept that we must repeat the RF excitation multiple times is essential background for an understanding of the way in which we can modulate T1 contrast.

Change the Starting Point

In our discussion of transverse relaxation above, we started with two tissues with the same M_0. Immediately after the 90° RF pulse, $M_z = 0$ and $M_t = M_0$. We then wait until TE and sample the signal. Signal arising from the two tissues will differ in proportion to the difference in T2 of the two tissues. In this scenario, T1 is irrelevant, having no impact on contrast.

Next, consider the case of multiple repetitions introduced above. If we repeat the excitation and signal sampling at TE multiple times with a delay between excitations (TR) that is several times longer than T1 of the tissues, what will signal arising from the two tissues look like? The signal we sample will in fact be essentially the same as that sampled after a single excitation. As we saw from Figure 3-1, this is so because M_z of each tissue has enough time to fully recover before the subsequent RF pulse comes around; M_z of each tissue is essentially in its fully relaxed, resting state. After an interval of 3 times T1, 98.9% of M_z will have recovered.

Things change if we deliver the RF pulse at a substantially shorter interval (Fig. 4-3). In this case, M_z only partially recovers before the next RF pulse is delivered. As a result, M_z is significantly less than M_0 at TR. Remember that the magnitude of M_z at the time the RF is applied (i.e., at TR) determines the amount of signal (M_t) that is generated. Because tissues recover at different rates (they have different T1), they will have different M_z at the time of the second RF. Consequently, we will detect differences in signal after the second RF that reflect these differences in T1. This is T1

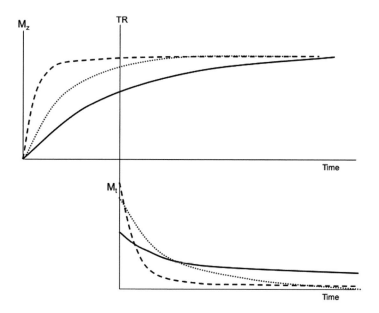

FIGURE 4-3. Short TR alters initial M_t. Each line represents a specific tissue. TR indicates the time at which the second (and subsequent) RF pulse is applied. Because M_z has not fully recovered, only a portion of the longitudinal magnetization M_z is present when this next RF pulse is applied. The amount of M_z present at TR determines the amount of M_t present in the lower graph of transverse relaxation at $t = 0$. If we sample M_t immediately (at $t = 0$), the difference in signal between tissues is due to differences in T1 that determined the amount of M_z recovered when the RF pulse was applied at TR.

contrast. No matter how long or short TE, the signal difference due to these T1 effects is built into the signal we sample.

To modulate the degree to which the signal ultimately reflects differences in T1, we modulate TR. We have already seen that, when TR is extremely long, we will see no evidence of T1 contrast. Shortening TR, however, increases the degree to which the signal reflects differences in the T1 of the tissues. It follows that in order to make an image that shows contrast that is based on T1 differences, we use a short TR. Although such short TR images are often referred to as "T1 weighted," notice that *any* image (unless TR could be infinitely long) contains information derived from differences in T1 of the tissues being sampled. By adjusting TR, we can only minimize or maximize T1 contrast, never eliminate it. To put it simply:

Maximal T1 Contrast: Short TR
Minimal T1 Contrast: Long TR

Figure 4-4 shows another series of MR images of the brain. Similar to those shown in Figure 4-2, all were obtained during one scanning session, each represents the same slice of tissue, and each was acquired using exactly the same parameters—these happen to be spin echo images—except, in this case, for TR. As indicated in the figure, TR varies from very short to very long. Varying TR varies the T1 contrast in the image. Notice how, as we progress from short to long TR, the image contrast completely changes. In fact, it inverts, with CSF changing from dark to bright and gray matter from lower signal relative to white matter at low TR to higher signal than white matter at longer TR. Modifying TR can have dramatic effects on image contrast through modification of the degree to which T1 contributes to image contrast.

Contrast Agents and Their Effect on T1

Paramagnetic contrast agents shorten the T1 of spins when unpaired electrons of the paramagnetic element are within 3 Å (angstroms) of the proton. Currently, all paramagnetic contrast agents approved for use in the United States employ gadolinium (Gd), which is highly paramagnetic, having nine unpaired electrons. Shortening of T1 decreases the time required for longitudinal relaxation to occur and can be viewed (Fig. 4-5) as shifting the T1 curve to the left. This effect brings out differences in tissues (e.g., liver and metastasis in our example below) due to differential shortening of T1; only tissues that take up the paramagnetic substance will "benefit" from this effect.

A classic example of the T1 shortening effect of paramagnetic contrast agents is blood-brain barrier breakdown in the setting of CNS pathology. Normal brain and various types of pathology are quite difficult to distinguish on images that depend on T1 differences for tissue contrast. In

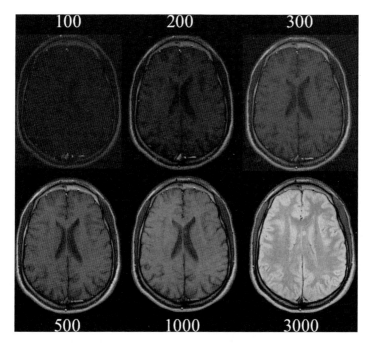

FIGURE 4-4. T1 contrast is modulated by TR. As TR (white numbers) is varied (all other parameters are unchanged), tissue contrast changes from one reflecting T1 differences (white matter with higher signal than gray matter and CSF very dark) to one reflecting T2 differences (white matter darker than gray matter and CSF that is not as dark). When using a short TR, differences in M_z are present when the RF pulse is applied, creating differences in signal immediately afterward. When using a long TR, however, such differences are eliminated as M_z has fully recovered for all tissues by TR. Notice also that signal to noise increases with TR because more M_z recovers before each subsequent RF pulse. The more M_z, the more M_t (signal) generated by the RF.

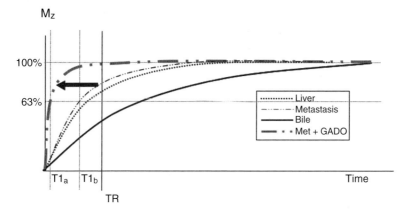

FIGURE 4-5. T1 shortening effect of contrast agents. In this case of a liver metastasis (tumor), M_z of the metastasis and liver tissue are very similar and would, therefore, be difficult to distinguish. The T1 of the metastasis ($T1_b$) becomes shorter ($T1_a$) when gadolinium-containing contrast material accumulates due to tumor vascularity. The change in T1 shifts the T1 curve of the metastasis to the left. Thus, at TR, M_z for the tumor and normal tissue are very different. As a result, signal from the tumor will be much higher and detection will be enhanced. Met, metastasis; GADO, gadolinium.

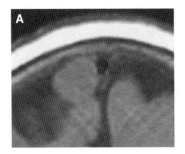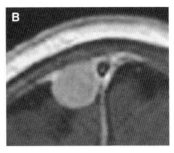

FIGURE 4-6. Contrast enhancement. Both images of this meningioma were obtained using identical parameters. (A) Before the contrast infusion, the tumor has signal indistinguishable from normal brain tissue. (B) T1 shortening accomplished by adding the contrast agent leads to a dramatic contrast between signal from the tumor and normal tissue.

Figure 4-6, the meningioma has identical signal intensity to and is nearly indistinguishable from adjacent brain on the images obtained without administration of contrast material. The distinction between tumor and brain becomes obvious on the contrast-enhanced images. Normal brain does not "enhance" because the contrast agent does not cross the blood-brain barrier and, therefore, has no effect on brain T1. Pathology (such as tumor, infarction, etc.) that breaks down the blood-brain barrier allows uptake of the contrast agent with subsequent shortening of T1 in the pathologic tissue. *Voilà*, we have dramatic tissue contrast!

Contrast agents also cause a modest shortening of T2. However, because the relative shortening of T2 is small and the absolute time T2 is always (in tissue) very short relative to T1, the absolute shortening of T2 caused by paramagnetic contrast agents is minimal and generally not clinically relevant. As we will discuss in Chapter 18, paramagnetic contrast agents, in high local concentration, can cause substantial disruption of B_0 homogeneity leading to T2' effects with dramatic shortening of T2*.

Proton Density Contrast

All of our examples have begun with the premise that both of the tissues being sampled have the same M_0. Although it makes for convenient example cases, this is not the case in the real world. M_0 is the net magnetization derived from the sum of magnetization vectors from all of the spins in the sample; more spins yield greater M_0. It follows that, if we examine equal volumes of two different tissues, the M_0 of each will depend on the number of spins within the volume of tissue. That is, M_0 depends on the density of spins in the tissue. Because M_0 determines the magnitude of signal (M_t) that is generated by the RF pulse, we will observe differences in signal between tissues because of their different proton densities. This is proton density (sometimes called spin density) contrast.

Contrast due to differences in proton density is always inherent in the MR signal. Although we can minimize contrast due to T1 by making TR very long or minimize contrast due to T2 by making TE very short, no adjustment of parameters can alter contrast due to proton density. It is always there. If we make TR very long and TE very short, contrast due to T1 and T2 will be minimized (but never completely eliminated!) leaving an image with contrast predominately due to proton density differences.

Putting Things Together to Control Image Contrast

Based on the effects described above, a few salient observations about contrast modulation are shown in Table 4-1.

Any MRI examination will be composed of several different image types, each with a unique contrast. This approach adds significant diagnostic power to the MRI exam when compared with CT, for example, where only one type of image contrast can be obtained. Additionally, however, employing multiple different contrasts helps ensure that we avoid a potential pitfall. Say we observe the relaxation curves of two tissues, perhaps a kidney tumor and the normal kidney parenchyma in which it is growing. If the tumor happens to have longer T1 and T2 than normal tissue, but similar proton density, we may see an effect such as that depicted in Figure 4-7. Using a moderately short TR, we will have higher signal from normal tissue than from tumor after each RF pulse once we are in a steady state. Because of the differences in T2, we will detect higher signal from normal tissue than from tumor at TE_1, but higher signal from tumor than from normal tissue at TE_3. The problem will be if we sample signal at TE_2. At this point in time, tumor and normal tissue have identical signal intensity and will be indistinguishable. If only to avoid this potential pitfall, it is worth acquiring images with various contrasts.

TABLE 4-1. Contrast modulation by TE and TR.

Dominant contrast	TE	TR
T1	Short	Short
T2	Long	Long
Proton density	Short	Long

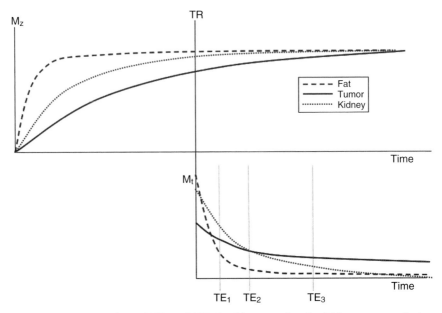

FIGURE 4-7. Interaction of TR and TE. In this example of a kidney tumor, choice of TE has a dramatic effect on detection of the lesion. The TR and all three example TEs are long, creating images that are all somewhat T2-weighted. At TE_1 and TE_2, tumor and normal tissue have different signal, but the direction of the difference varies. At TE_1, tumor is lower signal than kidney, whereas tumor signal exceeds that of normal kidney at TE_3. Notice that, at TE_2, the two are indistinguishable. To avoid this pitfall, we always acquire several images with different contrasts.

One last comment: Why is it that Table 4-1 does not describe a contrast created by employing a long TE and short TR? Such an image would feature both T1 and T2 contrast and might be useful. The downside, however, is that both long TE and short TR diminish the signal amplitude at TE. Thus, such an image, though it could be created, would have poor signal-to-noise ratio.

5
Hardware, Especially Gradient Magnetic Fields

Why This Chapter?

I am often asked why I bother to teach about the "nuts and bolts" of the MRI scanner system. After all, with the exception of physicists and engineers who are specifically interested in dealing with and perhaps modifying the hardware components of the scanner, virtually every MR user will leave the upkeep of the system to professional service personnel. Because these system components are generally not user modifiable, the user will rarely interface with the hardware. Even MRI technologists who sit at the console day in and day out have little practical use for technical knowledge about the magnet that creates the B_0 magnetic field, for example.

In case you are considering skipping this chapter. . . .

The reason this chapter appears at this point is because *understanding the gradient magnetic field is essential to understanding spatial localization* and the rest of this book. You can feel relatively free to leave the other sections within this chapter until later, but the section on the gradient magnetic field is a must!

Nonetheless, there are several reasons to have a basic understanding of the MRI system components, how they interface with one another, and how the components can impact system performance and image quality. First, performance of specific system components can have a major impact on overall system performance and, ultimately, on the type of imaging the system is capable of. Second, recognizing and dealing with scanner problems and artifacts is facilitated by knowledge of the MRI system. Finally, anyone who may be in a position to weigh in on the purchase of an MRI scanner will benefit from knowing which components merit the expenditure of additional capital and which may not be as worthwhile, despite the insistence of energetic salesmen.

The B_0 Magnetic Field

Requirements

Building a useful magnet for human MRI requires attention to three key requirements. First, the opening within the magnet (called the bore or gap, depending on magnet configuration) must be large enough to fit the patient. Recently, scanners have been designed to image extremities only, allowing a smaller bore size to be used that accommodates only a knee or elbow. Second, a very strong magnet is required to generate a static magnetic field suitable for human MRI. With increase in the strength of the static magnetic field, signal increases. Keep in mind, however, that even the weaker magnets on the market are very strong. The 0.3-Tesla magnets used in many open MRI scanners, for example, have strength equivalent to the types of crane-mounted magnets used to move scrap automobiles around the junkyard. Increases in signal are linearly related to field strength at the range of field strengths (less than 7 Tesla) likely to be encountered in human imaging. At extremely high field, however, partial plateau of this increase in signal begins to manifest. Finally, a very homogeneous magnetic field contributes to signal strength and minimizes artifacts. Whereas achieving a very strong magnetic field with high homogeneity is possible, achieving both at once with a bore size suitable for human imaging is challenging; at higher field strength, homogeneity becomes more difficult to achieve across large distances.

Magnet Designs for Generating B_0

Resistive electromagnets are used extensively in MRI but almost never to create the strong static magnetic field B_0. They will be discussed when we deal with the time-varying magnetic fields essential to MRI (gradient and radiofrequency fields). Although in principle, a resistive electromagnet that employs continuous flow of current through a coil of conductive wire can be used to generate a strong and homogeneous B_0 field, the enormous cost of electricity required to maintain such a field had led to its disappearance from production.

What determines the magnet configuration?

Typically, a distinction is drawn between open-design permanent magnet systems that employ a vertically oriented magnetic field and closed-design superconducting systems with horizontally oriented magnetic fields. This line of demarcation is an artificial one, however. The open-design vertical field is also used in systems based on superconducting, albeit lower field strength magnets. These "midfield" systems have field strengths ranging from 0.5 to 1.0 Tesla, are built using two plates, and produce a vertically oriented field. High-field superconducting open-configuration scanners have also been constructed with two donut-shaped "plates" side-by-side to allow access for "interventional MRI." Surgical procedures can then be performed under real-time MRI guidance. The patient slides through the "holes" in the donuts, and the surgeon stands between them. Cylindrical configuration "high-field" systems have also

Recently, the FONAR Corporation Upright MRI (Melville, NY) has been marketed employing a 0.6-Tesla resistive electromagnet. One advantage of this design is that the field can be eliminated by simply powering off the magnet coils. Barring this exception, however, only two principle magnet types are used to generate B_0 for human MRI systems at present: permanent and superconducting. A short comparison of the salient differences is shown in Table 5-1. Figure 5-1 is a cross-sectional diagram of the typical components contained behind the lining of the magnet bore on a typical clinical MR scanner.

been made for research use, allowing scans to be performed on a monkey sitting up in a chair that is raised into the vertically oriented cylindrical bore using an elevator. The one permutation you will not encounter is a closed-configuration permanent magnet system. The design and strength of permanent magnets simply will not support such a configuration.

Permanent Magnets and Vertical Fields

As the name implies, permanent magnets provide a "permanent" magnetic field. Think of them as large, sophisticated, and expensive versions of the magnets you use to post photos and memos on the refrigerator door. These magnets comprise two large disk-like plates composed of ferromagnetic elements embedded in a matrix. The two "plates" are generally placed one atop the other with an intervening gap (Fig. 5-2). It is into this gap that the patient is placed, becoming the "meat" of the sandwich and the two magnet plates the "bread," so to speak. The Upright MRI described above employs two vertically oriented permanent magnet plates. This design allows the patient to sit or stand during the examination.

Because of the stacked configuration of the magnet components, the B_0 field is oriented vertically, from floor to ceiling (Fig. 5-2). Because the sides of the magnet need not be enclosed, permanent magnets are used to create "open" MRI systems where the patient enjoys a much larger space and unobstructed view. The vertical orientation of the magnetic field also

TABLE 5-1. Contrasting permanent and superconducting magnet designs.

Characteristic	Permanent magnet	Superconducting magnet
B_0 strength	0.002–0.3 Tesla	0.7–11.0 Tesla
B_0 orientation	Vertical	Horizontal (sometimes vertical)
Gantry configuration	Open	Cylindrical (sometimes open)
SNR (signal-to-noise ratio)	Lower	Higher
Magnetic susceptibility	Relatively insensitive	Highly sensitive
Chemical shift	Small	Large
Spectral fat saturation	*Not* possible	Possible
Cost	$$	$$$$$

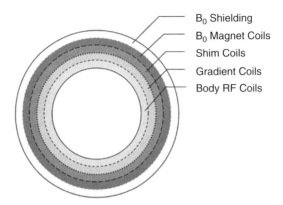

B$_0$ Shielding
B$_0$ Magnet Coils
Shim Coils
Gradient Coils
Body RF Coils

FIGURE 5-1. Components within the "magnet" bore. This diagram is a cross section of a superconducting MRI scanner. The patient lies in the center and sees a plastic liner. Behind the plastic lie the layers of hardware depicted in the diagram. Note that, although we may refer to this hulk as "the magnet," it contains many components besides the B$_0$ magnet coils.

facilitates RF coil optimization. The nature of permanent magnet designs, however, restricts them to relatively low field strengths (generally less than 0.3 Tesla), and, as a result, signal-to-noise ratio (SNR) is lower on permanent magnet systems, leading to less image quality compared with superconducting systems. At lower field strength, the chemical shift of fat and other metabolites relative to water (see Chapter 7) is relatively small. This may minimize certain artifacts (magnetic susceptibility) and allow

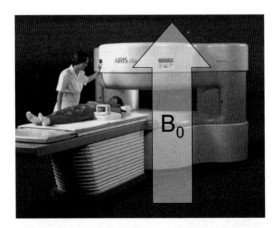

FIGURE 5-2. Permanent magnet open MRI. The patient slides between the two plates containing components of the permanent magnet. Note the vertical orientation of the 0.3-Tesla B$_0$. (Photograph courtesy of Hitachi Medical Systems North America, Inc.)

acquisition of images with minimal distortion in patients with metallic hard-ware. However, the limited chemical shift precludes the performance of spectral fat saturation and spectroscopy at these low field strengths.

Superconducting Magnets and Horizontal Fields

Electromagnets consist of a coil of wire (called a solenoid) through which electric current is passed. The flow of current generates a magnetic field parallel to the long axis of the solenoid with the polarity of the field determined by the direction of flow of current. The "right-hand rule" (Fig. 5-3) indicates that, if you curl the fingers of your right hand in the direction of current flow, your thumb will indicate the orientation of the field. Such electromagnets are used to generate the gradient magnetic fields used in MRI but are generally no longer used to generate the static magnetic field, B$_0$.

At temperatures above absolute zero, all metals conduct electricity with resistance. This means that a portion of the current that enters the conductor will be dissipated as heat. As a result, continuous conduction of electricity requires continuous supply of current. Electromagnets must always be attached to a supply of electric current or their fields will rapidly dissipate. The excessive cost associated with keeping such a resistive electromagnet at high field strength is the reason this technology for creating the B$_0$ field in MRI has been abandoned.

As temperature approaches absolute zero (less than 4 K to 9 K), certain elements and compounds become superconducting. This means that they conduct electricity without any resistance. If current is not dissipated as heat, it can, in theory, flow forever *without an external supply of current.* Superconduction allows a very large amount of current to flow through the magnet coils without the need for a constant supply of expensive electric

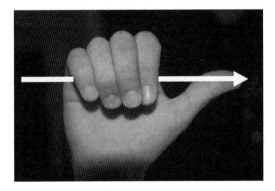

FIGURE 5-3. The right-hand rule. When Tamar curls the fingers of her right hand in the direction of current flow, the orientation of the resultant magnetic field is indicated by her extended thumb.

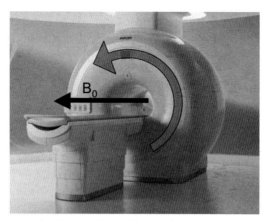

FIGURE 5-4. Superconducting horizontal-bore MRI. The patient lies on the table and is slid into the bore along the direction of B_0 (black arrow). The gray arrow indicates the direction of current flow within the superconducting coils that generate B_0 at 1.5 Tesla. (Photograph courtesy of Philips Medical Systems America, Inc.)

current. Superconducting alloys of niobium (niobium-tin and niobium-titanium) are used to make the solenoids for superconducting magnets utilized in MRI scanners. The solenoid coils are cooled to 9 K or less (see text following), and current is supplied to the coils until the desired field strength is reached. At that point, the external current is disconnected, and, assuming temperature stays within range, the magnetic field strength will persist without any measurable change for years.

The design of superconducting magnets allows very high and very homogeneous fields to be achieved, avoiding many of the limitations of permanent magnets . . . except for space; the bore of the "closed" MRI is still a put-off to claustrophobic patients (Fig. 5-4). To try to minimize the disadvantages of "open" permanent magnet systems and "closed" superconducting systems, several vendors have developed open configurations employing two superconducting magnets stacked one atop the other with an intervening space for the patient. These designs look, superficially, much like permanent magnet systems, employing a vertically oriented magnetic field and affording the open MRI configuration. They also allow field strengths up to 1.0 Tesla (Fig. 5-5). Exploiting the combination of higher field strength with superior coil designs that are feasible only in vertical field systems produces excellent image quality that approaches that of some "closed" MRI scanners.

Keeping Your Cool: The Cryogen System

Because extremely low temperatures are essential to the maintenance of superconduction, extensive engineering effort has gone into designing the

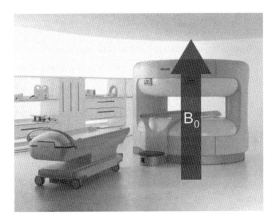

FIGURE 5-5. Superconducting magnet open MRI. Similar in configuration to the open MRI depicted in Figure 5-2, the plates of this 1.0-Tesla scanner contain super-conducting coils. As with other open-configuration scanners, the orientation of B_0 is vertical. (Photograph courtesy of Philips Medical Systems America, Inc.)

container in which the magnet coils reside. In brief, a metal vacuum bottle called a dewar is built to house the solenoid and is then filled with liquid helium (boiling point 4.22 K). Some means are required to prevent the rapid boil-off of the liquid helium reservoir. Older magnet designs (many still operational) employ a second dewar surrounding the one containing the helium-bathed coils. This container is filled with liquid nitrogen. As boil-off of liquid nitrogen is rapid (up to 15 or more liters/day), it needs replenishing every few weeks. Although this is a significant expense, liquid nitrogen is a lot cheaper than liquid helium.

Newer magnet designs forego the nitrogen layer and instead mount a pump at the top of the helium chamber. This pump traps helium gas as it boils off and compresses it to return it to the liquid state. (Remember Boyle's law?) This "cold head" is responsible for the sound of an idling steam locomotive in the scanner room.

Losing Your Cool: Magnet Quench

If the temperature of the magnet coils rises above the superconducting range (>9 K), the coils shift from superconduction to resistive conduction. This results in rapid heating, which induces even more rapid boil-off of helium. As the liquid helium becomes helium gas within its sealed metal container, pressure rises dramatically. A pressure release is always built into the container to allow dissipation of pressure and avoid an explosion. The helium gas is also vented outside of the building through a dedicated high-capacity duct.

If all goes well, a quench involves a very loud noise (like a freight train rolling through the magnet room), a drop in the ambient temperature in the room, and only a little "smoke" (helium vapor), with the helium gas vented successfully to the outside. If the ventilation system fails, however, helium (and nitrogen if it is in use) will fill the room as a gas, displacing breathable oxygen and posing a risk of rapid asphyxiation. For this reason, the room should be evacuated immediately. If the room is closed, however, the buildup of pressure from the expanding helium may make opening of inward swinging doors impossible. It may be necessary to break a window to relieve the pressure. The pressure buildup can also cause the helium and nitrogen gases to condense, forming puddles of liquid cryogens. These puddles pose a frostbite hazard.

Shimming

We have all sat in a cheap (or not so cheap) restaurant at a table that wobbles from side to side. How do you fix the annoyance? Fold up a piece of paper or cardboard and slide it under the table leg that is too short. That piece of paper is a shim.

Although a great deal of effort goes into designing a magnet that will generate a homogeneous magnetic field, nothing is perfect. Even the best design and manufacturing will result in a magnet with a less than adequate field homogeneity. This problem is also solved using shims. In this case, small bits of magnetic field are added so that the net magnetic field is homogeneous. Remember that B_0 is represented as a vector. The goal of shimming is to detect the same magnitude and orientation of the B_0 vector at every location within the usable portion of the magnet bore.

Shims come in three main varieties:

1. *Passive shims* are pieces of metal that are deliberately placed in the magnetic field at the time the magnet is installed. These cause minor distortions of the magnetic field in an effort to force it back to its ideal configuration.

2. *Superconducting shims* are additional superconducting magnets, separate from the one that creates B_0. These are adjusted, also at the time of installation, to further refine the field homogeneity.

3. *Room-temperature (gradient) shims* are gradient magnetic fields that are adjusted at the time of each scan preparation to fine-tune the field homogeneity. These shims principally compensate for variability in B_0 caused by the heterogeneous make-up of the patient; different tissues have slightly different magnetic susceptibility leading to this effect.

Magnet manufacturers generally specify a threshold for magnetic field homogeneity in parts per million (ppm) as this is a fraction of the field strength. This specification is quoted over a specific volume centered at the isocenter of the magnetic field. The term *isocenter* indicates the physical location of the most homogeneous portion of the static magnetic field B_0.

For example, a tolerance of 10 ppm over a 50-cm spherical volume for a 1.0-Tesla magnet would mean that the field cannot vary more than 0.00001 Tesla over this 50-cm region.

Another factor that can affect magnetic field homogeneity is temperature. In fact, change in temperature over time, even within one scanning session, can alter the shim and, subsequently, image quality. On permanent magnet systems where no superconducting shims are available, small heaters embedded within the magnet plates are used as shims.

Radiofrequency Transmission

Once we have a B_0 magnetic field, we are ready to generate signal. As we discussed in Chapter 3, signal is generated using a rotating magnetic field, B_1 or RF. The RF is generated using an electromagnet that is driven by an RF amplifier. The amplifier receives specifications of frequency, phase, bandwidth, power, and duration and delivers appropriate power to the coil. The RF coil can be part of a movable surface or volume coil such as the head coil. Often, such coils are used for both RF transmission as well as signal reception. Alternatively, RF can be transmitted using the body coil that is built into the magnet bore (Fig. 5-1). This approach is becoming universal on newer scanners from many vendors.

Radiofrequency Calibration

Once we have hardware in place to transmit RF, we will want, perhaps, to generate a 90° RF pulse. How do we do it? What determines the flip angle that will result from a given combination of RF power and duration? The simple truth is that this must be determined by trial and error for each patient. Because of differences in size and density from person to person, a different amount of power will be required to generate the 90° flip in each. RF calibration is an integral part of the "prescan" that is performed at the outset of every MRI pulse sequence or at least every examination. In the most straightforward approach, using a very fast and simple pulse sequence that generates signal, but no image, the signal magnitude is measured at various RF power/duration settings. The one that returns the greatest signal is, by definition, the amount of RF power required to generate a 90° flip of M_z. From this point, calculations can yield the fraction of power required for other smaller or larger flip angles.

The Gradient Magnetic Field

As we will learn in the next chapter, gradient magnetic fields are absolutely central to MR imaging. The "gradient" is a linear change in magnetic field strength along one linear direction within the scanner. Gradient magnetic fields are generated using resistive (not superconducting) electromagnets that are turned on and off rapidly during MRI. This ability to switch gradients on and off rapidly is a key performance characteristic of the MRI hardware and one that vendors tout in their brochures and sales pitches . . . and charge for!

Spatial localization of the MR signal will require gradient magnetic fields in each of the three orthogonal directions. For our discussions, we will consider a typical horizontal-bore superconducting MRI scanner where the patient lies on a bed to be slid into the bore. We will call the direction parallel to B_0 the z dimension, the plane parallel to the floor the xz plane, and the plane perpendicular to the floor *and* parallel to B_0 the yz plane.

Where does the noise come from?

For anyone who has been in or around an MRI scanner, one of the most memorable parts is the loud buzzing, banging, and clanking. What creates this varied and often very loud noise? Recall that when we power-up a gradient magnetic field or turn on the RF, we create an electromagnet. As with any two magnetic fields, the gradient or RF field will interact with the B_0 field, and the weaker (gradient or RF) will tend to align with the stronger (B_0) field. As a result, the magnet hardware (coils) will also torque to align with B_0. The noise we hear is mechanical noise created when these time-varying magnet coils exert stress on their mountings. Rapidly repeated stresses occur when the gradients and RF are switched on and off, leading to vibrations. The rate—call it frequency—at which the gradients and RF are switched on and off and the amount of power delivered to the coils determines the pitch (frequency) and intensity of the noise.

These designation, though commonly used conventions, are essentially arbitrary. Any direction can be termed x, y, or z or A, B, or C for that matter. The concepts also apply equally to vertical B_0 "open" systems and vertical-bore superconducting MRI scanners such as those used in research with monkeys.

To illustrate the basics of a gradient magnetic field, let us consider the z dimension. As shown in Figure 5-6, two circular coils are present, one at each end of the scanner, equidistant from isocenter. The coils actually surround the bore, integrated into the lining of the scanner within the diameter of the coils of the main magnetic field B_0 and the shim coils (Fig. 5-1), so that the patient slides through the center. This design is called a *Helmholtz coil pair*. In a real scanner, the two parts of the Helmholtz pair might actually be composed of multiple coils of wire (a solenoid), but for simplicity we will only show one loop.

If current is run through both coils simultaneously, but in opposite directions, two magnetic fields are generated of equal magnitude, but in opposite directions. Because magnetic field strength declines with distance from the

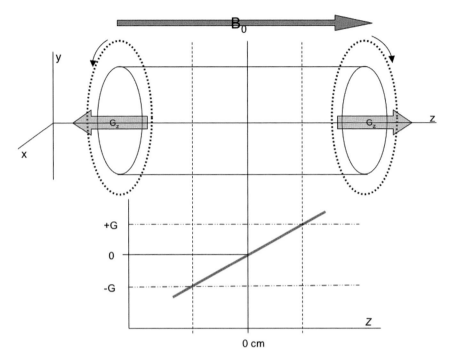

FIGURE 5-6. Gradient magnetic field along z. The dotted-line circles at each end of the scanner diagram represent the two gradient coils. The curved arrows indicate the direction of current flow, each in the opposite direction of the other. The wide gray arrows show the direction of the magnetic field generated by each coil. The plot below the diagram displays the linear change in the net G_z. Because G decreases with distance from the coil and both coils are equidistant from isocenter, net G_z is zero at isocenter and increases symmetrically to the right and left with distance from isocenter, but with orientation to the right on the right side and to the left on the left side of isocenter.

source of the magnetic field, the field strength is higher near either of the coils and lower near isocenter. At isocenter, the vectors describing the field generated by the two coils are equal in magnitude but point in opposite directions. Thus, the vector sum, call it G_z, of the gradient magnetic fields is 0 at isocenter. As we move from isocenter along the same direction as B_0 (to the right in Fig. 5-7), G_z increases in magnitude with the same direction as B_0. We have two magnetic fields, G_z and B_0, with identical direction. Their vector sum B_{net} is $B_0 + G_z$, which is greater than B_0. If we now measure the field strength an equal distance from isocenter, but in the opposite direction along B_0 (to the left in Fig. 5-7), G_z will have the same magnitude but will now have a direction opposite B_0. Thus, B_{net} ($B_0 + G_z$) will be less than 0. The graph in Figure 5-4 shows that when we measure B_{net} at all

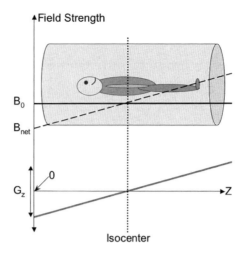

FIGURE 5-7. Net field strength is a function of gradient strength and direction. The graph at the bottom of the figure shows the strength and orientation of G_z along the z dimension, as was shown in Figure 5-6. Above, the horizontal solid line represents B_0, which does not change strength with location; it is the *static* magnetic field. The dashed line plots the net magnetic field strength (B_{net}) at each location along z. This is the vector sum of B_0 and G_z.

locations along the z dimension, we will find a linear change in B_{net} due to a linear change in G_z, such that B_{net} is equal to B_0 at isocenter. This is termed a *symmetric gradient magnetic field*. Although we could generate an asymmetric gradient magnetic field by providing unequal amount of current to each gradient coil, in practice, asymmetric gradient magnetic fields are not widely used in clinical MR imaging.

To generate a gradient magnetic field perpendicular to B_0, the same principles apply, but a different design is required for the gradient magnetic field coils. Considering the y dimension gradient magnetic field G_y, what would happen if we used a Helmholtz coil pair like that used for the z gradient? We would still have no net effect at isocenter and increasing strength of G_y as we move away from isocenter. However, because the orientation of G_y will be perpendicular to B_0, the vector sum of $B_0 + G_y$ will cause a very slight shift in the orientation of B_{net} relative to B_0 (Fig. 5-8A). In order to avoid this problem, we must alter the gradient hardware. Placing a pair of coils at each side of the bore along the y dimension, equidistant from isocenter, we can generate a magnetic field on each side that is parallel to B_0 such that there is a gradient of the magnitude of G_y along the y dimension, but the net magnetic field G_y is always parallel to B_0 (Fig. 5-8B). Thus, we have a gradient of field strength along the y dimension with no alteration in the orientation of B_{net} relative to B_0. Toward the top of the diagram,

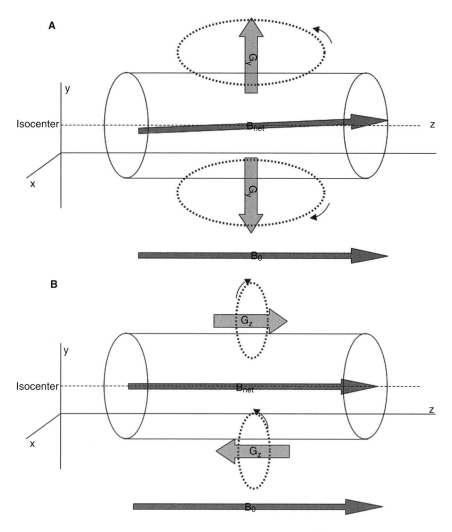

FIGURE 5-8. A potential problem with x and y gradient design. (A) If the coils used to generate the two components of the x or y gradient magnetic fields are oriented so they produce magnetic fields orthogonal to B_0, net gradient strength will indeed be zero at isocenter where the two components cancel each other. At a distance from isocenter, however, the vector sum of the net gradient magnetic field and B_0 will result in B_{net} that is not parallel to B_0. (B) To keep B_{net} parallel to B_0, the coils used to generate the gradient magnetic field components are oriented so that the magnetic fields that they produce are oriented parallel to B_0 but with opposing direction along the z dimension. Thus, these magnetic fields add to or subtract from the magnitude of B_0 but do not affect its orientation.

$B_{net} = B_0 + G_y$, at isocenter $B_{net} = B_0$, and toward the bottom of the diagram, $B_{net} = B_0 - G_y$.

Designing a gradient magnetic field for the x dimension is done using the same type of hardware design as the y gradient. We now have three *independent* gradient magnetic fields, one in each orthogonal direction. Remember that each of these gradient magnetic fields is generated by a unique dedicated hardware setup such that the gradient system for an MRI scanner actually has three gradient subsystems. As we will see at the beginning of the next chapter, we will use a gradient magnetic field to determine the orientation of the imaging plane (slice). One of the many advantages of MRI is the ability to image in any oblique plane. Such oblique imaging requires gradient magnetic fields along oblique trajectories. To generate such oblique gradients, however, we do not require any additional hardware. Considering the gradients as vectors, we can see how turning on two or three gradients simultaneously will generate an obliquely oriented gradient magnetic field. It is the magnitude of each component that determines the orientation of the gradient, so we just adjust the amount of current pumped into each gradient coil to generate the desired oblique gradient magnetic field.

The RF Coils

RF coils perform two essential functions in MRI. First, they are used to transmit the RF pulses that generate signal. Second, they function as receiver antennae during signal sampling. Conveniently, because RF transmission and signal sampling occur, by definition, at different times (see Chapter 8 on pulse sequences), we can use the same piece of hardware for both purposes. Additionally, because the RF and signal both have, by definition, the same frequency (ω_0), no adjustment of the coil is required for efficient execution of both functions.

We alluded to the receiver coil in Chapter 3, calling it an antenna. That is, essentially, all a receiver coil is—a loop of conductive material connected to a device that detects voltage. Coils come in a wide array of shapes and sizes, many optimized and contained in specialized, often flexible, covers to fit specific body parts. It is not unusual for an MRI suite to have six or more specialized coils for different body and musculoskeletal applications in addition to a head coil. All solenoid design MR scanners and several open design scanners also contain a whole-body coil that is built into the lining of the bore of the scanner. This coil is used for RF transmission. Although it can be used for reception, we will see that it is not often employed for this purpose.

The details of coil design are well beyond the scope of this book, but there are several characteristics of receiver coils that are helpful to be familiar with, even if you will never design an RF coil. We will address the following items:

- Tuning
- Impedance matching
- Sensitivity: Surface coils
- Penetration: Quadrature design coils
- Coverage: Phased array coils

Tuning

Any antenna will be a more sensitive detector if it is designed in proportion to the wavelength (determined by frequency) of the signal to be detected. This is true whether we are dealing with a mobile telephone, sonar, a radio telescope, or MRI. The need for excellent coil tuning is magnified by the fact that the signal to be detected in MRI is so small. Just as televisions were once (before cable and satellite TV) tuned by adjusting a mechanical knob or dial on the TV set, MRI coils were originally tuned by adjusting mechanical rods or knobs attached to the coil housing. The adjustments (which actually adjust capacitors in the coil circuit) are made while transmitting a signal of appropriate frequency. Adjustments are made until the received signal is maximized. On all commercial human MRI scanners currently on the market, coils are pretuned for specific field strength or tuning is accomplished automatically during the prescan.

Keep in mind that because ω_0 is determined by magnetic field strength (B_0), RF coils are *not* interchangeable between scanners using different strengths of B_0.

Impedance Matching

RF transmission is most efficient when the impedance of the coil is matched to the impedance of the RF amplifier providing power to the coil. When there is a mismatch in impedance, RF will be reflected rather than absorbed, leading to inefficient excitation, suboptimal signal, and poor image quality. In addition, the RF power required to achieve excitation may rise to unacceptably high levels that pose a patient safety problem. The size, shape, and density of tissue within the coil (e.g., the size and shape of the patient's head) alter coil impedance. In order to optimize RF transmission, these variations in coil loading between patients must be compensated. To adjust coil impedance, reflected signal is observed while RF is transmitted until the reflected signal is minimized. Similar to coil tuning, the impedance matching process was originally performed manually but is now automated as part of the prescan process. For some applications, such as adult head imaging, there is little-enough variation between patients so that fixed impedance coils may be used.

Surface RF Coils and Coil Sensitivity

The main factors that determine the ability of a properly tuned and matched coil to detect small amounts of signal are the proximity of the coil to the signal source and the diameter of the coil. This is the basis for the use of surface coils in MRI: the closer the coil is to the body part of interest, the stronger the detected signal. In fact, the only instance in which we will not use a surface coil for signal detection is where the thickness and size of the body part being imaged is so great that distance from the center of the object to the coil results in signal drop-off at the coil. In this situation, we will resort to quadrature design, described in the next section.

An important consideration in the use of surface coils is positioning. In addition to placing the coil as close as possible to the body part of interest, the coil must be situated so that it is perpendicular to the plane through which the RF rotates. This is because M_t can only induce voltage in the coil when its vector, or at least a component of its vector, is perpendicular to the plane of the receiver coil. Thus, if we place a single surface coil parallel to B_0, M_t will have a component perpendicular to the coil at all times except when M_t is exactly parallel to the plane of the coil. If the coil is positioned orthogonal to B_0, however, M_t will never be orthogonal to the plane of the coil, and we will never detect any signal.

Quadrature RF Coils

Although surface coils are maximally sensitive and optimal for signal detection and it is technically possible to accomplish RF transmission using them, maximum efficiency and penetration of the RF energy into the tissue are achieved when RF can be transmitted from multiple orientations. Similarly, sampling with coils oriented at multiple angles allows for more robust detection of signal arising within the central portions of the patient that will be, by definition, distant from the surface coil (Fig. 5-9).

Quadrature (also known as circularly polarized) coil design employs two separate coils, typically oriented at 90°. We record signal from both coils simultaneously, yielding two signals that are out of phase by 90°. By convention, one of the signals is termed "real" and the other "imaginary." Both signals are, however, just as real. We could call them Ying and Yang or Laurel and Hardy just as well, but conventions are conventions. Because we know the phase difference between the two signals, we can use the magnitude of the signal detected at each coil to compute the net magnitude of the signal arising from the sample using simple 10th grade geometry (Fig. 5-10).

The quadrature design enhances RF transmission and signal detection because, as the component of the RF or M_t perpendicular to one of the coils is declining, the component perpendicular to the other coil is increasing. In addition, when imaging a thick body part like the head, we have two

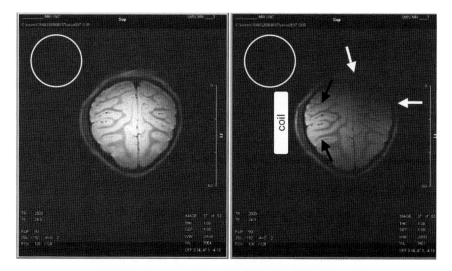

FIGURE 5-9. Volume versus surface coil reception. Two images were obtained using a volume coil (left) and a surface coil (right). The volume coil provides more homogeneous signal throughout the image, including areas within the depths of the slice. Using the surface coil (white rectangle), however, results in uneven signal intensity with high signal (black arrows) near the coil and lower signal (white arrows) farther from the coil. The more prominent noise (white circles) in the volume coil image also attests to its lower sensitivity.

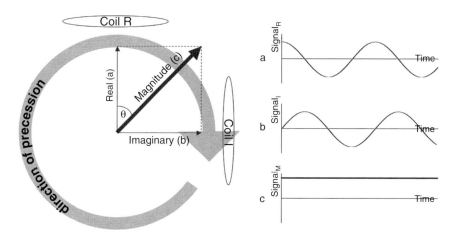

FIGURE 5-10. Quadrature receiver coil. Two separate coils are oriented at 90° with respect to each other. As a result, the signals induced in the two coils (a and b) by M_t (thick black arrow) rotating through a plane perpendicular to both coils are out of phase by 90° (sine curves to the right). The sum of the two sine functions yields a constant amplitude function (c). *Real* and *Imaginary* (thin black vectors) are the components that sum to yield *Magnitude* (thick black vector). These three vectors form a right triangle. Thus, we can compute the magnitude from its components ($M^2 = R^2 + I^2$) and determine the absolute phase of the magnitude vector as well.

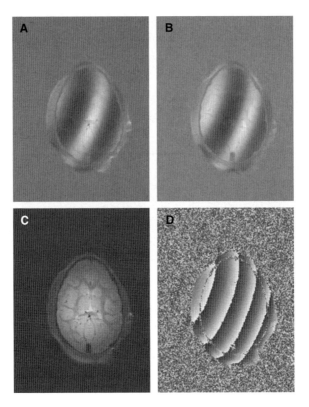

FIGURE 5-11. Reconstruction of the quadrature signal. Reconstructing the signal from only one channel at a time yields images from the (A) real and (B) imaginary signals. The phase image (D) shows the phase orientation of the signal (M_t). Image quality is poor as only a portion of the signal seen in the magnitude image (E) is present.

coils receiving signal from two different "viewpoints." If we generate a signal from only one channel, real or imaginary, we will essentially have a surface coil image with a substantial loss of image quality (Fig. 5-11). Another advantage of the quadrature coil arrangement, though not commonly used, is the ability to compute the phase of the signal (Fig. 5-10). This allows the creation of so-called phase images where the pixel intensity represents the absolute phase of the MR signal.

Phased Array Coils

Because surface coils are the most sensitive for signal detection, it would be ideal to use them whenever imaging tissue close to the skin surface. However, we must also recognize another limitation of surface coils.

Because coil sensitivity is also inversely related to the diameter of the coil, very large surface coils are not efficient. As a result, only a small area can be sampled with a single surface coil. Phased array coils were developed to overcome this limitation and retain the sensitivity advantage of the surface coil design.

A phased array coil is essentially a group of surface coils (called coil elements) arranged to cover a large body area such as the spine, head and neck or torso. Overlap of the coil elements and special preamplifiers are used to ensure continuous coverage and minimize interactions between the coil elements that could lead to signal loss at the coil element interfaces. It is the fact that the coil elements each feed their signal to unique receiver channels that allows the integration of signal from multiple coil elements to form a single image without any loss of signal.

The Receiver (A2D)

When we speak of the receiver of the MRI system, the device or group of devices we are describing is the electronics that samples the MRI signal and converts it from an analog to a digital signal. The analog signal is the continuously precessing net M_t that, when sampled in an analog mode such as with an oscilloscope, looks like a decaying sine function (Fig. 5-12) called

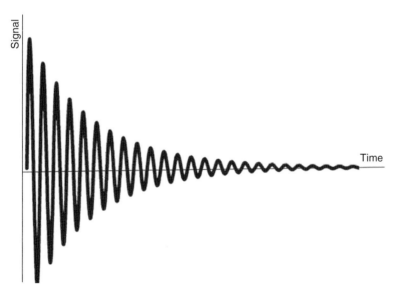

FIGURE 5-12. Free induction decay (FID). Signal (M_t) as detected by one receiver coil. The oscillation of the signal represents its rotation toward and away from the coil. When the curve crosses zero, M_t is parallel to the plane of the coil.

a *free induction decay* (FID). In order for the MRI scanner computers to deal with the signal, however, it must be a digital signal. To transform the signal from analog to digital form, we employ an analog to digital converter (A2D).

The A2D repeatedly samples and records signal amplitude for discrete time periods of duration T_s. Its performance is described by two main characteristics: (1) the general frequency range in which the receiver is designed to sample and (2) the sampling rate. For clinical MRI, for example, frequencies in the MHz range (roughly 12 to 120 MHz, depending on field strength) must be sampled, whereas for laboratory spectroscopy techniques at very high field, even higher frequencies are encountered. Sampling rate is important because it determines the highest frequencies that can be sampled accurately. Thus, the sampling rate T_s determines the receiver bandwidth. This relationship and the significance of bandwidth are described in detail in Chapter 7. For now, suffice it to say that a high-bandwidth receiver is one that samples very rapidly. (T_s is very short.) Such a high-bandwidth receiver is desirable, particularly for certain high-speed-imaging applications. As the signal is sampled, it is stored temporarily in high-speed, high-capacity memory. The capacity of this memory determines how many images can be acquired without need for a pause in scanning to allow time for image reconstruction. High-speed receivers and large amounts of memory are often options that, of course, add to the cost of the MRI system.

The Computer

We will learn in Chapter 6 that the timing of events in an MRI pulse sequence is critical to effective imaging. It is the computer system that directs the orchestra that is MRI and makes sure when and how each event occurs. Not too long ago, most commercial MRI systems employed arcane computer architecture that would be unfamiliar (and unintelligible) to most MR users. Recently, however, commercial vendors have been employing very standard PC hardware and operating systems (Windows XP, LINUX) to build the MRI scanner console computer. The MR operator sits at a rather ordinary flat-panel display and uses a standard PC mouse and keyboard to operate the scanner through an interface that resembles that of a common PC.

Although the shell and interface of the computer system look familiar, the guts of the system still contain sophisticated proprietary hardware that is essential for running the system. Figure 5-13 shows a schematic of the MRI system components. When the MR operator enters the scan parameters in the console computer interface, this information is downloaded to a computer board that sets up the instructions to be delivered to the scanner hardware components. This board functions, in essence, as an extremely

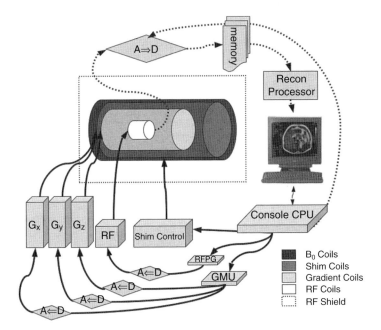

FIGURE 5-13. Schematic diagram of the MRI scanner system. Solid arrows indicate the steps involved in signal generation. Broken arrows indicate the steps involved in signal reception and image reconstruction. The key at lower right details the components of the scanner bore. Gray prisms at the lower left represent the amplifiers that drive the various coils.

accurate timer, dispatching instructions to the gradients, RF, and receiver in the right order and on a precise schedule.

Either built into the console computer or as subservient modules, two specific hardware components are used to appropriately trigger the gradient and RF amplifiers. These "amplifiers" are simply the devices that supply power to the gradient and RF coils. They are "supervised" by the gradient management unit (GMU) and RF pulse generator (RFPG). Just as the MR signal is an analog signal, the gradient and RF pulses are analog functions. In order for the digital computer to generate these analog pulses (also known as waveforms), a digital to analog converter (D2A) interfaces between the GMU or RFPG and the gradient and RF amplifiers.

After supervising generation of the MR signal, the computer system plays a central role in sampling and processing the signal. First, signal sampling by the receiver is triggered by the same console computer. After the signal is written to memory, specific computer components—often dedicated CPU and memory hardware—are used to reconstruct the MR images from the sampled signal. These special computer components perform the digital Fourier transform (DFT) that we will learn about in Chapter 6.

Finally, the reconstructed images are written to more permanent storage on a hard disk drive. On most commercial MR scanners, the original raw data are not stored permanently after the images are reconstructed. MR systems functioning in a research mode may provide an option for retention of this raw data, but the data will not be of much use to the clinical MR user.

The amount of memory available for storing raw MR signal data and for performing the DFT as well as the speed of the reconstruction computer determines how rapidly images can be reconstructed. Many scanners contain multiple reconstruction computers working in parallel to accelerate image reconstruction. The performance and abundance of this reconstruction hardware is what determines whether images appear on the screen in real time or if you have to wait for several seconds (or even minutes) after the scanner has completed the scan for image reconstruction to finish. Reconstruction speed, once again, also affects the price of your MRI system.

Though not a part of the actual scan acquisition hardware, the MRI console may also provide an array of software tools for image archival, printing, and image processing as well as the means to write data to removable media such as CD-ROM or DVD.

Shielding

Design and construction of the container that houses the MRI magnet and gradient coils as well as the building and room the scanner is installed in require a great deal of care and attention to detail. The design must provide specific measures to control several potential problems:

- B_0 fringe field
- Eddy currents
- RF noise

B_0 Fringe Field

As we saw in Figure 1-1, any magnetic field is described by magnetic field lines that emanate from the source of the magnetic field. In general, an unshielded magnetic field will decrease with the inverse square of distance. That is, the magnetic field strength at a distance x from a field of strength B_0 will be B_0/x^2. The magnetic field extending away from the source is called the fringe field. It is important for several reasons. First, patients such as those with pacemakers might be unsafe in the fringe field. Objects that are ferromagnetic might also be attracted toward the MRI scanner if they are brought into a substantial fringe field. In general, anywhere the fringe field exceeds 5 gauss is considered a potentially hazardous location. Second, distortion of B_0 may occur, leading to poor shim and image distortion. Think of the interaction of ferromagnetic objects with the magnetic field as a two-way street. Just as the field may interact with the object, attracting it and creating a safety problem, any metallic object can interact with the fringe field, causing distortion of field lines that lead to poor image quality. This problem is bad enough if there is a stationary ferromagnetic object in the fringe field such as a steel beam. Things become even more complex if moving metallic objects (even if they are not ferromagnetic) traverse the field lines. Field lines can and do extend beyond the confines of the scanner room and even outside the building, particularly in the case of very high field strength magnets. Anything from a wheelchair to an elevator or a tractor trailer can cause these effects if they cross the path of the fringe field.

Both of these problems can be addressed with one or both of the same two solutions. First, access to the fringe field can be restricted. By building a large room or building or even putting up a fence, both safety and interference concerns are addressed. Where real estate is at a premium, however, a better solution is needed. This comes in the form of magnetic field shielding. Simply put, magnetic fields are set up that oppose the fringe field. Remember that magnetic fields are simply vectors, and opposing vectors of equal magnitude sum to zero. These opposing magnetic fields truncate and contain the fringe field. This can be done using ferromagnetic material such as steel plate. Newer commercial MRI scanners are generally actively shielded. Additional magnet coils are built into the scanner's exterior layers that oppose, truncate, and contain the fringe field. Although this does not eliminate the fringe field entirely, it permits siting in a reasonably small room which, with no or minimal additional passive shielding, will fully contain the potentially problematic portions of the fringe field.

Location still plays a significant role when siting an MRI scanner. Proximity to elevators and other large moving metallic objects must be taken into account. In addition, when multiple MRI scanners are installed in close proximity, their B_0 fields may interact as well. To minimize this interaction, adjacent scanners are generally situated so that their non-like poles abut each other.

Eddy Currents

During imaging, gradient magnetic fields are turned on and off at rather high rates. What we have then is a time-varying magnetic field. From Faraday's law of induction, we can predict that this time-varying magnetic field will induce current in any nearby conductor. Further, once we have current flowing through that conductor, it in turn will generate a unique magnetic field. Thus, we have our gradient magnetic field *plus* an additional magnetic field induced by the gradient magnetic field. These, of course, sum to a net gradient magnetic field that is different from the linear gradient we expect to be applied. As a result, our spatial encoding, which depends on linear predictable gradients of magnetic field strength, is corrupted, leading to image artifacts.

The eddy current problem is addressed in two ways. In the first approach, the gradient coils are designed with active shielding. Just as with B_0 shielding, additional magnetic fields are generated. The fields are not constant (as with B_0 shielding) but come on in sync with the gradient magnetic field and attenuate the gradient magnetic field between the gradient coils and the outer metallic portions of the scanner, reducing induced eddy currents. Imaging is unaffected because the region within the diameter of the gradient coils toward the patient is unaffected. In the second approach, the gradient magnetic fields are deliberately distorted so that the eddy currents they induce sum with the predistorted gradient magnetic field to yield the uniform gradient that is desired. This process is called preemphasis and is possible because eddy currents, once characterized, will always manifest in the same way because they are a function of the scanner hardware.

RF Shielding

You may have had the experience of speaking on a portable telephone when suddenly an unexpected voice is heard on the line. What happened? Quite simply, someone nearby is talking on another portable phone that uses the same frequency as yours. The telephone receiver cannot tell which voice is which, so any signal with the same frequency makes it into your earpiece. Similarly, the receiver coil used in MRI is tuned to be sensitive to a specific frequency range. It does not know how to distinguish MRI signal from police or CB radio traffic, and the coil will pick up any signal that is in its sensitive range. This may lead to significant image artifacts that are discussed in Chapter 10.

To prevent contamination of the MRI signal, the scanner room must be shielded to exclude all signals that are within the frequency range measured in MRI. This is done by enclosing the room in a Faraday cage. The Faraday cage is simply an electrically continuous envelope of conductive material that is connected to ground. Commonly used materials include copper sheet and mesh and steel plate. The key is to be sure that every joint including the door and window openings have excellent electrical connections so that there is no breech in the RF shield. It is also important to keep the door closed during scanning, as it is a key component of the shield as well.

Any cables made of conductive material that enter the Faraday cage must enter through a special "penetration panel" where the current they carry is filtered to remove unwanted RF signals (noise). In order to allow non-conductive tubing, fiberoptic cables, and so forth, to enter the MRI room, *waveguides* are placed through the penetration panel or wall. These are conductive tubes that attenuate any RF noise in much the same way that your FM car radio signal is attenuated and vanishes when you drive into a tunnel of sufficient length relative to its width. Similarly, waveguides must be of appropriate length-to-diameter ratio so that they attenuate any RF signal that might be present outside the room. It is important to be careful not to run any conductive material such as wires through the waveguides unless the cables are properly filtered. Such a wire violates the shield, effectively serving as a broadcast antenna that brings any RF signal outside the Faraday cage right into the room.

The Prescan Process

Chapter 8 will pull together all we have discussed to this point and present the material as a cohesive and functional "pulse sequence." Before that pulse sequence ever happens, however, a series of steps must be taken to prepare and calibrate the scanner hardware. These steps are typically performed before each and every scan and are all automated as part of an auto-prescan procedure found on all commercial MRI scanners. We have already discussed most of these items in detail, but we will fill in some information as well as review the whole process here. Note that while it may seem like an annoying delay before the "real scanning" starts, without the prescan, we would have only a very poor quality image, if any at all. The first portion of the prescan process (Table 5-2), coil tuning and matching, was discussed previously as were shimming and RF calibration. The remaining steps that comprise the prescan are discussed in the sections that follow.

Center Frequency Determination

Determining the center frequency accurately finds ω_0 for the patient. Because of slight fluctuations in B_0 as a result of, for example, temperature or tissue composition, ω_0 cannot be predicted but must be determined by experiment. A signal is acquired from the tissue without any spatial localization (no gradient magnetic fields). If that signal is sampled and subjected to the Fourier transform (see Chapter 6, third box), we will obtain a range of frequencies, each associated with signal amplitude. ω_0 is simply the frequency at which we measure the greatest signal. The difference between

TABLE 5-2. The prescan procedure.

Coil tune and match
Shimming of B_0
Center frequency determination
RF calibration
Receiver gain setting

this "observed" ω_0 and the ω_0 calculated based on the expected strength of B_0 is termed the *observer offset* or *frequency offset* and is used to set the correct frequency of the RF. The typical offset, which reflects the precision of the calibration of B_0, ranges up to several thousand hertz.

Receiver Gain Adjustment

Receiver gain determines the strength of the signal that will be transmitted to the A2D. Typically, we adjust the degree to which this signal is attenuated before being passed through to the A2D. This step is important because excessive amplitude results in truncation (clipping) of the data, degrading image quality. If we do not provide enough signal amplitude to the receiver, on the other hand, signal to noise will suffer. Just like Goldilocks, we like it just right!

Part II
User Friendly: Localizing and Optimizing the MRI Signal for Imaging

6
Spatial Localization: Creating an Image

What Is an Image?

Let us be clear about our discussions to this point: we have not generated anything that even remotely resembles an image! The preceding chapters discuss in detail how we can generate, measure, and manipulate an NMR signal. Yet, if asked where in the patient the signal measured in the previous chapters *comes from*, we can only answer that it comes from each and every bit of tissue that is within range of the RF receiver coil. We cannot be more specific than that because the RF receiver coil cannot be focused on a specific physical location in order to only receive signal from that one location; any and all signal from all locations will be detected. What will be detected if we place the patient in the scanner so that his or her abdomen fills the RF receiver coil? Certainly, the feet and ankles are too far outside the coil to generate any signal. However, the measured signal does come from the entire abdomen, and there is absolutely *no* way to differentiate signals arising from the kidney, adrenal, bowel, liver, and so forth, or, for that matter, signals arising from cancer and signals arising from healthy tissue. Again, unlike CT where the x-ray beam is shone only on the body region of interest (a slice), the coil cannot be focused on, say, the left kidney to the exclusion of all other signal. The NMR technique, as described to this point, is well-suited to measuring the properties of a homogeneous sample such as a test tube containing a protein in solution, but it is virtually useless for detecting *localized* abnormalities in a sample as heterogeneous as the human body.

To be clinically useful, MRI must provide measures of signal coming from discrete locations in the body. Ultimately, the images will be most useful if we can distinguish very small portions of tissue that are very close together. Keep in mind that, at the end of the day, MRI is nothing more than differentiating two tissues—normal or pathologic—based on their T1, T2, T2*, proton density, diffusion, et cetera (see previous chapters), *and* their location. Consider a human liver containing a metastatic tumor. If the signal measured from tumor and normal liver tissue is indistinguishable, we will fail to detect the presence of the metastasis. As we have seen, this *can* occur if the MRI parameters (TE, TR, etc.) are selected in a way that, intentionally or not, minimizes these differences. Similarly, if the tumor and healthy tissue generate different signals, but the MR signal we measure contains signal from both tumor and healthy tissue, the result is a *single signal measurement that reflects a composite of the two tissues and fails to differentiate them.* In practice, we refer to this as a partial volume effect, or partial volume artifact.

Image Geometry

What is the nature of the image we are trying to create? The MR image—similar to CT, ultrasound, and PET images—represents a slice of tissue; MRI is a tomographic imaging method. When viewed on a computer display, the image is shown as a two-dimensional grid of squares (actually, they could be rectangles as well) called *pixels* (for picture elements). The slice of *tissue* that the image represents is, of course, three-dimensional; it has a real thickness. Therefore, each pixel actually represents a prism-shaped chunk of tissue that we refer to as a *voxel* (for volume element). The grayscale image intensity displayed within the pixel representing a given voxel is proportional to the MR signal measured at that location in the patient. Spatial resolution, of course, is a function of the number of voxels that are employed to create the image.

All we need to do is parse the signal acquired from a volume of tissue into that arising from individual slices and then further separate it into that arising from discrete locations (voxels) within each of those slices. Generating images from NMR data is no simple matter, however. The NMR effect was discovered toward the end of World War II, and NMR measurements (spectroscopy) were used extensively in chemistry and physics throughout the 1950s, 1960s, and 1970s. It was not until the late 1970s, however, that scientists succeeded in making an (albeit crude) MR *image.* Clinical MRI did not arrive until the 1980s. There is a well-known dispute regarding who "developed" MRI. While the earliest MRI images of the human body were generated independently in 1977–1978 by groups led by Raymond Damadian and Sir Peter Mansfield, the field focused (FONAR) method used by Damadian did not turn out to be an efficient means for practical imaging. Even Damadian's FONAR Corporation today manufactures MRI scanners that use the approach developed by Mansfield's group. Mansfield's approach was based on the principle of frequency encoding (see the "Frequency Encoding" section in this chapter) developed by Paul Lauterbur. The 2003 Nobel Prize in Medicine was awarded to Mansfield and Lauterbur for the advance of *imaging*, separate from the discovery of NMR; that one went to Bloch and Purcell in 1952.

Understanding and Exploiting B$_0$ Homogeneity

Before we actually start to describe the formation of an MR image, we must return to the concept of B$_0$ homogeneity and the gradient magnetic field. Until now, everything that we have considered was based on a key assumption: the externally applied magnetic field, B$_0$, is constant. That is, at every point within the MRI scanner and, therefore, at every point within the patient, the strength of B$_0$ is exactly the same. In the real world, of course, it is not possible to create such a perfectly homogeneous magnetic field. Though we acknowledge reality, in order to further our endeavor to understand MRI, we have made a leap of faith and assumed that B$_0$ is the same magnitude and direction at every location in the scanner.

The Gradient Magnetic Field: A Review

To generate an image, we will begin by destroying B$_0$ homogeneity! The key point, however, is that although we make B$_0$ heterogeneous, we will always do so in a transient, orderly, and predictable manner. This corruption of B$_0$ homogeneity is accomplished by applying a linear gradient magnetic field. Gradient magnetic fields and the hardware used to generate them are discussed in greater detail in Chapter 5. For now, it is important to recall some basic concepts. The gradient magnetic field differs from the B$_0$ field in several important ways:

- It is generated by a resistive electromagnet;
- It is only turned on at specific points during image acquisition;
- It is much weaker than B$_0$;
- Most importantly, its strength *varies* along a linear path either parallel or perpendicular to B$_0$.

Gradient Magnetic Fields Are Linear

The linear change in gradient strength is depicted in Figures 5-6 and 5-7 in the previous chapter. As an example, consider a gradient magnetic field parallel to B$_0$ that we will call the z gradient, or G$_z$. As we move toward the center of the scanner bore, the strength of G$_z$ declines until we reach isocenter. This location where the strength of G$_z$ = 0 is the isocenter. Continuing in the same direction away from isocenter, the strength of G$_z$ will increase. At a given distance on either side of isocenter, the magnitude of G$_z$ is the same; however, its orientation is opposite. This symmetry in magnitude and direction of G$_z$ is central to understanding the effect of the gradient magnetic field. This symmetry is also the reason that G$_z$ = 0 at isocenter; equal and opposite components of G$_z$ cancel each other at isocenter.

Location Is Frequency

In 1973, Paul Lauterbur described the concept that modulation of precessional frequency by a gradient magnetic field can be used to localize NMR signal. This concept forms the foundation on which all modern MRI is based and led to Lauterbur's Nobel Prize in 2003. When the gradient magnetic field is on, what does a proton "see"? Simply, the applied magnetic field (B_{net}) becomes the sum of B_0 and, in this example, G_z; $B_{net} = B_0 + G_z$. Thus, as shown in Figure 5-5 in the previous chapter, the location of a proton along the z dimension determines the *net* magnetic field that it experiences and, consequently, the precessional frequency of that proton. We have now varied the strength

> **Notice the subtle introduction of a key concept:** Location is always described in terms of distance from isocenter and the location relative to isocenter. Because it confers unique field strength, B_{net} can be described by frequency of precession. From here on, our mantra will be: "Frequency *Is* Location." Learn it, love it, live it. . . .

of the applied magnetic field—we now speak of B_{net}, not B_0—along *one dimension* of the MRI scanner. What next?

A First Look at Signal Localization

At the beginning of this chapter, we recalled how, given a perfectly homogeneous B_0, the signal detected will arise from all portions of the patient within range of the coil. We also discussed why this is not particularly useful information (i.e., partial volume effects) and the need to look at a slice of the patient. In the presence of G_z, however, protons will experience a different B_{net} depending on their location along G_z. As a result, the precessional frequency (ω) will vary; at isocenter where $B_{net} = B_0$, $\omega = \omega_0$, but as distance from isocenter increases, ω will change according to G_z.

Now, in the presence of a gradient magnetic field, we will observe that, although signal detection cannot be manipulated in order to only "listen to" a certain portion of the patient, we can control *the part of the patient from which we generate signal in the first place*. If only spins within a specific slice of tissue, perhaps through the midportion of the abdomen, are excited by the RF, then signal comes only from that slice.

Slice Selection Using the Gradient Magnetic Field

With the gradient magnetic field G_z on, protons will experience a different B_{net} and therefore, a different ω depending on their location along G_z. If B_1 is transmitted with a frequency of ω_0 while G_z is on, only protons with $\omega = \omega_0$—those located precisely at isocenter and experiencing B_0 without additional field strength due to G_z—will have resonance with B_1. Remember that $G_z = 0$ at isocenter. Because G_z varies along the z dimension, but *not* along the x or y dimensions, all spins at the isocenter of G_z achieve resonance with the applied B_1 regardless of their x-y location. We have defined a plane perpendicular to B_0 and have excited only the spins residing within this plane. The signal detected now comes only from an axial slice (transverse to B_0). Of course, for slice selection to work, G_z *must be on during the time that B_1 is on.*

Slice Thickness

As we emphasized earlier, a slice has real thickness. Measurement of signal only arising from spins lying on a plane (i.e., infinitely thin) is an impossibility. Similarly, it is physically impossible to transmit B_1 at a single frequency. The RF transmitter hardware is not and never will be that precise. B_1 is always transmitted as a limited range of frequencies or RF bandwidth.

Caution: The use of the term *bandwidth* at this juncture may lead to confusion when we discuss receiver bandwidth in a later section. The two are entirely distinct parameters.

When a range of frequencies centered on ω_0 is transmitted as the RF pulse, all spins resonant with any of those frequencies will become excited. This group of excited spins represents a range of frequencies residing on either side of isocenter (Fig. 6-1). That is, a slice has been selected; when signal is measured, it comes only from this slice centered at the isocenter of G_z.

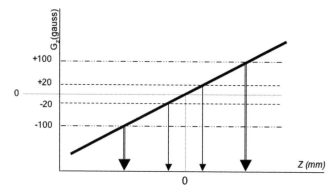

FIGURE 6-1. Range of RF frequencies modulates slice thickness. When a given range of RF frequency is transmitted, all spins experiencing a field strength ($B_{net} = B_0 + G$) that confers a frequency of precession within that range will become excited. This defines the slice. In this example, a slice with thickness defined by the thin arrows is excited by transmitting a narrower range of frequencies than the one defined by the striped arrows.

How is slice thickness determined? The scan operator fills in a field on a computer screen to specify the slice thickness, but what happens to ensure that the slice will, in fact, be 5 mm thick and not 1 mm, 2 mm, or 25 mm thick? Using a gradient magnetic field for slice selection leads to two possibilities for determining the thickness of the slice. As indicated above, transmitting a narrower range of frequencies will result in a thinner slice, whereas a broader range of frequencies will yield a thicker slice (Fig. 6-1). Ultimately, it is not the absolute range of frequencies transmitted but the match between the frequencies transmitted and the range of precessional frequencies that exist in the patient. The range of frequencies in the patient is a function of the range of magnetic field strength, B_{net}, across a given distance in tissue. B_{net} is determined by the gradient magnetic field G_z, which can be set to yield a greater or lesser range of gradient magnetic field strength over a fixed distance by adjusting its strength (read slope). When more power (electric current) is put into the gradient coils, the slope of the gradient magnetic field increases. As a result, G_z and B_{net} change a greater amount over a fixed distance. Similarly, when power input to the gradient coils is decreased, the field will change less over that same distance. Thus, any range of field strength (and consequently any range of precessional frequency ω) will occur over more or less distance depending on the gradient strength. If we transmit RF at a fixed bandwidth, the thickness of the slice of tissue that becomes excited will vary with the gradient strength; more power to the gradients (steeper slope) will lead to a thinner slice and less power (shallow slope) to a thicker slice (Fig. 6-2).

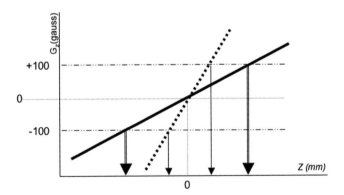

FIGURE 6-2. Gradient strength modulates slice thickness. Two slices are selected: one defined by the thin solid arrows and one defined by the striped arrows. In both cases, the same range of RF frequencies is transmitted. By altering the strength of the slice select gradient, we modify the spatial extent of tissue (slice thickness) over which B_{net} ($B_{net} = B_0 + G$) confers ω, matching the frequencies transmitted by the RF. Steep (stronger; thick broken line) gradients limit the range of frequencies to a thinner slice (solid arrows), whereas shallower (weaker; thick solid line) gradient strength "spreads" the same range of frequency across a thicker slice (striped arrows).

So how thin a slice can we image? Setting aside the issue of signal to noise, the previous discussion leads us to a physical limitation on the minimum slice thickness. (Maybe we should be calling it slice thinness?) To generate the thinnest possible slice, we will make the RF bandwidth as narrow as possible (excite only a small range of frequencies) and, at the same time, make the gradient magnetic field as strong (steep) as possible (keep the range of frequencies to be excited within the smallest distance along the gradient magnetic field). How steep we can make the gradient magnetic field (how strong our gradients are) and how narrow we can make the RF bandwidth (how precise our RF amplifier is) determine the absolute minimum slice thickness for a given MR system's hardware. Examining the specifications for a typical clinical MR system will show that the minimum slice thickness is generally in the range of 0.1 mm! Because of signal-to-noise limitations, we could never generate a useful image of that thickness. However, understanding the basis for this curiosity may be the best test of our understanding of slice selection.

Slice Location

The preceding example will not get us too far in performing clinical MRI exams. Only acquiring slices that are centered on isocenter would be too limiting, requiring us to move the patient for each successive slice. In practice, we simply adjust the transmitted RF frequency to match ω at the location of interest (Fig. 6-3). Knowing the nature of the gradient magnetic field used for slice selection allows us to know B_{net} at any location and adjust the RF transmission frequency to correspond with ω at that location.

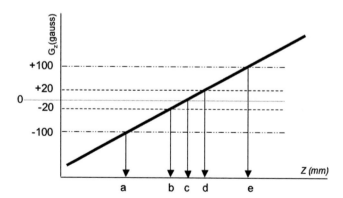

FIGURE 6-3. RF frequency determines slice position. When the RF frequency is centered on ω_0, we have selected a slice centered at isocenter (position c). Varying this central RF frequency results in slices located on either side of isocenter (a, b, d, e). Location is determined by ω (determined by $B_{net} = B_0 + G_z$) present at that location.

Plane of Section

Another unwelcome limitation of our example is the restricted plane of section. When using the z gradient magnetic field for slice selection, slices will always be transverse to the patient (orthogonal to z). One of the great advantages of MRI, of course, is its ability to image in any plane of section, certainly not only the transverse plane. Just as transverse images are selected by using the z gradient magnetic field that is orthogonal to the plane of the transverse slice, using a different gradient magnetic field will generate images perpendicular to that dimension. If the x gradient magnetic field runs left to right, using it for slice selection will yield sagittal images. If the y gradient magnetic field runs floor to ceiling, using it for slice selection will generate coronal images.

What about oblique slices? Remember that gradient magnetic fields are represented by vectors that describe their magnitude and orientation. As vectors, if more than one is present at the same time, they will sum to a single resultant vector. This means that a single obliquely oriented gradient magnetic field will be present. Simultaneous application of multiple gradient magnetic fields will generate images perpendicular to the vector sum of those gradient magnetic fields. The orientation of the slice is determined by the gradient magnetic fields used, which ones, and how much power is supplied to each. *Voilà!* An infinite array of oblique images can be generated. Recognize how much is going on "behind the scenes" when the MR technologist is rotating graphical lines over a scout image to prescribe the required oblique image.

Localizing Signal Within the Plane of the Slice: Background for Frequency and Phase Encoding

Dividing a Single Signal

The signal we acquire when employing the method for slice selection described above is a composite signal arising from all spins at all locations *within the slice*. While we do know that the signal is coming from a specific location (the slice), only a single measurement of signal intensity can be retrieved from that slice. Often students ask: What does the image look like at this point? If we define the image as an array of 256×256 pixels, but we only have this single measurement of signal, the same shade of gray representing the signal intensity acquired will have to be put in each and every pixel.

Organs, tissues, and disease within the slice cannot be separated or localized. We really haven't come much closer to imaging than when we collected a signal from the whole body without slice selection. At this point, we need a method that will determine what part of the signal coming from this slice belongs in each different location within the slice. Recall that our slice is an array or matrix of pixels, each representing a voxel at a specific location in the slice of tissue being imaged.

The starting point is indeed a single signal coming from all of the spins within the slice. Individual voxels or individual portions of the slice are *not* imaged separately and then put back together as in CT or SPECT (single photon emission computed tomography). In MRI, this single signal arising from the *whole slice* is separated into a number of component signals, each from a specific location. The sum of these component signals, it turns out, will yield the original signal we measured from the whole slice. As a crude analogy, MRI is like listening to a symphony (a composite signal from a whole slice) and deducing what instruments (tissue types) are playing and where on the stage (location in the plane of the slice) each type of instrument is located. The symphony example is really quite a difficult task, even for an experienced listener. If asked to determine only the types of instruments in the orchestra, most of us would do pretty well. Similarly, if there was only one instrument type, it would not be hard to tell where specific parts of the symphony come from: solos from identifiable discrete locations, ensembles from larger or multiple locations, and, of course, the whole symphony. However, determining instrument type and location simultaneously would be quite challenging; it amounts to solving an equation with two unknowns.

Setting Up for Spatial Localization

To the engineers, audiophiles, and associated geeks, it is clear that MRI amounts to nothing more than (albeit complex) signal analysis. There is more to it, however. In MRI, the signal we analyze is not a complete unknown akin to signals received by a radiotelescope. For spatial localization in MRI, we stack the deck, specifically setting up predictable variations in the signal that depend on the location the signal arises from. Armed with this foreknowledge, the location of the component signals can be determined. Our equation now contains only one unknown—signal intensity— which reflects tissue type. Spatial location, we will see, is no longer a variable because we cause signal to vary by location in a known and predictable manner.

Localization Within the Slice

Spatial localization within the plane of the slice is a two-step process. First, we will perform localization along a single dimension using a method called frequency encoding. Once signal has been separated according to its location along that first dimension, we will *subsequently* separate the signal from each location along the first dimension into separate components, each from a different location along the second in-plane dimension.

Remember our mantra: *Frequency Is Location*. If this is not clear, please review this concept as discussed earlier in this chapter and know it well before continuing.

Frequency Encoding: The *Next* Stage

Once the spins within the slice have been excited, the slice select gradient is turned off; it has completed its function and is no longer needed. The spins are now precessing, at least in part, in the transverse plane with a precessional frequency of ω_0. Their precessional frequency is ω_0 because, with no gradient magnetic field on, the only magnetic field they experience at this time is B_0. Next, while the spins in the slice still have net transverse magnetization (and before we record any signal), a gradient magnetic field is turned on in a direction orthogonal to the slice select direction. For our example where the z direction is used for slice selection, let's say that the x gradient magnetic field is now applied. What is the effect? The net magnetic field strength experienced by the spins, B_{net}, now varies along the x dimension in a linear manner (Fig. 6-4). As a result, the precessional frequency of spins in the slice now varies in a linear manner along the same x dimension. Note that spins at the same x location will experience the same B_{net} and have the same ω regardless of their location along the third (y) dimension.

At this point, there is measurable difference between spins that depends on their location along the x dimension: frequency of precession. The signal is *frequency encoded*. How can we exploit and measure that difference to

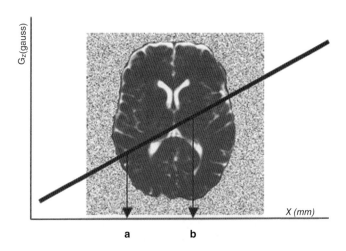

FIGURE 6-4. Frequency encoding. Once we have selected the slice, applying a gradient magnetic field (G_x) along one dimension (x) causes spins to precess with different frequencies depending on their location (a, b) along this frequency-encoding dimension.

separate signal based on location? We could tune our receiver coil (like tuning your car's FM radio) to be exclusively sensitive to specific frequencies and then measure signal intensity for each of those frequencies. This would yield signal intensity arising from the locations in the slice where ω matches the sensitive frequency of our receiver. In this manner, we could systematically measure the signal at each of many locations along the x dimension. However, the limit of the frequency difference that we can detect and, it follows, our spatial resolution, will depend on the precision with which our receiver can separate small differences in frequency, locations very close together along x. In spite of the fact that the minimum spatial separation along x required to yield a frequency difference is infinitely small (i.e., frequency changes with every micron or even smaller increment in location), the spatial resolution would be quite poor using this approach because the precision of receiver hardware is comparatively very poor relative to the spatial resolution we require to generate a useful image.

Separating Frequencies with the Fourier Transform (Don't Be Afraid!)

To fully exploit the high spatial resolution that lies within this *frequency-encoded* signal, we require a method that can extract signal intensity for very many small increments of frequency. Enter the Fourier transform, a full mathematical treatment of which is beyond the scope of this text. More importantly, such an intimate understanding is unnecessary to understand spatial localization in MRI. The following description of Fourier analysis as used in frequency encoding (and later, phase encoding) is simplistic, but truthful. Although we will look at the Fourier transform as, essentially, a "black box," the actual function and limitations of Fourier analysis will not be distorted.

The easiest way to grasp the concept embodied by the Fourier transform is to first examine what is known as the inverse Fourier transform. Simply stated, if we have several signals (sine functions), each with a unique frequency and amplitude, we can find a single signal that represents these individual signals as a group. How? Simply add the sine waves together (Fig. 6-5). That is the inverse Fourier transform. The forward Fourier transform does the converse: given a single signal, it can identify the components that were added together to form that *composite* signal. That's all! The internal workings of the Fourier transform, as we just said, are not prerequisite to our understanding of spatial localization in MRI, and we will not examine them at all.

Signal from the excited spins within the slice is measured as a single complex function (signal amplitude changing over time) with a frequency and amplitude that is the sum of signals arising from each of the spins within the slice. We take multiple samples of this complex signal over time, each a measure of signal amplitude taken at a point in time. The Fourier transform analyzes these samples and returns a list of frequencies and

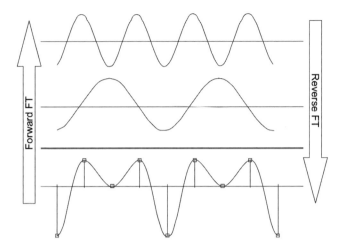

FIGURE 6-5. The Fourier transform. In this simplified example, two sine functions can be added together point-by-point to yield a single composite function. This is the *reverse* Fourier transform. When we sample the composite signal, the Fourier transform can extract the two component signals.

corresponding signal amplitudes. These frequencies are the individual components that make up our composite signal.

Fourier Analysis Applied to the Frequency-Encoded Signal

In the presence of the frequency-encoding gradient along x, the signal sampled and input to the Fourier transform is composed of a range of frequencies determined by the frequency-encoding gradient magnetic field. Each sample has only one characteristic: signal amplitude. The series of measurements is recorded in computer memory in the form of an array that we can think of as a single row in a spreadsheet, one cell for each sample. Again, signal amplitude is the quantity entered into each cell. Once these data have been recorded, it is fed into the Fourier transform, our "black box." The Fourier transform receives two types of information: (1) measures of *signal amplitude* and (2) a discrete *number of samples* in the *order in which they were collected*. These data are the MRI *raw data*, also referred to as *time-domain data* and sometimes as *k-space data*. The designation of the data as *k*-space data at this point is somewhat erroneous, but we will have plenty to say about *k*-space later on. In any case, the number of samples is, as we will see, key to spatial resolution.

The Fourier transform, given the data input described above, returns a number of sine functions, each with its own frequency and associated signal amplitude. Our row of raw data (signal amplitude sampled over time) has been transformed into measures of signal amplitude for each of a number of frequencies. These are the components of the composite signal that was sampled by the MRI scanner. If we now work backward and add the component functions (sine waves) together (the inverse Fourier transform described above), we will end up with a single sine wave that *approximates* the composite signal we started out with. We say approximates because only with an infinite number of samples over time will the Fourier transform exactly replicate the source signal that was sampled. From this fact, we understand that the greater the number of samples fed to the Fourier transform, the greater the fidelity of the results. We will discuss this more when we cover the truncation artifact in Chapter 10.

How Many Samples Do We Need?

One fine point: In MRI, because we are analyzing digital data, a specific implementation of the Fourier transform is employed called (surprise!) the digital Fourier transform (DFT). The only reason to be aware of this is that the DFT will only handle a number of samples that is a factor of two (2^n). It will return the same number of amplitude-frequency combinations. This explains why MRI images always seem to come with certain pixel dimensions like 64, 128, 256, 512, and so forth. This is due to the nature of the adaptation of the Fourier transform for digital data. The details are beyond the scope of our discussion and, frankly, will not help you understand diagnostic MR images.

Finally, what use is it to know the signal amplitude associated with each item on a list of component frequencies? Remember that the Fourier transform of the signal from our slice would yield only one frequency (ω_0) if the frequency-encoding gradient were not present. By applying this frequency-encoding gradient magnetic field, the spatial location of different portions of the aggregate signal amplitude is determined: *Frequency Is Location.*

For those that are really on their toes, this statement will be very unsettling. If we provide the Fourier transform with multiple samples, how can it possibly yield a single frequency? The answer, of course, is that there indeed will be multiple frequencies. The source of those frequencies lies in the differences in ω conferred on spins by their molecular environment. The electron clouds of different molecular environments will generate local magnetic fields that cause subtle variations in B_0. Alas, we return to the fact that absolute homogeneity of B_0 is impossible. This inherent variability in B_0 leads to multiple frequencies that form the molecular signature detected in MR spectroscopy. Because the frequency differences relative to ω_0 are so small relative to the frequency differences that result from the gradient magnetic field used for frequency encoding, it is only *in the absence of gradient magnetic fields* that these molecular differences can be detected. Spectroscopy will be discussed in more detail in Chapter 19.

Frequency Encoding: The Bottom Line

In summary, the signal (a composite of signal from all spins in the slice) is sampled over time; multiple measurements of signal amplitude are made at separate but continuous points in time. *During the time we are sampling*, a constant gradient magnetic field is continuously present, causing a linear variation in precessional frequency along the dimension of this *frequency-encoding gradient*. The multiple samples of signal amplitude acquired over time are recorded in order in computer memory (Fig. 6-6). Each of these samples contains signal derived *from the entire slice!* We next feed these data into the Fourier transform, yielding one component frequency and an associated signal amplitude for each data sample processed. Thus, *time-domain*

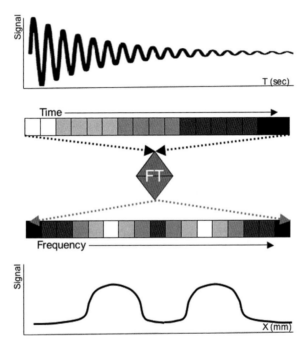

FIGURE 6-6. Basic operation of the 1DFT. The FID shown at the top is the signal we are sampling. Each of the boxes in the two rows of shaded squares represents a sample of signal amplitude; the lighter the shade of gray, the greater the measured signal amplitude. In the top row, each is a sample recorded over time (T) and recorded in time order from left to right. Signal is higher early on because signal is diminishing over time with T2* in this example where we are sampling an FID. The Fourier transform returns a list of frequencies, recorded in increasing order from left to right in the bottom row. Each box contains the signal amplitude that is associated with that frequency. In this example of signal acquired from an axial slice through the legs, we see higher signal (whiter) where there is more tissue. The plot at the bottom is a simple graph of location (x, determined by frequency) along the horizontal axis and signal amplitude plotted along the vertical axis. The two humps represent the two legs from which we have detected signal.

data are transformed into *frequency-domain data*. Because we can determine the location of specific frequencies based on the slope of the applied frequency-encoding gradient, we can assign signal amplitude to the location in the image from which it arose. Once again, *Frequency Is Location*.

The One-dimensional Image

What do we have at this point? An image? Not exactly. We know the distribution of signal intensity across one dimension of the slice only. Let's say we have selected a transverse slice through the lower legs. Graphing location along x (the left-right dimension) on the horizontal axis and signal intensity along the vertical axis, we get an "image" like the one at the bottom of Figure 6-6. There is signal where the body parts (legs) are and no signal outside of them. This is sometimes called a one-dimensional image, and the process that generated it is a one-dimensional Fourier transform (1DFT). Whereas this method may be employed during calibration of the scanner as part of the prescan, it does not create an image that is useful for diagnosis.

Often students ask: What does the image look like at this point? If we define the image as an array of 256 × 256 pixels, but we only have a single measurement of signal for each point along one dimension, the same shade of gray representing the signal intensity at each location along x will have to be put in each and every pixel along y. Organs, tissues, and disease at each x location cannot be separated or localized along y. The "image" would look like a row of stripes oriented perpendicular to the x dimension (Fig. 6-7), but of course this is not truly an image at all.

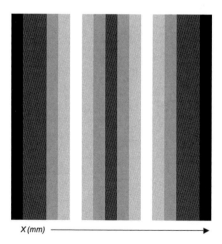

X *(mm)*

FIGURE 6-7. The "image" produced by the Fourier transform of a single row of data. In reality, the Fourier transform only provides us with a single list of frequencies and corresponding signal amplitudes; it is a one-dimensional "image." If we define our image as a two-dimensional array of pixels and "force" the data to fill this space, we can only put the same value of signal intensity in every pixel along "y" (vertical dimension) for a given location along y.

We are only marginally closer to imaging than when we collected a signal from the whole body without slice selection and certainly have not yet generated a useful medical image. At this point, we need a method that will determine what part of the signal at each point along x (separated during frequency encoding) comes from individual locations along the second in-plane dimension (in our example, y).

Phase Encoding and the Two-dimensional Fourier Transform

This is a good time for a strong cup of coffee, as we are venturing into the challenging but rewarding study of phase encoding, the final step in spatial localization that actually generates a real two-dimensional image. Fasten your seat belts!

Of course, we cannot apply *both* gradient magnetic fields at the same time in order to accomplish frequency encoding along two dimensions; the simultaneous application of two gradient magnetic fields is equivalent to applying a single obliquely oriented gradient magnetic field. Applying both gradients at once will result in frequency encoding along the oblique direction described by the resultant vector of, in this example, x and y. In the description of projection techniques in the text that follows, the gradients are applied at two separate points in time, collecting two separate signals, one during the application of each gradient magnetic field.

How We Don't *Do It*

Our frequency-domain data—a list of signal amplitudes each with corresponding frequency that refer to specific locations along the x dimension—contain definitive information regarding location along x. For each of these locations along x, we must now separate signal along y. The most common suggestion students offer for achieving this goal is to merely frequency encode again using the y dimension gradient instead of x. (You know how the saying goes: If your only tool is a hammer, every problem becomes a nail!) Truth be told, this could be done. Frequency encoding twice along each of two orthogonal directions would yield two arrays of frequencies and associated amplitudes. These data could be put through a mathematical algorithm to interpolate the acquired signal to the matrix of locations in the slice. The mathematical method is called *back projection*, and it is the method used to reconstruct CT images from multiple passes of an x-ray beam. However, using two orthogonal frequency-encoding directions is like merely taking frontal and lateral radiographs of the chest and trying to reconstruct a chest CT image. For this multiple frequency-encoding approach to be useful, many more "views" are required. The CT scanner shines its beam on multiple small detectors, making many passes through the body from many different directions. An MRI technique was developed to use multiple (many more than two) frequency-encoding directions for reconstruction of an MR image. The back-projection method was described by Paul Lauterbur in 1973 and was, perhaps, the first technique capable of generating an MR image. He called his technique Zeugmatography. Although acquisition of a true NMR image was certainly a major advance, the projection approach is inefficient and has gone the way of the leisure suit. Nonetheless, a single array of data acquired using frequency encoding is still sometimes referred to as a *view*.

Why Phase Encode?

Based on the concept of frequency encoding described by Lauterbur, Richard Ernst developed a much more robust means for encoding and reconstructing an MR image. This approach that Ernst originally termed "NMR Fourier zeugmatography" in contrast with Lauterbur's (projection) zeugmatography is now called two-dimensional Fourier transform imaging (2DFT) and is the basis for all modern MRI. The main difference between the two approaches is the use of the Fourier transform in Ernst's method. The hallmark of his method is phase encoding. Phase encoding allows us to extract locations along the second (y) dimension efficiently and with better signal-to-noise ratio than the projection method described earlier. The essence of phase encoding is an incremental change in phase of spins (all spins) in the slice such that the amount of change in phase varies with distance from isocenter.

First, let us address the manner in which gradient magnetic fields affect phase. As a spin precesses about B_0 at a fixed frequency ω_0, its absolute orientation will change with a fixed periodicity such that it will repeatedly return to its "starting" orientation after the same time interval (called a *period*). If we briefly accelerate the precession of this spin and then slow it back down to precess again at ω_0, it will now return to a point further along in its path every period (Fig. 6-8). This "phase shift" was induced by the change in frequency. Thus, by *briefly applying a gradient magnetic field, frequency will be changed only transiently, but a permanent change in phase will occur that persists long after the gradient magnetic field is turned off.* Spins seeing higher gradient magnetic field strength will have larger changes in phase. Notice that it is not the absolute gradient strength that matters but the change relative to the baseline (B_0) frequency of precession.

If we compare the phase shift of spins relative to their phase under B_0 alone, spins subject to a greater magnitude of G_y will have a greater (albeit transient) increase in frequency and, therefore, a greater permanent shift in phase relative to spins subject to less magnitude of G_y. Which spins are subject to greater magnitude of G_y? Farthest from isocenter, the magnitude

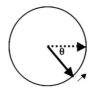

FIGURE 6-8. Phase shift induced by the gradient magnetic field. In this top-down view of spin precessing in the transverse plane, the solid arrow indicates the point to which the spin returns every period while experiencing B_0; the spin, in this example, makes a full revolution (360°) each period. Adding the additional phase-encoding gradient causes the spin's precession to accelerate. It now arrives at the location of the broken arrow during one period, having traveled a bit more than 360°. Next, the phase-encoding gradient is turned off. The spin again experiences only B_0 and travels 360° during each subsequent period. The phase shift θ remains.

of G_y will be greatest, and those spins far from isocenter will experience greater shift in phase. Remember that at isocenter G_y is, by definition, 0 and has no effect on phase. Also note that our description of phase is always relative to some point of reference, in this example relative to phase in the absence of G_y under B_0 alone. Phase cannot be measured as an absolute; we do not observe the phase of any spin, only its effects.

How Can Phase Be Detected?

Consider the effect of this phase-encoding gradient not on one spin's phase but on the phase of a group of spins. Because any two or more spins cannot be in the same place at the same time, they cannot experience the same magnitude of the phase-encoding gradient and cannot experience the same degree of phase shift. Based on our assumption that, absent gradient magnetic fields, all spins experience identical magnetic field strength, B_0, it follows that all spins will precess at the same frequency, ω_0, and, therefore, precess in phase. This phase coherent precession (what we achieve by applying the RF pulse B_1) is the condition under which we measure maximum signal from a group of spins. Phase coherence implies that, at any point in time, the vector sum of the transverse magnetization of a group of spins (i.e., net transverse magnetization = signal intensity) will be maximal. Under the effect of the phase-encoding gradient, however, each spin is at a slightly different location along the gradient magnetic field, is subject to a unique magnetic field strength $(B_0 + G_y)$, and has a different frequency of precession, ω, than adjacent spins. The spins will now begin to precess *out of phase*. The result, of course, is that, at any point in time, the vector sum of the transverse magnetization of a group of spins will be less than maximal due to the more random phase of the spins in our group. We will detect less net M_t in the presence of the gradient magnetic field than in the presence of B_0 alone. Furthermore, distance from isocenter will determine the degree of difference in signal under the gradient magnetic field compared with B_0 alone; increasing distance from isocenter confers a greater difference in applied field strength relative to B_0 and a consequent increase in phase dispersion and *decrease* in signal intensity.

How "Rapidly" Does Phase Change?

We can now identify a difference between spins occupying different locations along y based on phase under the phase-encoding gradient compared with phase at baseline (i.e., under B_0 alone). Differences in measured signal intensity (less with the phase-encoding gradient than without) reflect differences in phase, but how can the phase information be extracted to separate and localize the MR signal along y? The solution lies in a creative understanding of the nature of phase change caused by varying the strength of the phase-encoding gradient. When comparing phase of the spins without applying the phase-encoding gradient (B_0 only) to phase under a single strength of the phase-encoding gradient, a variation in the magnitude of phase change (detected as signal change) occurs that varies with location relative to isocenter; greater phase change occurs farthest from isocenter and vice versa.

What results if we now transiently apply the phase-encoding gradient multiple times, each time at a different strength? Stronger applications of the phase-encoding gradient will result in more phase shift and, as a result, less signal. Now consider the change in phase (detected as signal loss) induced by one application of the phase-encoding gradient relative to the others, *and* look at how the change in phase between gradient applications at a single location along y compares with other locations along y that are nearer or farther from isocenter. Looking at Figure 6-9, compare the change in gradient strength (arrows) that is proportional to phase change at points a, b, and c. Clearly, the change is greatest as we move farther from isocenter. As we cannot directly measure phase, what we are observing, in essence, is the rate of change of phase from one (phase-encoding) gradient application to the next. This parameter can be measured as change in signal intensity, but only *in comparison* with the signal of spins at other locations along y. Farthest from isocenter, we observe the highest rate of change of phase across multiple gradient applications. At isocenter, of course, there is no gradient change, and the rate of change of phase of all spins is the same (i.e., $= 0$).

Because we "measure" phase (as decrease in signal amplitude due to the effects of the phase-encoding gradient) at each of several points in time, we now have multiple measures of signal amplitude collected over time. (Sound familiar?) Further, the signal is spatially encoded. As described earlier, different rates of change of phase (manifest, of course, as different rates of change of signal intensity) exist when comparing signals acquired

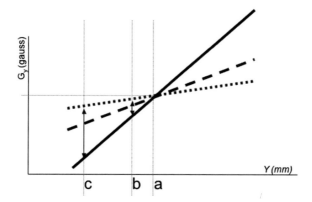

FIGURE 6-9. Change of gradient strength varies with distance from isocenter. The three thick lines represent three applications of the phase-encoding gradient magnetic field, each at a different strength (slope). Each gradient application is performed at a separate point in time and precedes a *separate measurement* of the MR signal. These three gradient strengths are *not* applied simultaneously and are shown together in this diagram only for demonstration. At isocenter "a," by definition, all gradient magnetic fields are 0. Spins located at isocenter experience no change in B_{net} ($B_{net} = B_0 + G$) as each gradient is applied and no change in phase. At "b," adjacent to isocenter, different gradient strength is experienced under each of the three applications of the phase-encoding gradient magnetic field. The magnitude of change in gradient strength is indicated by the thin double arrows. This change in gradient strength confers a change in phase at a given location (y) between spins experiencing, for example, the gradient represented by the solid line versus the dashed line. At "c," furthest from isocenter, the greatest change in gradient strength and, as a result, the greatest change in phase is observed.

under the multiple applications of the phase-encoding gradient. Those rates of change of phase are linearly arrayed along y; lowest is closest to isocenter, and highest is farthest from isocenter. All we need is a method to extract this "rate of change of phase" (read frequency) information.

Filling in the Data

What does the data look like at this point? We acquire signal after each transient application of the phase-encoding gradient (Fig. 6-10). Remember that signal measurement involves collecting multiple separate samples over time while the frequency-encoding gradient is on. We place the data in computer memory that we can conceptualize as a single row of a spreadsheet. This process is repeated once for each of multiple different strengths of the phase-encoding gradient with *no* change *other* than different amplitude of the phase-encoding gradient. The result is one linear array of amplitude values acquired over time *for each unique strength of the phase-encoding gradient*. This generates multiple rows in our spreadsheet. Each

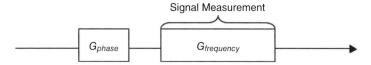

FIGURE 6-10. Temporal sequence of spatial encoding. Phase encoding entails the transient application of the phase-encoding gradient magnetic field. After this gradient magnetic field is *shut off*, signal is measured *while the frequency-encoding gradient magnetic field is on.*

contains measures of signal amplitude acquired over time. We now have a spreadsheet with multiple columns *and* multiple rows. This spreadsheet is called the *raw data* or *time-domain data*, otherwise affectionately referred to as *k*-space (Fig. 6-11). We will use the term *k*-space from here onward.

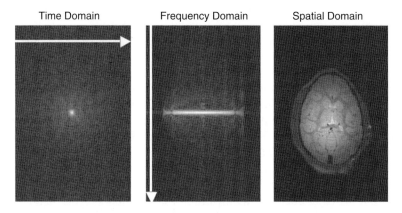

FIGURE 6-11. From raw data to image. This example shows an axial image of the brain acquired using a spin echo technique in which frequency encoding is left to right and phase encoding is top to bottom. The white arrows indicate the direction of the Fourier transform: first horizontal and second vertical. The time-domain data (left, also termed *raw data* or *k*-space) in no way resembles the image (right). Signal intensity is highest in the center of *k*-space because we are sampling spin echoes that peak in the middle of our sampling period. TE, in fact, is at the midpoint of the left-right dimension of *k*-space. The frequency-domain data (middle image) contains some spatial information; signal is correctly localized along the right-to-left direction. Because signal at any point from left to right cannot yet be localized along y, the frequency-domain "image" only shows a vague outline of the brain. The high signal horizontal band across the middle of the frequency-domain "image" corresponds with signal encoded with the lowest strength phase-encoding gradient applications, where signal attenuation is least. The upper and lower portions of the frequency-domain "image" have increasingly lower signal as we move toward the edges. This corresponds with the increasing strength of the phase-encoding gradient used to encode these signals. After the final top-bottom Fourier transform, the actual image is revealed (spatial domain, right).

Each cell contains a single measurement of signal amplitude, nothing more, each value containing signal from *the entire slice*. The columns represent the time at which each sample was acquired, and the rows each represent a different strength of the phase-encoding gradient.

Exactly as described under frequency encoding, we Fourier transform the data in *k*-space along the length of each row (left to right). This 1DFT is performed *separately* for each spreadsheet row and yields, for each row, a new row of cells containing amplitude data where the columns correspond with frequency rather than time. At this point, we have performed a 1DFT separately on multiple rows of *k*-space and have a spreadsheet called the *frequency-domain data* that reveals a crude outline of the image (Fig. 6-11). Columns now represent frequency, and, as discussed under frequency encoding above, those frequencies correspond with actual locations along the dimension of the frequency-encoding gradient. The rows, however, still only represent different strengths of the phase-encoding gradient, *not* location in the slice from top to bottom. At a given left-right location in our data, values from each and every row contain information (signal) from *everywhere* along the up-down dimension in the slice at that left-right location.

What information in *k*-space is contained within each cell of a single column, that is, at the same location left-right? Because the amplitude data in each cell of a given column have the same frequency (on the frequency-encoding dimension), that signal all comes from the same location along this dimension, x in our example. The variation in signal intensity between these cells (i.e., from row to row) is a function of the strength of the phase-encoding gradient applied before the measurements of signal amplitude are made *and* the location of spins along the phase-encoding dimension. This variation in signal encodes the location of components of the signal along the phase-encoding dimension. When comparing signal acquired under different phase-encoding gradient strength, spins far from isocenter undergo a greater rate of change of phase and generate less signal, and spins closer to isocenter have a lower rate of change of phase and generate more signal. Rate of change of phase, of course, refers to the magnitude of phase change from one phase-encoding gradient application to the next and is reflected in the change in signal amplitude that results from dephasing under the influence of the phase-encoding gradient. We are dealing with change in signal amplitude over time; conceptually, this is the same as our temporal sampling of the signal during the application of the frequency-encoding gradient. Just as the Fourier transform could extract the component frequencies and their associated amplitude components along the frequency-encoding dimension, it can extract the "frequency" (i.e., rate of change of phase) components along the phase-encoding dimension.

This final step, then, involves feeding all the cells of each column into the Fourier transform. The output of the Fourier transform will be a series of frequencies (rates of change of phase) and their corresponding signal amplitude. Because *frequency is location*, we have now localized signal correctly along the phase-encoding—in our example y—dimension. Remember that the signal was already localized along the frequency-encoding dimension—in our example x. We now have a true image (Fig. 6-11). The image is merely a spreadsheet in which each cell contains signal amplitude and the columns and rows represent *frequency*. Because *frequency is location*, this is one and the same as our image.

The number of these "frequencies" extracted from the Fourier transform, corresponding with locations along the phase-encoding dimension, is determined by the number of samples over time that we feed into the Fourier transform. This, of course, is the number of lines in our data, each representing signal acquired with a unique strength of the phase-encoding gradient. Note that for *each* additional line of *k*-space we must (1) excite the slice, (2) transiently apply a new, unique strength of the phase-encoding gradient, and (3) sample the signal *in the presence* of the frequency-encoding gradient. Be mindful that increasing spatial resolution along the phase-encoding dimension increases imaging time; doubling the number of locations in the image along this dimension doubles the time required to acquire a complete image.

Some Comments Regarding *k*-Space

Why indeed have we bothered to plow through this difficult and seemingly esoteric material? The goal at the outset, after all, was to improve our ability to interpret and use MRI in *clinical* imaging. It turns out that there are many aspects of image quality and imaging efficiency that are determined by what is going on in *k*-space.

What Location in the Image Does a Point in k-*Space Represent?*

Where in the image does the signal found in any one location in *k*-space come from? Taking a given line of *k*-space (time-domain data), each sample of signal amplitude collected over time contains information coming from the entire slice. All spins in the slice were excited, so all produce signal. For a given line in *k*-space, each location in that line contains information that arises from *every* location along the frequency-encoding dimension of the image. Because, for a given location along the frequency dimension, each line of *k*-space contributes to *all* locations along the phase-encoding dimension in the image, it follows that *every location in the k-space contributes information to every location in the image*. This is why corruption of a single point in *k*-space will lead to an artifact that propagates throughout the image. This will be covered in more detail later.

Because each point in k-space contains signal from the entire slice, we can generate a "similar" image of our slice from many or few phase-encoding steps (lines of k-space). Likewise, because each sample along the frequency-encoding direction in k-space contains signal from the whole slice, we can generate a similar image of the slice with only a few samples (frequency-encoding steps). The number of frequency-encoding steps (number of samples over time) will not alter the spatial extent (field of view) of the slice, just the spatial resolution.

Topology of k-*Space*

Although each location in the time-domain data does contain signal originating from all locations in the slice, each location in this raw data does not contribute equally to the image. Notice that signal amplitude in both the time-domain and frequency-domain data varies significantly. Highest signal amplitude resides in the center of our spreadsheet, and extremely low signal amplitude occupies the periphery. What cannot be seen in these "images" of the raw data are variations in frequency. Based on the fact that the lowest gradient amplitudes are represented in the center of k-space, low frequencies occupy the center of the spreadsheet and high frequencies are at the periphery. Because higher-gradient amplitudes cause greater dephasing and signal loss, it follows that the highest signal amplitude is found in the center of k-space.

Tissue contrast is defined as a difference in signal amplitude between two tissues. Therefore, the highest signal components of k-space, at its center, contribute most significantly to image contrast. Spatial resolution, on the other hand, depends on high-frequency information to sharply distinguish *spatial* transitions in signal intensity (i.e., edge discrimination). This information is encoded in the periphery of k-space where amplitude is low but a great deal of important information resides, nonetheless. In Figure 6-12, we have reconstructed the same image using different portions of k-space while discarding others. These examples drive home the manner in which different portions of k-space modulate different aspects of contrast and spatial resolution.

In certain applications, tissue contrast may change during sampling of the MR signal. For example, during bolus administration of a contrast agent for MR angiography (MRA), overall signal intensity changes rapidly with transit of the contrast bolus. Consequently, all lines of data cannot be acquired during the short time that intravascular contrast concentration is maximal. However, we can acquire the central lines of k-space during the peak of the bolus. In this case, the difference in signal between vessels and background will be greatly enhanced by carefully timing the acquisition of those essential central lines of *k-space* to coincide with the peak of the bolus. This is the basis of contrast-enhanced MRA, discussed in more detail in Chapter 16.

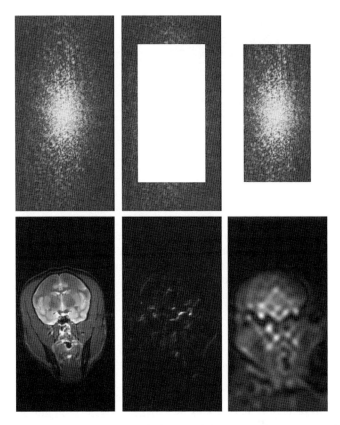

FIGURE 6-12. Contrast, spatial resolution, and *k*-space. The top row shows the portion of *k*-space used to reconstruct each corresponding image shown in the bottom row. At bottom left, the full image is generated using all of *k*-space. In the bottom middle panel, only the periphery of *k*-space is used to reconstruct the image. Sharply defined edges and the outlines of the image are present, but overall signal and contrast are poor. On the bottom right, only the center of *k*-space is used to reconstruct the image. As a result, contrast is present, but edges are markedly blurred.

k-space demonstrates a phenomenon called conjugate symmetry. Looking at *k*-space (Fig. 6-13), we see that there is both up-down and right-left symmetry, but the degree of symmetry present is even more than meets the eye. For every point in *k*-space, the signal amplitude in the corresponding location diagonally opposite it is virtually identical. Thus, if we only acquire 51% of the lines in our raw data, following the first Fourier transform, we can, using this diagonal symmetry, interpolate the bottom half of *k*-space that we did not actually acquire. The resulting image will be virtually indistinguishable from an image reconstructed from a fully

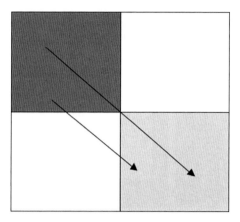

FIGURE 6-13. Conjugate symmetry of k-space: Interpolation of data points not actually collected (light gray) from the data acquired that reside in the diagonally opposite quadrant of k-space (dark gray) can be accomplished by exploiting the conjugate symmetry of k-space (arrows).

"acquired" k-space. Signal-to-noise will suffer because we have only collected 51% of the signal compared with a full k-space image, but imaging time drops by nearly 50%.

Distribution of contrast and spatial information in k-space and the performance improvements enabled by partial k-space imaging are just two examples of how understanding spatial localization can directly impact and improve clinical applications of MRI. More to come. . . .

7
Defining Image Size and
Spatial Resolution

In the previous chapter, we gained an understanding of how the MR signal that comes, of course, from the entire slice can be localized to individual locations along the length and width of that slice. It might seem that the number of locations, determined by the number of phase- and frequency-encoding steps, determines the spatial resolution of the image. This, however, is only partially true. As we defined in the very first chapter, spatial resolution is a function of voxel size. Voxel size is determined by not only the number of voxels in the image but also by the dimension of the image along which those voxels are arrayed. Two images of different size, but with the same number of voxels along each in-plane dimension, will have different voxel size and, therefore, different spatial resolution.

How Much Area Will Be Included in the Image?

Let's look at an example. For an imaging study of the pancreas, the scan operator has prescribed an axial slice through the abdomen at the level of the pancreatic head using 256 frequency-encoding steps. Based on our understanding of slice selection, the signal received at the coil will come from the entire slice. In the presence of the frequency-encoding gradient, which, of course, is on at a fixed strength during the time we sample the signal, spins will see a different B_{net} depending on their location along the frequency-encoding dimension. Thus, a specific range of frequencies will contribute to the aggregate signal that we sample at the coil. It turns out that the range of frequencies that make up the aggregate signal is determined by the size of the patient along the frequency-encoding direction. In our example, if frequency encoding is performed from right to left, the width of the abdomen will determine the distance along the frequency-encoding gradient the signal is derived from. The longer this distance (i.e., the larger the patient), the greater the range of B_{net} that is "seen" by the spins and the broader the range of frequencies that will contribute to the aggregate signal that we will sample and feed to the Fourier transform:

remember that "frequency *is* location." That range of frequencies will then, via the Fourier transform, resolve to 256 pixels covering the *entire* width of the abdomen. If, however, we are only interested in the pancreatic head and wish to maximize spatial resolution at that location in order to detect a small carcinoma, is there a way to array our 256 voxels only over the region of the pancreatic head to make an image of only this small region?

Specifying the Field of View

Continuing with our example, observe that frequency of precession is determined by location. The closer the spins are to isocenter, the lower their frequency of precession and vice versa. Just as we can tune the receiver of our FM radio to be sensitive to a specific frequency (actually a narrow range of frequencies), we can also specify that the receiver in our MRI scanner only accept frequencies within a specific range. Specifying a range of frequencies that corresponds with the distance of interest along the frequency-encoding direction (e.g., the region of the pancreatic head) will yield an image that displays signal from *only* that region (Fig. 7-1). Or will it?

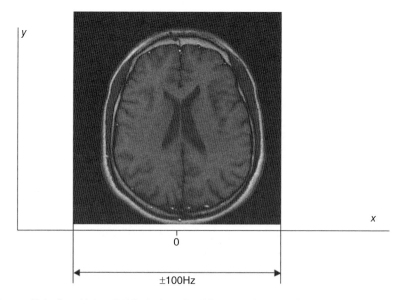

FIGURE 7-1. Specifying field of view. In this example, x is the frequency-encoding dimension. Spins precess at different frequencies depending on their location along x. Setting the receiver to detect a range of 100 Hz on either side of the center frequency (ω_0; 0 on the x axis) will detect all signals arising from the brain slice being imaged.

How Do We Detect Specific Frequencies?

It is certainly true that we can specify that the scanner only "listen" to a specific range of frequencies and ignore all others. However, this does not necessarily translate to sampling signal from a specific spatial location within the patient. The distinction lies in recalling the nature of digital sampling and understanding its limitations.

As discussed in Chapters 5 and 6, when sampling the MR signal, we employ a digital receiver (analog-to-digital converter, or A2D). This device records total signal amplitude over discrete periods of time to generate the time-domain data that we record in k-space and ultimately Fourier transform to create an image. The parameter that defines our digital sampling is the sampling time (T_s). Given that we sample for a fixed time T_s and that there is no "down time" between samples, the number of samples and T_s define the total time for sampling the signal.

Aliasing and Its Fixes

Sampling Rate, the Nyquist Rule, and Undersampling

An important limitation of our signal processing approach must be introduced at this point: The sampling time, T_s, affects our ability to accurately sample the signal. How so? It turns out that, as depicted in Figure 7-2, we must obtain at least two samples for every cycle of the signal that we are trying to sample. If we satisfy this condition, the result will be an accurate depiction of the original signal. If not, we will generate a result with the same amplitude but with a lower frequency than the original. This phenomenon, described by Harry Nyquist in 1927, is known as the Nyquist-Shannon theorem or more commonly as the Nyquist rule. In order to satisfy the Nyquist rule, the A2D must be set to sample at least twice as fast as the highest-frequency component contained within the aggregate MR signal. If not, we will "undersample" the signal.

And so what if we undersample? What does it mean for the resultant image? Remember that "frequency *is* location" as explained in Chapter 6. The Fourier transform returns a range of frequencies, each with associated amplitude. For correctly sampled frequencies, the appropriate amplitude component will be associated with its true frequency and placed in the location within the image from which it actually derived. Components of the signal that are undersampled will be assigned frequencies lower than the actual signal component they derive from. Because these lower frequencies correspond with locations closer to isocenter, their associated signal will be placed incorrectly within the prescribed field of view (Fig. 7-3). This consequence of undersampling is known as aliasing and produces the so-called wraparound artifact (Fig. 7-4).

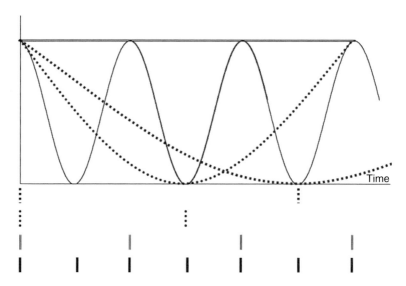

FIGURE 7-2. Sampling rate. The solid sinusoid represents the actual signal being sampled. Each of the other lines represents the signal measured at different rates of sampling. The short vertical lines at the bottom of the figure show the time interval for samples used to generate each of the resultant signals. Only when sampling is fast enough to return two samples for each cycle of the signal will we accurately replicate the signal. In all other cases, a lower-frequency signal results.

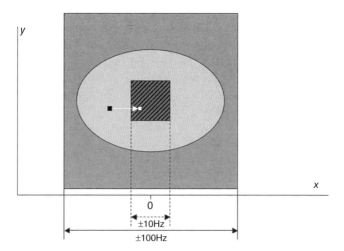

FIGURE 7-3. Aliasing in concept. If we sample fast enough to only represent signal between the dashed lines, any signal arising outside of this region will be undersampled. Because it is detected as a lower frequency, it will be placed in the image at the location corresponding with that lower frequency: closer to isocenter.

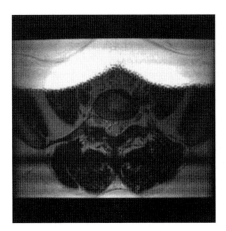 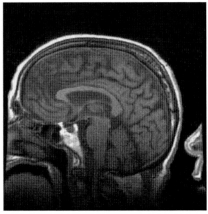

FIGURE 7-4. Aliasing in real life. On the left, the anteroposterior dimension of the field of view is smaller than the patient's actual anteroposterior thickness. The bright signal superimposed on the abdomen is actually fat from the buttocks, which resides outside the field of view. On the right, the anteroposterior dimension of the field of view is inadequate for the patient's nose. No, there is no one else in the scanner smelling his cologne.

Avoiding Aliasing: Oversampling

Aliasing can be a quite troublesome artifact. As seen in Figure 7-4, aliasing looks much like a double-exposed radiograph. Because different parts of the patient are superimposed on one another, the diagnostic utility of the affected portions of the image will be reduced or negated entirely. Fortunately, the workaround to avoid aliasing is rather simple: oversample! How so? We have a problem when we try to apply our 256 voxels to the small field of view covering the pancreatic head only. What if we instead acquire 512 phase-encoding steps to generate 512 voxels spread over double the field of view? Spatial resolution will be the same because our voxel size has not changed; we have double the field of view but double the number of voxels to cover it. The accuracy of our spatial localization, however, will improve. The larger field of view extends farther from isocenter along the frequency-encoding direction, contains higher-frequency components, and, therefore, must be sampled at a higher rate (shorter T_s). In doing so, we accurately sample a larger field of view at the same high resolution. Even though we acquired more samples in the frequency-encoding direction, because we sampled faster, total sampling time (and imaging time) can be the same. Now we can discard the voxels outside of our desired small field of view and only display the small field of view covering the pancreatic head, at the desired high resolution and without the troublesome aliasing. This is oversampling, and because oversampling in the frequency-encoding direction does not affect imaging time, it is, on clinical MR scanners, always done as a default.

How About the Phase-Encoding Direction?

As you are probably all too aware, aliasing is also a problem in the phase-encoding direction. In fact, thanks to oversampling in the frequency-encoding direction, many of us have never and will never actually see aliasing occur in the frequency-encoding direction. Thinking back to our discussion of spatial localization, remember that phase encoding is analogous to frequency encoding as we similarly obtain multiple samples over time, but, in the case of phase encoding, the "time" is the interval between phase-encoding steps. Just as with frequency encoding, too few samples will lead to undersampling the aggregate signal and the Fourier transform will assign signal to erroneously low frequencies, leading to aliasing or "wrap-around" in the image. Also similar to frequency encoding, we can eliminate aliasing by oversampling. By acquiring enough phase-encoding steps, we can accurately sample all signal, even beyond the desired field of view, and still maintain the desired spatial resolution. Finally, just as when we oversample in the frequency-encoding direction, we can display only the desired field of view and discard the unwanted and irrelevant information.

As we can see, aliasing and its cure (oversampling) are the same whether we are discussing the phase- or frequency-encoding direction. But there is a difference: imaging time. Remember that the total imaging time is a function of TR, number of phase-encoding steps (N_p), and number of signal averages (NSA):

$$Time = TR \times N_p \times NSA$$

Adding additional frequency-encoding steps does not extend the total imaging time because it occurs within the TR. Further, by sampling faster, we can acquire more frequency-encoding steps without any increase in total sampling time. Each and every phase-encoding step, however, increases the total time to generate the image. It is this time penalty that turns aliasing in the phase-encoding direction into such a problem.

How Does My MRI Vendor "Stop" Aliasing?

Virtually all of the MRI scanner vendors offer an option to stop aliasing in the phase-encoding direction. By merely checking off an option on the scanner console with a catchy name like "no phase wrap," "anti-alias," "anti wrap," or "foldover suppression," aliasing will be banished from images even if the field of view is smaller than the body or part thereof being imaged, and with *no* increase in imaging time! Like most "magic," however, this trick is nothing more than some sleight of hand. As we would expect, oversampling is employed to solve the aliasing problem. But how does the imaging time remain unchanged? It turns out that for imaging time to remain the same, the number of signal averages is decreased in proportion to the increase in phase-encoding steps. If, for example, the number of phase-encoding steps is doubled, the number of signal averages will be halved. Thus, aliasing is eliminated, imaging time is unchanged, but signal-to-noise declines by half! This explains why all sharp MRI technologists know that they must double the number of signal averages if they are going to employ this handy option. Once again, we see that MRI parallels life: there is no such thing as a free lunch!

Refining the Field of View

Based on our understanding of aliasing, it should become apparent that defining the field of view in terms of a specific distance, say 22 cm for the head, is quite removed from what the scanner actually does to set that field of view. The range of frequencies that we sample *accurately* is the true definition of field of view. In fact, the MR system is so obstinate that, even if we specify a field of view, it will tell us that we are wrong by placing (inaccurately sampled) signal from outside our chosen field of view right in the middle of the image.

Gradient Strength Determines Field of View

The parameter that determines what range of frequencies corresponds with the field of view that we wish to image is gradient strength. Over a fixed distance, a stronger (steeper) gradient magnetic field will induce a greater range of frequencies and will induce higher frequencies at the extremes of that distance than in a case in which gradient strength is lower. Thus, field of view (FOV) is inversely proportional to gradient strength (G):

$$\text{FOV} \; \alpha \; 1/\text{G}$$

Sampling Rate Determines Field of View

Whereas gradient strength determines the range of frequencies that will be represented along the dimension we choose as field of view, it is the sampling time, T_s, that determines whether we can accurately sample that range of frequencies. If the field of view we choose contains a range of frequencies ±25 kHz, for example, we must sample at least twice that rate. It follows that the faster we sample (the shorter T_s), the greater the range of frequencies and the larger the field of view we can sample accurately. Thus, field of view is also indirectly proportional to T_s:

$$\text{FOV} \propto 1/(GT_s)$$

Receiver Bandwidth

The receiver is the A2D that samples the MR signal. As we have seen, the speed with which the A2D can sample is *the* direct determinant of the range of frequencies that can be sampled accurately. This range of frequencies is termed the *receiver bandwidth*. Receiver bandwidth is essentially a measure of receiver performance. Higher-bandwidth receivers are able to sample very rapidly and, as a result, can correctly sample very high frequencies. Because rapid sampling means that T_s is very short, the bandwidth (BW) is the inverse of T_s:

$$\text{BW} = 1/T_s$$

Receiver Bandwidth and Field of View

Putting it all together, we now see that the field of view—the range of frequencies that we can accurately sample—is directly proportional to bandwidth:

$$\text{FOV} \propto 1/T_s$$
$$\text{FOV} \propto \text{BW}$$

Nonetheless, the bandwidth does not necessarily determine field of view. Modulation of gradient strength can narrow or widen the field of view at a specific bandwidth:

$$\text{FOV} = \text{BW}/G$$

How Do We Specify Field of View in Real Life?

When you sit down at the MRI console to set up a scan, the computer interface will provide a field or menu for specifying the FOV, usually in units of centimeters or millimeters. Bandwidth, if it is in fact user-modifiable, is specified by making an entry in a different field. As we now understand, given a specific bandwidth, gradient strength must be modified to set the field of view. The scanner interface does not ask you to specify the gradient strength: It is calculated by the console computer based on the field of view and bandwidth you have specified.

How Small Can the Field of View Be?

In light of the relationship between field of view, receiver bandwidth, and gradient strength, we can observe a physical limitation on field of view. To minimize field of view, we need to maximize bandwidth (that is, minimize T_s) and maximize gradient strength. Both parameters have physical limits determined by engineering considerations and how much money you spent on your gradient system and receiver hardware. As a result, the minimum field of view will be somewhere around $0.1\,cm^2$. We, of course, would never be able to generate a useful image even at 10 times that field of view. However, understanding the basis for this hardware limitation of the MR system underscores the nature of field of view in MRI.

A Footnote Regarding Receiver Bandwidth

If you observe a sharp MRI technologist, you will notice that they will always try to minimize the receiver bandwidth. Why? If we step back and think about what the receiver bandwidth implies, we notice that a narrower bandwidth means that only a smaller range of frequencies must be sampled accurately. The narrower the range of frequencies that must be sampled, the lower the highest frequency components will be, allowing T_s to be longer. Because T_s is the time during which we record signal, the longer T_s, the more signal we record per sample. Thus, signal to noise increases in proportion to T_s. Because $BW = 1/T_s$, the narrower the receiver bandwidth, the greater the signal to noise.

8
Putting It All Together: An Introduction to Pulse Sequences

Putting It All Together

This chapter is, in a large part, a review of what we covered regarding spatial localization in Chapter 6. We will now "put it all together" and view the chain of events required to produce an MR image in its entirety. *Pulse sequence diagrams* will be used to graphically depict this sequence of events.

What Exactly Is a Pulse Sequence?

The execution of a pulse sequence is much like a symphony. As we saw in Chapter 6, a series of time-varying magnetic fields (gradient and radiofrequency) as well as the receiver (A2D) are turned on and off in precise sequence. In an orchestra, each instrument must turn on at the correct note (frequency) and volume (amplitude) at the correct time and, of course, become silent at exactly the right time. In the MR pulse sequence, the time-varying magnetic fields (radiofrequency and gradient) and receiver are the instruments. Each is activated at a specific frequency and amplitude for a specific period of time. The epochs during which the time-varying magnetic fields are on are termed *pulses*. The *sequence*, of course, is the order in which the various pulses occur. *Voilà*, we have a pulse sequence.

Interestingly, some MR scientists use their spare time to program the scanner so that the sounds of switching gradients and RF will actually play music! Each time we

As of this writing, you can hear Scott Joplin's "The Entertainer" implemented on the MRI scanner by James Wilson at http://www.fmrib.ox.ac.uk/~wilson/bin/mritunes/ scott.mp3.

110

turn on a gradient magnetic field, for example, the gradient coils will attempt to align with B_0. The vibration produced makes the hardware function as a musical instrument. The pitch, duration, and intensity of the "music" can be controlled by modifying the frequency, intensity, and duration of gradient switching. The MRI scanner is, in a sense, just a very expensive electronic synthesizer. It thus comes as no surprise that the pulse sequence is, in many ways, similar to sheet music.

The Pulse Sequence Diagram

Music is "written" on a series of parallel lines called a *staff*. Moving from left to right along the staff is the flow of time. The musical notes written on the staff are graphical symbols that indicate when an instrument should be silent and when it should make music. The notes and other markings further indicate the note (frequency) to be played as well as the tone, tempo, and intensity. For a symphony, different staves with different arrangements of notes are required for each instrument.

It's Just a Timeline

The pulse sequence diagram (Fig. 8-1), though it strikes fear into many beginning to learn about MRI, is conceptually the same as music notation, but perhaps much simpler. A pulse sequence diagram is merely a staff, a set of parallel lines. Each is a timeline detailing what role each component of the MR system will play in generating the image. In the examples used in this chapter, there are six such parallel timelines. The top displays operation of the RF, the next three each display the operation of one of the three orthogonal gradient magnetic fields, the fifth shows the receiver, and the bottom displays the MR signal.

Notation

Just as music can be displayed as a series of notations, the pulse sequence diagram has its own notation system. When the RF or gradient is turned on, you will see an oval-shaped notation (open arrow in Fig. 8-1). What does the form of this notation indicate? Think of the diagram as a graph. The horizontal line is the x axis in units of time, usually seconds or milliseconds. There is also a vertical axis, but it is generally not drawn in the pulse sequence diagram. The vertical axis represents amplitude.

At the point in time when the gradient or RF is turned on, the leading edge of the polygon will begin to ascend. Because gradient and RF hardware cannot physically turn on to full strength instantaneously, there

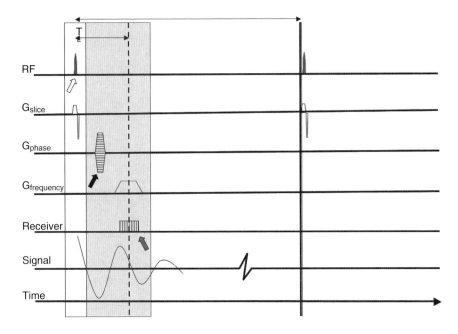

FIGURE 8-1. Generic pulse sequence. This schematic shows the basic components of a pulse sequence that samples the FID. For clarity, no echoes are shown. The open box delineates the excitation module including the RF pulse (open arrow) used to generate signal. The gray box delineates the readout module. Short double-arrow and dashed line: TE. Long double-arrow and thick line: TR. Horizontal striations within the G_{phase} symbol (large black arrow) indicate different strengths of the phase-encoding gradient. Note that only one strength is applied per TR. Vertical striations in the Receiver symbol (large gray arrow) indicate multiple samples obtained in sequence over time.

is a slope along this leading edge. Once the required amplitude is reached, the top of the box flattens, and, when the gradient or RF is turned off, it descends along a slope. Again, the "turn off" cannot occur instantaneously. Thus, the height of the box indicates the amplitude of the gradient or RF, the width indicates the duration for which it is kept on, and the slope at each end indicates the rate at which the gradient or RF turns on and off.

There are aspects of the time-varying magnetic fields that are not depicted in the pulse sequence diagram. For example, the frequency of the RF is not indicated in the notation. This factor might be added as a superimposed notation or as a footnote.

Building the Pulse Sequence

Before diving into the details of different pulse sequence types, there is another important way to view what is going on. For MRI, each pulse sequence *must* contain two elements that we will call modules:

1. An excitation module (clear box in Fig. 8-1), including the slice selection gradient and the RF pulse employed to generate the signal. This component also accomplishes the first stage of spatial localization: slice selection.
2. A readout module (shaded box in Fig. 8-1) comprises phase and frequency encoding and signal sampling (often referred to as *readout*). Many different types of readout modules can be employed. These will be introduced soon. Readout modules account for a large part of the variety in pulse sequences.

Beyond these two essential modules, additional modules can be added to the pulse sequence. For example, we will learn about saturation techniques in Chapter 12. As we will see, these saturation techniques can be viewed as preparatory modules that are added to the front end of any pulse sequence.

Figure 8-2 shows a restaurant menu featuring various "courses" (pulse sequence modules) that can be combined to develop a customized "meal" (pulse sequence). Choices from the "Entrees" section are, of course, required, whereas the other courses are optional. Many of the optional offerings on this menu will not be introduced until later chapters. When they are introduced, it will be helpful to refer back to the menu to see how the components fit together and what options are available.

The Spin Echo Pulse Sequence: A First Example

As we discussed in Chapter 3, to generate a spin echo, an 180° RF pulse must be applied *while* the spins have net transverse magnetization. As a result, net transverse magnetization lost due to T2′ effects will begin to be recovered beginning at the time of the 180° pulse. We can sample the maximum signal (maximum recovery of T2′ information) when the 180° pulse is positioned symmetrically in time between excitation and signal recording (TE).

As its name implies, this pulse sequence is distinguished by the presence of a 180° RF pulse between the initial RF excitation pulse (90°) and TE. You may soon notice that the spin echo pulse sequence differs from the gradient echo pulse sequence we will discuss next *only* by the presence of the 180° pulse.

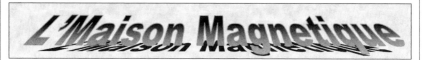

Appetizers

ϒ Inversion Recovery
ϒ Spectral Saturation
      -- Choice of fat, water or silicone
ϒ Diffusion Sensitization
      -- Small (3 simultaneous directions)
      -- Large (6+ individual directions)
ϒ Spatial Presaturation – *any style*
ϒ Magnetization transfer

Entrees

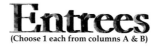

(Choose 1 each from columns A & B)

A

     ⟋ Standard Full Flip Angle
     ⟋ Partial Flip Angle
     ⟋ TONE Pulse

B

     ⟋ Gradient Echo
     ⟋ Spin Echo –*single or multiple*
     ⟋ Fast Spin Echo
     ⟋ Echoplanar
     ⟋ Spiral
     ⟋ Propeller

Specials

     ⌣ Multi Slice
     ⌣ Flow Compensation

Desserts

     ☞ Filtering
     ☞ Time Intensity Analysis
     ☞ MPR
     ☞ 3-D Rendering (MIP, Volume, SSD)

<u>In a rush?</u>

     ⏱ Convert any choice in column B marked with ⟋ to single shot (additional charge)
     ⏱ Add SENSE to any selection "on the house"

<u>Hungry?</u>

     🍽 🍽 Double (triple, quadruple…) portions available at an extra charge

FIGURE 8-2. The pulse sequence menu. Choices from both columns A and B in the "Entrees" section must be made. Additional options are at the customer's discretion. Many will not be introduced until later chapters.

TABLE 8-1. Features of the spin echo pulse sequence.

Module	Action	Function
Excitation module	RF and slice select gradient are turned on simultaneously	Signal generated within a single slice
Readout module	Phase-encoding gradient is turned on briefly and then turned off	Phase encoding
	180° RF pulse with slice select gradient the *same* as during excitation	Phase of spins within the slice is inverted
	Frequency-encoding gradient is turned on and then off	See gradient recalled echo (GRE) pulse sequence
	Frequency-encoding gradient is turned on while signal is sampled	Frequency encoding and signal sampling

The Spin Echo Pulse Sequence in a Nutshell

Salient components of the spin echo pulse sequence are summarized in Table 8-1 and the pulse sequence diagram (Fig. 8-3).

Timing is set up such that the midpoint of the sampling time-period occurs at TE. Note that this ensures that the maximum signal amplitude

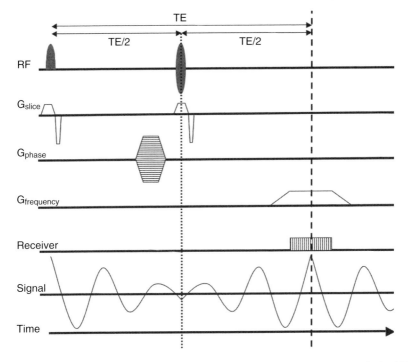

FIGURE 8-3. Spin echo pulse sequence. The hallmark of this pulse sequence is the 180° RF pulse applied midway between the 90° RF pulse and TE (at TE/2). The result is an initial decline followed by regrowth of signal until the maximum signal is achieved (the spin echo) at TE. After TE, notice that signal again declines, relaxing with T2*. (For an explanation of the striped and solid symbols, see Figure 8-1.)

(the peak of the echo) is sampled while we are filling the central time points in each line of k-space. This is important, as the central portion of k-space dominates image contrast, which is dependent on signal magnitude (see Chapter 6). Notice, however, that because nothing can be accomplished instantaneously, signal sampling occurs both before and after maximum refocusing when signal is less than maximal. Such is life in the real world!

What Happens After TE: Multiple Echoes and Multiple Slices

In the examples we have been discussing, TE is much shorter than TR. This distinction is salient throughout all standard MR pulse sequences until we begin to discuss fast imaging methods in Chapter 13. As you can see from the pulse sequence diagram in Figure 8-1, this leaves a large span of dead time after the signal has been sampled and recorded in k-space until it is time to give an additional RF pulse and sample the signal again. This wait is necessary because the delay between RF pulses is the TR and it modulates the contrast of the image. If we decide to shorten our imaging time by delivering the second RF pulse immediately after TE, we have essentially made TR very short and dramatically altered the contribution of T1 differences to the image contrast (see Chapter 4). There are, however, two ways we can make good use of this dead time instead of merely waiting around for the end of TR. Notice in the following sections that, because we are using time that would have been required anyway, the additional information we gain by using this dead time is essentially free; we can generate additional images without the cost of additional imaging time. More in the two sections that follow.

Multislice Imaging

We all know that multiple slices are required to image any body part and generate a useful amount of information. One slice just can't show it all. On the other hand, we know that the time to generate an image is dependent on filling each line of k-space—one line for each pixel we want in the phase dimension of the image—during a separate TR. Thus, the time to image a slice is $N_p \times TR$. If we are using 256 phase-encoding steps (a common spatial resolution in clinical practice) and a TR of 500 milliseconds (typical for a spin echo pulse sequence with T1 contrast), the time to generate one slice will be 128 seconds, or 2.13 minutes. It follows that, if we require 25 slices, the imaging time will be 25 times ($N_p \times TR$), or 40 minutes! Good luck holding still for that scan! Because patients routinely exit the MR scanner after 20 to 30 minutes having undergone several pulse sequences of many slices each, there must be a trick.

The trick is to use the dead time. Remember that we excite only one slice at a time. After we excite slice no. 1 and sample its signal at TE, we must wait until TR before delivering RF *that excites that slice again*. This is because the spins within slice no. 1 are recovering longitudinal magnetization after the RF pulse. However, this slice-selective RF pulse did not excite the rest of the patient. All tissue outside slice no. 1 is fully relaxed, including tissue residing in the location of adjacent slices. If we apply a second RF pulse immediately after TE, with the slice select gradient and RF tuned to excite a different slice, the relaxation of slice no. 1 will continue unaffected while slice no. 2 is excited. We then sample signal after a time TE after the second RF. This signal is recorded in a new data file, forming the first line of *k*-space for slice no. 2. After this second TE, we can immediately excite slice no. 3, sample the signal after an additional time TE, and record the signal in another data file forming the first line of *k*-space for slice no. 3. Continuing in this manner, it will be possible to excite additional slices until the time TR after the first RF has been reached. At that point, we *must* revert to exciting slice no. 1 in order to retain the image contrast the TR dictates.

How does this use of dead time affect total imaging time? The time to image slice no. 1 is unchanged ($N_p \times$ TR), but we are now able to obtain multiple slices within the same time required to generate just one. This is multislice imaging (Fig. 8-4), and it is an integral part of virtually all MR pulse sequences other than certain fast-imaging applications. The duration of TR determines the number of slices we can obtain without requiring additional imaging time, determined by how many periods of length equal to TE we can fit within one TR.

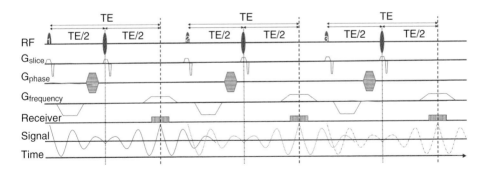

FIGURE 8-4. Multislice spin echo imaging. Slices 2 and 3 are excited during the time between signal sampling for slice 1 and TR (to the right; not shown because it is beyond the limits of the diagram) when slice 1 must be excited again to generate data to fill an additional line of *k*-space. Multislice imaging is not restricted to use in spin echo pulse sequences. It can be and is used in gradient echo and other approaches. (For an explanation of the striped and solid symbols, see Figure 8-1.)

Let us now return to our example of a pulse sequence with TR = 500 milliseconds and 192 phase-encoding steps. Perhaps the TE in this case is 15 milliseconds (typical for a spin echo image with T1 contrast). During the TR, we can excite up to 32 slices one after the other. Instead of 40 minutes for 25 slices, we will obtain all 25 slices in 1.6 minutes. Not only that, but we can even get an additional eight slices without any additional imaging time! What if we actually needed 40 slices? One option is to run through the pulse sequence once to acquire the first 32 slices and then repeat the *entire pulse sequence* again just to get the additional seven slices. This, of course, doubles the total imaging time. Another approach that is a favorite trick, even a reflex, of experienced MR technologists is to increase the TR somewhat. In our example, increasing the TR to 600 would just about let us squeeze in the 40 slices. Using this approach, the imaging time would also increase, but only by 100 milliseconds, not by a factor of two. One note of caution: Increasing the TR does allow us to squeeze in more slices without a large time penalty, but it also changes image contrast. Remember that nothing is completely free in the world of MRI.

One final issue: We learned earlier that the MR system does not allow us to selectively sample signal from a specific location such as a slice. The coil will detect any signal that is present. In that case, when we sample signal after the second RF that excites slice no. 2, isn't there residual signal from the first RF pulse? Won't it "contaminate" our signal from slice no. 2? Although this is a potential problem, remember that T2 is generally much shorter than T1, so transverse magnetization dissipates much more rapidly than longitudinal magnetization recovers. When we sample the signal at TE after the second RF pulse, the signal (i.e., transverse magnetization) of slice no. 1 has fully decayed, and the only measurable signal derives from slice no. 2. When residual signal from the previous RF pulse is a problem, it can be resolved with spoiling techniques. These will be discussed in Chapter 13, as they do indeed present a problem for fast imaging.

Multiecho Imaging

In this variant use of the dead time after TE, but before TR, instead of immediately exciting another slice, we will generate several images of the same slice with different contrasts (Fig. 8-5). The signal recorded at TE— we will call it TE_1 at this point—will of course be entered into k-space. Next, before applying any additional RF pulses, we will turn on the frequency-encoding gradient again and sample the signal. Notice that no additional phase encoding or slice selection is performed. The time at which we sample the signal this second time will be termed TE_2, and it will be recorded in a new k-space. Each time we repeat the RF pulse at TR, we will again record signal at TE_1 and TE_2, recording each in its respective k-space. Notice that within a given TR period, signal from each TE has

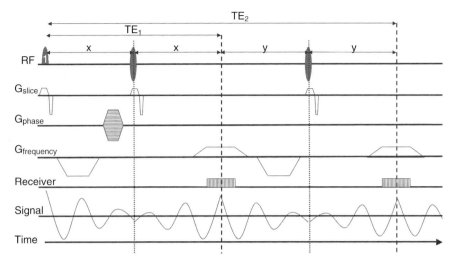

FIGURE 8-5. Multiecho spin echo imaging. Signal is recorded after a single 90° RF pulse but refocused multiple times by applying 180° RF pulses to generate multiple spin echoes. TE_1 must occur at a time after the first 180° pulse equal to the time between the initial 90° and 180° pulses. Subsequently, TE_2 must occur when the time between the second 180° RF pulse and TE_2 is equal to the time between TE_1 and the second 180° pulse. (For an explanation of the striped and solid symbols, see Figure 8-1.)

identical spatial localization (slice, phase, and frequency encoding), but it is recorded at a different time after the RF and in a separate *k*-space. Fourier transform of each *k*-space will yield a unique image: the image acquired at TE_1 will have a contrast determined by TE_1, and the image acquired at TE_2 will have its contrast determined by TE_2, but *both will be images of the same slice*. The contrast of the two images will differ in the degree to which they show contrast based on T2. Typically, the multiecho technique is used with spin echo pulse sequences, a relatively long TR (several seconds) and one short and one rather long TE (perhaps 20 and 120 milliseconds). The result is two images: one with contrast mostly based on proton density (long TR and short TE) and one based on T2 (long TR *and* TE).

The Gradient Echo Pulse Sequence: Gradient Recalled Echo, Fast Field Echo, Fast Low Angle Shot, and So Forth

Now that we have understood the spin echo pulse sequence, gradient echo is easy! Simply write the pulse sequence *exactly* as we did for the spin echo pulse sequence, but *leave out the 180° pulse*. That's it. A gradient echo pulse sequence is merely a spin echo pulse sequence *without the spin echo* (read 180° pulse). What then does the term *gradient echo* signify?

Those readers with prior knowledge of MRI may ask about the flip angle employed during the excitation module. It is true that partial or modified flip angles are commonly used in gradient echo imaging, but this need not be the case. We will initially assume the flip angle is 90°, just as in the spin echo pulse sequence. Once the elements of the gradient echo pulse sequence are delineated, we will address the issue of other flip angles.

What Is a Gradient Echo?

First, let's define the term *echo*. Because, in the case of a spin echo, the signal declines and then, after the 180° pulse, increases in strength, someone thought it was similar to

> As you can see, the canonization of the term *echo* was really arbitrary. It could have been called a resonoid, a fluke, a Jerry, or whatever.

an echo. When you stand in a tunnel and scream "echo," the sound dissipates and then echoes back; it increases in strength after a delay. In the tunnel, the echo is caused by the walls of the tunnel that reflect sound waves. In the case of the spin echo, the natural precession of spins subject to varying field strengths (remember T2*) leads to an increase in signal after the phase of the spins is inverted, so to speak, by the 180° pulse. Review Chapter 3 if the mechanism of the spin echo is unclear.

An echo is merely an increase in signal after a delay during which signal declines. This applies to any increase in signal after signal decline, exactly what a gradient echo is.

Before we deal with the gradient echo itself, consider the following: Whenever we turn on a gradient magnetic field for any purpose, spins experience varying field strength depending on their location along the gradient, and this leads to dephasing and signal loss. The same is true when we turn on the frequency-encoding gradient during signal sampling. We *must* turn that frequency-encoding gradient on in order to localize signal within the image, but signal is lost in the process. Consider it a necessary evil. Importantly, however, the signal loss is *predictable and reproducible*. This is because we induce the signal loss by application of a *linear* gradient magnetic field.

A gradient echo is essentially a means for minimizing the signal loss incurred during signal sampling under the frequency-encoding gradient. To form a gradient echo, we first turn on the frequency-encoding gradient magnetic field (Fig. 8-6). This, of course, leads to signal loss. After this gradient is switched off, spins are out of phase, and signal has been lost in proportion to the strength of the gradient magnetic field and how long we leave it on. If we now turn on the same gradient magnetic field with the same strength but opposite polarity, the spins will undergo further "dephasing," but enough dephasing actually leads to rephasing (Fig. 8-6)! This is a gradient echo.

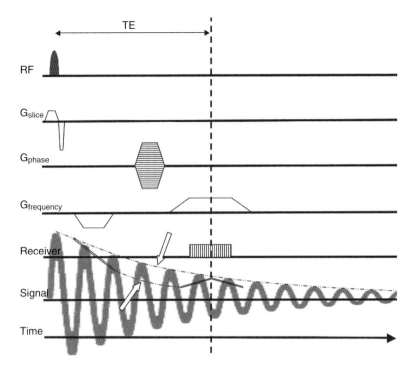

FIGURE 8-6. Gradient echo pulse sequence. First, notice the absence of the 180° RF pulse. The undisturbed signal that would be measured in the absence of any gradient magnetic field is shown in gray. The broken lines (open arrows) depict periods where signal decays with T2*. Double lines indicate periods where signal change accelerates due to the presence of a gradient magnetic field. Initially, signal declines and then grows back due to reversal of the polarity of the gradient magnetic field. The actual signal intersects the T2* curve (and has the same amplitude as the undisturbed signal) at TE; this is the gradient echo. (For an explanation of the striped and solid symbols, see Figure 8-1.)

As with the spin echo, maximum rephasing will only occur at an instant in time while signal sampling occurs over a period of time. The application of the dephasing and rephasing portions of the frequency encoding gradient must be balanced so that rephasing is as complete as possible at TE, the midpoint of signal sampling. Keep in mind, however, that, absent the 180° pulse, signal is lost according to T2* from the time of the initial excitation, and T2′ effects are *not* recovered. Thus, the overall signal sampled during a gradient echo pulse sequence is *less* than during a spin echo pulse sequence.

In MR terminology, the first application is called the *frequency-encoding gradient* and the second may be called the *readout gradient*. Some say that you must "read-out under the same gradient used for frequency encoding." If the terminology is confusing, just skip it, review the concepts, and call the

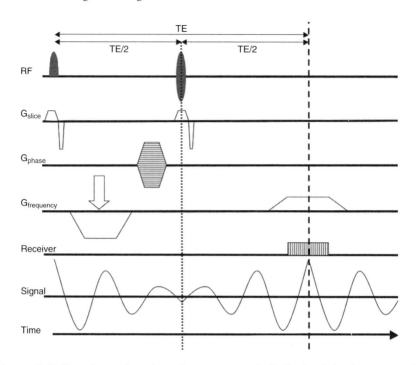

FIGURE 8-7. Complete spin echo pulse sequence. A dephasing lobe (open arrow) has been added to the frequency-encoding gradient. This preempts signal loss that would otherwise occur due to the effect of the frequency-encoding gradient. (For an explanation of the striped and solid symbols, see Figure 8-1.)

components by whatever names you wish. At this point, notice that the spin echo pulse sequence we discussed (Fig. 8-3) seems to be missing the first application of the frequency-encoding gradient. In fact, it was merely glossed over for clarity. Figure 8-7 shows the complete spin echo pulse sequence with the first application of the frequency-encoding gradient. Note that this spin echo pulse sequence in fact contains a "gradient echo." If it did not, the amount of signal remaining at TE and the signal of the image would suffer.

The Gradient Echo Pulse Sequence in a Nutshell

Salient components of the gradient echo pulse sequence are summarized in Table 8-2 and the pulse sequence diagram (Fig. 8-6).

Importantly, *while the frequency encoding gradient (AKA readout gradient) is on*, the signal is sampled such that the midpoint of the sampling time-period occurs when rephasing due to the gradient is maximal. This time point is TE.

TABLE 8-2. Features of the gradient echo pulse sequence.

Module	Action	Function
Excitation module	RF and slice select gradient are turned on simultaneously	Signal generated within a single slice
Readout module	Phase-encoding gradient is turned on briefly and then turned off	Phase encoding
	Frequency-encoding gradient is turned on and then off	Dephasing of spins
	Frequency-encoding gradient is turned on while signal is sampled	Rephasing of spins at TE, frequency encoding and signal sampling

What Makes Gradient Recalled Echo Different?

The absence of the 180° pulse confers several unique characteristics on the gradient recalled echo (GRE) pulse sequence. Whether these differences are advantageous or not, of course, depends on your point of view and the questions the pulse sequence is being used to answer.

The lack of the 180° pulse means that signal decays after excitation with the time constant T2*; signal losses due to T2′ from heterogeneity in the static magnetic field are not corrected. As a result, signal at TE will be lower than after a spin echo. Thus, the SNR of a GRE image will always be lower than a spin echo (SE) image. Accepting this lower SNR may be worthwhile, however, if we are looking to detect something that causes such heterogeneity of the static magnetic field. Blood products, for example, may be much more readily detected with GRE because the paramagnetic components in hemoglobin can accelerate T2* relaxation and lead to profound signal loss in GRE images that is all but undetectable on SE images. This topic will be covered in more detail in Chapter 18.

Because the 180° pulse is not used, the delays before and after the 180° pulse required for dephasing and rephasing of spins are also not necessary. Dephasing and rephasing using the frequency-encoding gradient can occur extremely rapidly by turning the gradient magnetic field on for a short time at very high amplitude. Remember, it is the *combination* of amplitude and duration of the gradient application that determines net dephasing or rephasing; with sufficient gradient amplitude, the process can be accomplished in a very short time. It follows, then, that TE can be much shorter in a GRE acquisition than in an SE acquisition because we do not require the time delays before and after the 180° pulse. In fact, the first fast-imaging methods were GRE acquisitions with very short TE. But we will learn more about that in Chapter 13.

The ability to use a short TE is also important because signal decays much more rapidly in GRE, with T2*, remember? A shorter TE allows sampling

TABLE 8-3. Typical times for TE and TR.

Image contrast	Spin echo TE (ms)	Gradient echo TE (ms)
T1 weighted	8–14	2–4
T2(*) weighted	80–120	15–20

before the signal has vanished. It turns out that the range of "usual" TEs in GRE imaging is much shorter than in equivalent contrast SE imaging (Table 8-3).

Table 8-4 lists some of the salient differences in GRE relative to SE and their implications.

Partial (AKA Modified) Flip Angles

Another hallmark of gradient echo imaging is the use of an RF flip angle (sometimes denoted by α) that is less than 90°. Although such modified flip angles are commonly used in GRE imaging, they can, in principle, be used with any type of pulse sequence. In fact, some commercial implementations of spin echo pulse sequences employ flip angles of slightly less than 90°.

Introducing Saturation

Why is it that we have used a 90° flip angle in all examples to this point? It is a convenient number to work with, but the real answer requires that we consider a real-life pulse sequence in which multiple successive applications of the RF at intervals of TR are required to generate an image. After TE, longitudinal magnetization slowly recovers. The T1 of the tissue and the time since the RF pulse determine the amount of longitudinal magnetization that will be available when we arrive at TR and excite the spins within the slice with the next RF pulse. If we deal with a situation where longitudinal magnetization will recover completely before TR, it turns out that a 90° flip angle will yield the greatest amount of signal (read transverse magnetization) when we apply the RF pulse. This will occur whenever TR exceeds about 3–5 times T1.

TABLE 8-4. Implications of differences between spin echo and gradient echo pulse sequences.

Difference in GRE	Effect	Practical implication
Absence of the 180° pulse	Measurement of T2* relaxation Shorter TE possible	Sensitive to heterogeneity in the static magnetic field Fast imaging

If TR is shorter, however, tissue magnetization will not be fully recovered when the second RF pulse is delivered at TR. Thus, the signal generated after the second RF pulse will be less than that generated after the first. The amount of longitudinal magnetization recovered after the third RF pulse will be even less. After about four successive RF pulses, the signal will achieve what is termed a *steady state*; the same amount of longitudinal magnetization will recover after all successive RF pulses. Because the steady-state magnetization is less than M_0, we say that the tissue magnetization is partially saturated. With a TR that is even shorter, the degree of recovery of longitudinal magnetization will be even less, and we will say that the degree of saturation has

It is generally advantageous to only fill *k*-space with signal acquired after a steady state has been achieved. As a result, the signal amplitude recorded in each line of *k*-space only differs based on the degree of phase-encoding gradient–induced signal loss. If signal from the first few echoes prior to the steady state are used, those first lines of *k*-space will have dramatically higher signal amplitude than those containing signal acquired after the steady state has been achieved. It is for this reason that most pulse sequences are *steady-state acquisitions*. This means that the signal from the first few echoes is discarded and only steady-state signal is recorded. Some cute MRI acronyms have resulted: GRASS stands for Gradient Recalled Acquisition in the steady state.

increased. Conversely, if we are dealing with a tissue with a relatively long T1, a greater degree of saturation will occur with the same TR.

The Ernst Angle

For a given tissue (and its T1), a longer TR will ensure maximum signal when we sample at TE. However, using an extremely long TR is generally impractical because it leads to very long imaging times and excludes T1 contrast from the image. If we wish to use a TR that is significantly shorter than 5 times the T1, the signal will inevitably be partially saturated. Is there a way to maximize signal at TE (i.e., minimize saturation)? It turns out that for a given combination of tissue T1 and TR, there is a specific flip angle that will yield the greatest steady-state signal. This angle,

For those who must know, the Ernst angle can be calculated from: $\cos \alpha = e^{-TR/T1}$, where α is the Ernst angle. Be advised that you do *not* need to know this equation. The graph in Figure 8-8 tells all.

described by Dr. Richard Ernst (Nobel laureate in chemistry, 1991), is termed the *Ernst angle*. As you can see in Figure 8-8, changing the TR alters the Ernst angle such that a shorter TR leads to a shift of

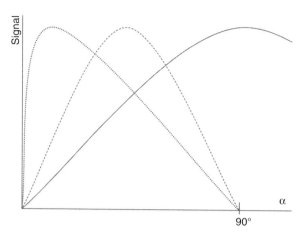

FIGURE 8-8. Optimal flip angle (α). These plots show how, for a given tissue, signal attenuation occurs as a function of flip angle depending on the TR. The solid line shows what would occur at very long TR: the maximum signal would occur with a 90° flip angle (Ernst angle). The dashed and dotted lines depict progressively shorter TR, where the Ernst angle becomes progressively smaller.

the peak of the curve to the left and longer TR leads to a shift to the right.

Identifying the Ernst angle allows us to maximize signal if we are using a TR that is short relative to the T1 of the tissue. This, by the way, is why some vendors have implemented the spin echo pulse sequence using flip angles less than 90°, but it is not the only effect of modifying the flip angle. Varying the flip angle can have major effects on image contrast.

Controlling T1 Contrast with the Flip Angle

Recall that T1 contrast will be greatest when tissues have large differences in M_z at the end of TR. At this point, the next RF pulse will turn the M_z into M_t (signal), and the initial difference in signal between tissues after the RF pulse will be due to the difference in M_z present prior to the RF pulse.

At a larger flip angle, more of M_z is turned into M_t. This leads to greater saturation as described earlier, but also notice that, as a result of the large flip angle, a larger amount of longitudinal magnetization remains to be recovered after the RF pulse. Two tissues with different T1 will have the greatest likelihood of showing different M_z at the end of TR when they will recover the greatest proportion of their M_z during TR. (TR, of course, defines the time during which the tissues can recover M_z). Because M_z at the end of TR determines the M_t (signal) after the RF pulse, signal will reflect T1 contrast when the flip angle is large, leading to more differentiation of M_z between tissues with different T1. Those differences are

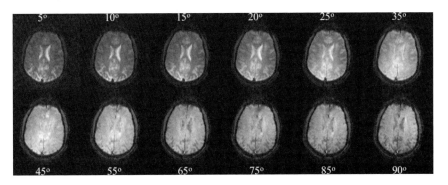

FIGURE 8-9. Contrast modified by flip angle. Increasing the flip angle (indicated above or below each image) suppresses T1 contrast despite the short TR (500 milliseconds) used to acquire all of these images. No parameters other than flip angle differ between images.

translated into differences in signal after the next RF pulse; signal differences that embody T1 contrast.

Contrast Modification in SE and GRE Imaging

Figure 8-9 shows how modifying the flip angle can dramatically change the contrast of the image; a very narrow flip angle can nearly eliminate T1 contrast from the image, leaving image contrast heavily dependent on T2. Because modifying the flip angle can deftly control the degree to which T1 differences contribute to image contrast, there is no longer a need to modify TR for this purpose. In spin echo imaging, we would set a very long TR in order to minimize contrast due to T1 differences and generate an image with contrast largely dependent on T2. With a narrow flip angle, however, T1 contrast is suppressed without need for a long TR. In fact, TR no longer plays a dominant role in defining image contrast. Whereas spin echo images with predominant T2 contrast are, by definition, time intensive due to the long TR required, similar T2 contrast can be achieved using a very short TR and a narrow flip angle. This point opens the door to fast imaging. In fact, modified flip angle gradient echo techniques were the first fast imaging techniques. Speed (short TR) can be achieved without any impact on contrast. More on this in Chapter 13.

9
Understanding, Assessing, and Maximizing Image Quality

What Is the Measure of a Good Image?

Medical technology is increasingly scrutinized as to its utility. In particular, there is increasing demand that demonstrable beneficial effects on patient outcomes be used to justify further investments in technology. This holds true whether you are a scientist competing for research funding who must show the potential significance of his or her work for human health or a clinician who must base diagnostic decisions on "evidence-based" practices. In light of this trend and the emphasis exerted by the FDA and insurance payers, among others, it is surprising that precious few of the imaging techniques in common use, including MRI, have been subject to, let alone have passed muster in, rigorous trials of their utility. Perhaps it is the gee-whiz technology sweeping us off of our feet: the introduction and adoption of new techniques may be regulated much more by market forces than by medical evidence.

What then defines a good or quality image? One approach, which seems quite prevalent, is to go for the aesthetically pleasing MR image. This certainly does impress observers and is important for marketing, but what does our (or a vendor's) *gestalt* impression of an image's beauty have to do with detection of disease? Are we studio photographers or *in vivo* imagers? As an example, most MRI vendors offer image-enhancement options such as filtering, smoothing, and zero-fill interpolation. Smoothing uses various algorithms, such as averaging adjacent pixels together, to generate an image with the appearance of less noise. By smoothing, you are essentially destroying spatial resolution in the interest of a prettier image! Beware: MR scanners may actually be set up with these options turned on by default.

The solution to the issues described above will not be found in this chapter. Only clinical research can provide the data, and only demand on the part of the consumers (or perhaps professional organizations, third-party payers, or the government) will stimulate the testing required to instigate that research. What we will explore in this chapter is the concept of image quality as well as some methods that are used to measure it. We will finish by discussing the importance of an ongoing quality assurance program.

What Is Noise?

The concept of noise is the foundation on which all measurements of image quality are built. Noise is simply signal that does *not* interest us. To keep the terminology simple, we will refer to the signal arising from the subject of our image (e.g., the patient) as the *signal of interest*. We will refer to noise as *signal of no interest*. Primary sources of noise include the sample and the MR scanner.

The sample (such as the patient) contains many potential sources of noise. Most basic is thermal noise. Assuming we are not working at absolute zero, molecules are moving. Random molecular motion leads to energy exchange between molecules, including water molecules, which modulates the MR signal in a random manner. When we deal with a living sample, physiologic changes in tissue content or location such as respiration, blood flow, and diffusion also create variation in the MR signal. Although such physiologic noise may not be random—it often has a regular or predictable pattern of variation (such as the cardiac cycle)—the fact we are not interested in these phenomena makes them signal of no interest (i.e., noise) nonetheless.

Perhaps a manifestation of our human limitations, despite best engineering efforts, the MR scanner hardware actually contributes noise that shows up in our images. The electronic systems used to generate RF and gradient magnetic fields, run the computer systems, and so forth, are less than 100% efficient. As a result, they generate electromagnetic fields that either modulate signal within the patient or are themselves detected as MR signal. One specific example of noise arising from the MRI scanner are eddy current effects, discussed in Chapter 5. Remember that shielding is employed to minimize the intrusion of noise (see Chapter 5).

Signal-to-Noise Ratio: Measuring Image Quality

Remember that in Chapter 1 we defined the goal of MRI as differentiating adjacent tissues based on differences in their MR signal. As we defined earlier, noise is simply signal of no interest. If the variations in signal due to noise exceed the variations in signal we are trying to detect, such as between brain and background, we will have trouble detecting those variations in signal.

Let's think about what we expect to see when looking at an MR image. At the most basic level, we expect to see signal where the object or patient we are imaging is located and *nothing* in locations where there is no object/patient. When looking at a brain image, for example, we expect to see signal only *inside* the brain. The reality, of course, is quite different. There will be signal, albeit low-level signal, in the background of the image as well. This signal of no interest is noise. Noise will be visible in the background if we adjust the window and level settings appropriately; it can be measured by obtaining signal intensity values from pixels in the background areas of the image (Fig. 9-1).

The noise that we see by adjusting the window and level settings of the image display does not exist only in the background, but it is present throughout the image. The more noise present in an image, the grainier it will appear. We can thus compare signal of interest measured from the body part we have imaged to signal of no interest measured from the background and derive a measure of how much of the signal of interest is contaminated by signal of no interest. In an extreme case in which the signal of no interest is extremely high relative to signal of interest, we might not even be able to discern the object we are imaging. Our measurement is called the signal-to-noise ratio (SNR). An image with very high SNR will appear to have no

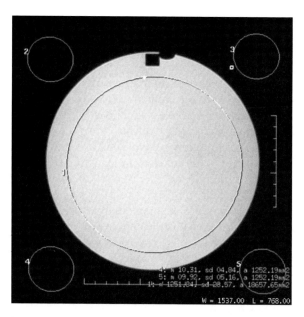

FIGURE 9-1. Phantom image for SNR measurement. This image transects a portion of the phantom containing pure fluid. Such a homogeneous region is ideal for measurement of signal (large circle within the phantom) to noise (smaller circles at the corners).

signal at all in the background and will look very "smooth," without graininess due to noise.

The SNR is measured by obtaining measures of signal intensity from two regions of interest: one placed in the image (signal of interest) and one placed in the background (signal of no interest). We examine relatively large regions of interest rather than individual pixels in order to minimize the effects of individual pixels containing extremely high or low signal intensity values. Whereas it might seem best to compare mean signal from each region of interest, remember that the aspect of noise that matters and makes our images grainy is the *variability* in the signal of no interest. If, for example, each and every pixel contained an equal amount of signal of no interest, our ability to detect variation in the signal of interest would not change. Because it is the variability in the signal of no interest that matters, we compare the mean signal of interest to the standard deviation (a measure of variability) of the signal of no interest. The most commonly used SNR measurement is calculated from these regions of interest as follows. Ideally, the noise measurement (σ_{noise}) should be computed as the average of the standard deviation in the background derived from several regions of interest (Fig. 9-1). The following equation may be used to calculate SNR:

$$SNR = \frac{0.66(\text{Mean}_{signal})}{\sigma_{noise}}$$

Because the variable signal due to noise is random and does not derive from a real source of signal, both positive and negative values can be found in the noise of an MR image. However, when we reconstruct a magnitude MR image (i.e., the usual way of displaying the MR image; see Chapter 5), we take the absolute value of all signal, negative or positive. To avoid overestimating noise, the scaling factor 0.66 is employed when computing SNR from such a magnitude image.

What Affects Signal to Noise?

Because high SNR is clearly a good thing, how do we maximize it? Simply put, there are two approaches: increase the actual magnitude of the signal or increase the sensitivity of the instrument (the MRI system) for detection of the signal. Table 9-1 details these possibilities.

Improvement in the magnitude of the MR signal can be accomplished by using four approaches. The first approach involves increasing the strength of B_0, which leads to larger M_z and, consequently, larger M_t (AKA signal). The second approach requires that we recall what exactly determines the signal we measure in an image. Most fundamentally, signal is measured on a voxel-by-voxel basis. This means that signal derived from a single voxel

TABLE 9-1. Factors leading to improved SNR.

Increase signal	Increase sensitivity
Higher field strength	Optimize coil
Larger voxel volume	Surface coil
Lower matrix	Phased array
Thicker slice	Lower SENSE factor
Signal average	Decrease receiver bandwidth
Optimize image	
Short TE	
Long TR	
Ernst angle	

is the sum of signal arising from all spins within that voxel. It follows that if our voxels contain more spins, then we will have more signal per voxel and, because noise is constant, higher SNR. Thus, any alteration of the image dimensions will lead to an increase in SNR (Table 9-1). Figures 9-2 and 9-3 show how signal to noise (and spatial resolution, of course) change with the image matrix and slice thickness. Altering field of view results in an alteration of voxel size without a change in image matrix. This change in the dimensions of the voxel will, of course, also modulate SNR (Fig. 9-4). Third, certain parameters of the MR pulse sequence modulate signal to noise. As described in detail in Chapters 3 and 4, increase in TR and decrease in TE and setting the flip angle to the Ernst angle augment signal magnitude and therefore increase SNR. These effects on SNR are shown in Figures 4-2, 4-4, and 8-9. Finally, signal averaging can be used to improve SNR (Fig. 9-5) without requiring any alteration in the pulse sequence. In signal averaging, we simply acquire multiple "copies" of the same image

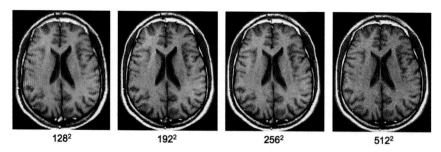

128²   192²   256²   512²

FIGURE 9-2. SNR as a function of matrix. As the matrix is increased (left to right, indicated at the bottom of each image), in-plane resolution improves, but SNR declines because of the decline in voxel size. Notice that the images become grainier, but edge definition improves.

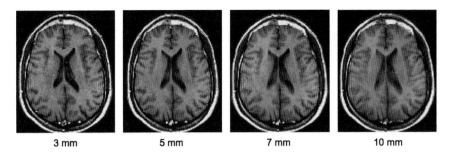

| 3 mm | 5 mm | 7 mm | 10 mm |

FIGURE 9-3. SNR as a function of slice thickness: The effects of increasing slice thickness (left to right, indicated at the bottom of each image) are analogous to those caused by change in matrix. Here, the thinner slices on the left are noticeably grainy due to lower SNR. Edge definition, however, is lost as we move to thicker slices.

and average signal pixel by pixel. Because noise is random, it is not augmented by the averaging procedure. Notice that improvements in SNR must be paid-in-full. That is, it will cost you spatial resolution (if voxel size is increased), time (if signal averaging is employed), or cash (to buy a higher field strength scanner) to improve this aspect of image quality.

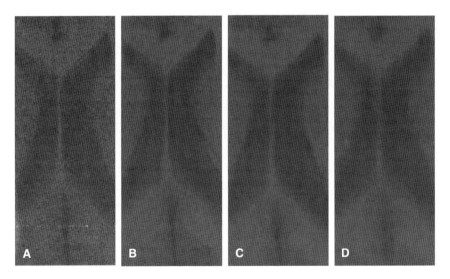

FIGURE 9-4. SNR as a function of field of view. To keep the playing field level, we have cropped these images. Field of view was progressively increased from smallest (A) to largest (D), without altering any other acquisition parameters. Once again, larger voxels (on the right) provide a smoother image. The smoothness is both because of higher SNR and the loss of edge definition. Notice the blurring of the brain-CSF interface.

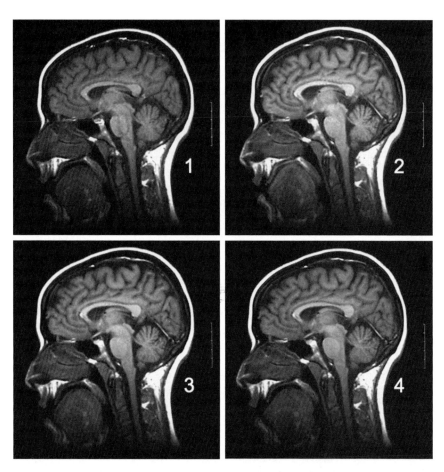

FIGURE 9-5. SNR as a function of signal averaging. The white numbers indicate the number of signals averaged to create each image. The improvement in SNR is obvious at four signals averaged. Notice, however, that edge definition does *not* change, because we have not changed voxel size. The cost of the improved SNR can be appreciated by squinting at the text in the lower left corner of each image; time increases from 1:30 to 5:10!

Contrast-to-Noise Ratio: Measuring Diagnostic Utility

No one will deny that high SNR is desirable and that some amount of SNR is absolutely necessary. What really matters, however, is how well an image will disclose differences in signal between tissues we are trying to differentiate. Consider an abdominal MRI examination performed to detect metastatic carcinoma. In order for the MRI image to be an effective means for detection, we must identify small metastatic lesions, perhaps because they exhibit higher signal on postcontrast images than surrounding normal liver parenchyma. If the noise in the image is so high, however, that the random variation in signal across the image is the same or greater than the difference in signal between metastasis and normal tissue, we will fail to detect the tumor.

Contrast-to-noise ratio (CNR) is a means for quantifying the degree to which the signal difference between two tissues we wish to distinguish will, in fact, be detectable in the image. The measurement of CNR, it follows, is specific to a given pair of tissues and can vary substantially depending on the difference in signal between these tissues. CNR is calculated as follows:

$$CNR = \frac{0.66(Mean_{lesion} - Mean_{normal})}{\sigma_{noise}}$$

Quality Assurance

As is probably apparent by now, the MR scanner is a very complex piece of equipment, and its proper function depends on many components working together with a high degree of precision. It follows, of course, that there is a pretty high likelihood of one or more components malfunctioning. There are two ways to find out if the system components are working properly. We could wait until image quality becomes degraded and then search for the cause. Alternatively, regular tests of system performance can be performed to detect problems, perhaps before they manifest as artifacts or poor image quality.

Many centers leave the quality assurance (QA) role to their service provider, most commonly the scanner manufacturer. Whereas many rely on this approach, our experience has been that our site-administered program of quality assurance often detects problems before the vendor's service team does. Recently, the American College of Radiology (ACR) has required a comprehensive QA program as a condition of MRI facility accreditation, though they do not specify that the program must be independent of the service provider. The keys to a good QA program include regular performance of a comprehensive array of standardized tests and tracking the measurements over time. By monitoring a plot of daily SNR measurements, for example, a drop in SNR can be detected even before noticeable changes in image quality occur.

Although a full treatment of MRI QA is beyond the scope of our discussion, we will take a brief look at the major areas that should be tested.

The Quality Assurance Measurements

In order for the results of the QA tests to be useful, measurements should be made in exactly the same manner each time they are performed.

Variations in such factors as position, pulse sequence, or regions of interest (ROI) placement could lead to spurious variance in the results that are greater than and obscure variance due to actual system problems. It is also wise to perform the tests at the same time of day and same day of the week (if they are not daily tests). This avoids daily variations as discussed below.

The Quality Assurance Phantom

The simplest phantom is merely a container filled with a solution designed to have proton density and relaxation parameters similar to tissue. Various solutions have been described, and the details are not really important for the average user. See Appendix 4 for sources of further information if you are interested in the details. In order to allow additional measurements, special phantoms are made containing embedded grids and high- and low-contrast objects. These items allow testing the accuracy of image geometry and contrast. A specific phantom was designed for and is required to achieve accreditation from the ACR (Fig. 9-6). This phantom provides all of the features required for a comprehensive QA program.

Every site should have a phantom dedicated to QA testing so that the same phantom is used every time testing is performed. It is equally important to position the phantom in exactly the same way each time testing is performed. Markings on the coil and a level are helpful in ensuring reproducible positioning. Measurements should be made at a fixed time of day to avoid variations that could be due to system usage, room temperature, and so forth.

It is generally advisable to use a phantom that is sized to fill the coil in the same way as it is filled during normal use. Most commonly, the head coil is used for phantom measurements. As a result, phantoms generally have dimensions similar to the human head. Special phantoms are available for testing coils of different sizes.

Signal-to-Noise Ratio

SNR is by far the most important parameter to monitor. For this reason, we make SNR measurements *daily* and continually monitor a plot of the daily measurements for any unexpected decreases. Measurements should be made on an image of a homogeneous portion of the phantom. ROIs are placed to occupy about 70% of the phantom area, and multiple ROIs are placed in the corners of the image (Fig. 9-1). The standard deviation from each of the background ROIs is averaged together and used with the mean signal from the phantom ROI to compute SNR as described above.

Uniformity

Recall our first words at the beginning of Chapter 1. We are attempting to differentiate adjacent tissues based on differences in signal intensity due to

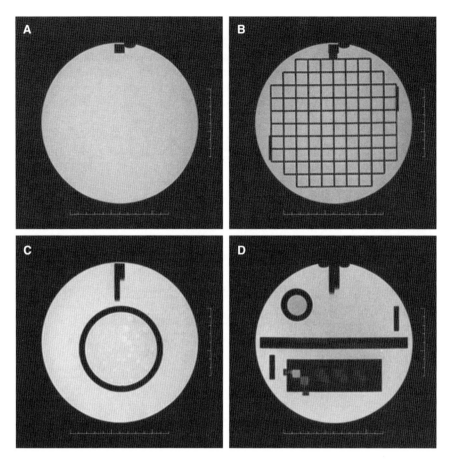

FIGURE 9-6. Phantom used for QA testing. (A) The homogeneous portion of the phantom, shown in Figure 9-1, used for measurement of SNR and uniformity. (B) Grid used to test for geometric distortion. (C, D) Embedded objects used to test contrast resolution.

the intrinsic differences in the tissue and not due to variability due to other causes. It follows that if we image a completely homogeneous object, signal intensity should not vary across that object. To test uniformity, we image a phantom containing a stable solution and measure the variability in signal intensity across a homogeneous portion of the phantom (Fig. 9-6A). Unacceptable uniformity may indicate many different problems, including poor B_0 homogeneity and coil sensitivity.

Geometry

As we will discuss in Chapter 10, magnetic susceptibility–related effects can lead to distortion of image geometry. These effects can result from problems with B_0 homogeneity, such as ferromagnetic debris (paper clips, hairpins, pocket knives, pens, and all kinds of stuff that should not be there) in the bore of the scanner. Problems with gradient calibration and eddy current effects can also disturb geometric reliability. To test and monitor the ability of the system to reliably depict geometry, a grid or series of objects with known dimensions and shape is embedded in a phantom (Fig. 9-6B). After imaging, measurements of the objects are made using the MRI console to ascertain that the sizes and shapes do not vary from expected values. Most commonly, measurements of the diagonals of the grid are made. Because the grid is square, measurement of each should yield the same value.

Contrast

Detecting the presence of disease depends on our ability to differentiate signal from one tissue from that of another tissue contiguous with the first. To test the MRI system's ability to generate images with sufficient contrast resolution, the test phantom contains several sets of low- and high-contrast objects (Fig. 9-6C, D). Images are assessed to determine if the expected number of objects can be discerned. In addition to QA testing, this component of the phantom is useful for testing new pulse sequences during development or for optimizing imaging parameters for best contrast resolution.

General Checks

Periodic checks of all of the MRI system components should be made. This can include checking for damaged or loose cables, table operation, ventilation, lighting, communication systems, and other components. It is wise to also check the penetration panel and doors regularly for loose contacts and connections and any conductive material that is passing through the waveguides.

10
Artifacts: When Things Go Wrong, It's Not Necessarily All Bad

Things Do Go Wrong . . . but It's Not All Bad News

Artifacts are common in all diagnostic imaging modalities, but nowhere is their study as much a field unto itself as in MRI. This is for a very good reason: MRI artifacts often convey important diagnostic information. They are not just nuisances. In the context of our study of MRI, artifacts are also important, an opportunity if you will, because they drive home many of the physical concepts we have been discussing. Finally, of course, artifacts can certainly be the first sign of trouble. Recognizing them allows the informed user to correctly identify the likely source(s) of the problem and even to determine if a user modification or a service call is necessary.

Motion

Motion artifacts occur when the subject/patient or part of it is not in the same location during all components of spatial localization. This can of course result from gross movement of the patients such as the nervous child, the demented grandmother, or the claustrophobic attorney. However, even if the patient is perfectly still, perhaps under general anesthesia, motion artifacts will occur. This is physiologic motion, be it respiration, the cardiac cycle, swallowing, peristalsis, and so forth. In fact, the only way to potentially generate an image free of all motion is to perform it postmortem or on an inanimate object. I say "potentially" because vibrations caused by the MR scanner hardware can induce motion artifacts when we image inanimate objects.

Recall that imaging time is a function of the number of phase-encoding steps (i.e., the number of voxels along the phase dimension) and does not generally depend on the number of frequency-encoding steps (i.e., the number of voxels along the frequency-encoding dimension). This is because each phase-encoding step requires repetition of TR. It follows then that the time between phase-encoding steps is rather long, measured in hundreds of milliseconds or even seconds. The time between frequency-encoding steps

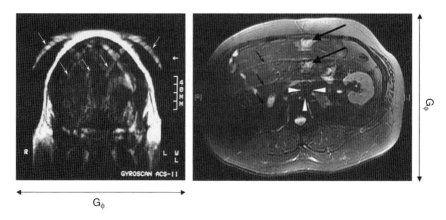

FIGURE 10-1. Motion artifact. Smearing of the image with incorrect placement of signal along the phase-encoding dimension is the hallmark of motion in MRI. Signal is encoded to varied locations because the subject is in a different location for each phase-encoding step. On the left, the artifact (arrows) manifests as multiple outlines of the head due to the patient moving the head right to left. On the right, respiratory motion leads to motion artifact (AKA ghosting; small black arrows). Motion of the aorta is due to motion from normal pulsatile blood flow. The true location of the aorta (right; white arrowheads) contains low signal, but multiple high-signal ghosts (right; large black arrows) traverse the left lobe of the liver. This artifact should not be mistaken for metastatic tumor within the liver.

(samples of the MR signal) by contrast is generally measured in hundreds of microseconds. Imagine you are a sports photographer. In order to take an action shot, you will choose a very short shutter speed—perhaps 1/2000 second—that is able to "stop" motion. So, too, in MRI: the time between frequency-encoding steps is so short that we can complete the readout of an entire line of k-space fast enough to beat even physiologic motion. During the delay between sampling of separate lines of k-space (TR), however, enough time elapses so that tissue is not in exactly the same location for each phase-encoding step. This difference between the time efficiency of frequency and phase encoding is the reason we tend to see motion artifacts propagate along the phase-encoding dimension but not along the frequency-encoding dimension (Fig. 10-1).

Although most MRI users reflexively state that motion artifacts only occur along the phase-encoding dimension of the image, it is not true that motion artifacts do not or cannot occur along the frequency-encoding dimension of an image as well. It is just that we generally do not see artifacts due to this motion because it occurs over a time frame much shorter than the entire sampling period. Similarly, fast-imaging techniques are able to virtually eliminate motion artifacts by acquiring all lines of k-space in a time shorter than the time frame of the motion. Because motion artifacts are nonetheless not seen along the frequency-encoding dimension of the image, we have a useful way to determine whether an area of signal abnormality is in fact a motion artifact. As an example, consider an axial slice through the upper abdomen where the aorta is posterior to the left lobe of the liver. The pulsation of the aorta commonly leads to motion artifacts where a silhouette of the aorta will repeat across the phase-encoding dimension. If the image is acquired with phase encoding along the anterior-posterior dimension, these "ghosts" of the aorta may show up in the liver and look like lesions (Fig. 10-1). If we acquire the same image again, but swap the phase- and frequency-encoding dimensions, the motion artifact will change its appearance and propagate along the new phase-encoding dimension. In our example, the ghosts will propagate from right to left, and the "lesion" in the liver will disappear.

Possible fixes for the motion artifact problem are shown in the box in this section. Immobilizing the patient and imaging faster are obvious approaches, but also remember that the source of the motion artifact can be addressed directly. Gradient moment nulling (AKA flow compensation; see Chapter 16) will actually minimize signal displaced due to flow. Spatial presaturation and crusher gradients can be used to destroy signal arising from a location where unwanted motion exists. Finally, gating methods can be used to time the start of the pulse sequence so that each TR begins at the same point in the respiratory or cardiac cycle.

Solutions to Motion Artifacts

- Control gross motion
  - Padding, restraints
  - Sedation, anesthesia
- Compensate physiologic motion
  - Gradient moment nulling
  - Crusher gradients
  - Spatial presaturation
  - Breath hold
  - Respiratory gating
  - Cardiac gating
- Image faster
  - Shorter TR
  - Longer echo train length (ETL)
  - Single-shot acquisition
  - Fewer signal averages

Undersampling (Wraparound Artifact)

We have already discussed the concept of undersampling and the wraparound artifact (Fig. 10-2) that results when we do not sample rapidly enough to correctly describe all signal arising from the object. We

Solutions to the Wraparound Artifact

- Increase FOV
- Oversample
- Spatial presaturation
  - Outer volume suppression
- Use wraparound elimination option
  - Foldover suppression, no-phase-wrap, etc.
  - Compensate with more signal averages
- Live with it!

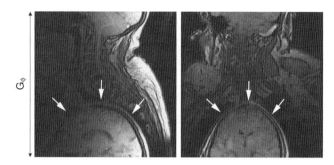

FIGURE 10-2. Aliasing (wraparound) artifact). Signal outside the field of view of the image is undersampled along the phase-encoding dimension (G_ϕ) and assigned a frequency corresponding with locations inside the too-small field of view. In this case, the top of the head (arrows) is superimposed on the chest when a small field of view centered on the neck is prescribed.

refer you to that discussion in Chapter 7 and will not repeat it here. We will, however, discuss some details regarding the wraparound *artifact* and its solution.

The most basic point to remember when considering wraparound (sometimes called foldover artifact) is that when we excite a slice (or volume) of tissue, *all* spins within that slice will yield signal that will show up in the image. If we wish to generate an image that only shows a restricted portion of the slice (i.e., a small field of view), there are two solutions. First, we can simply prescribe a small FOV, accepting the wraparound that will occur. This approach is a viable option when we are only interested in a very small portion of the FOV and the area into which wraparound intrudes does not extend far enough to enter the real area of interest (see box). Alternatively, we can oversample sufficiently to correctly place all signal arising from the slice. Oversampling is accomplished by prescribing a large FOV; the scanner will now set the sampling time (T_s) short enough to eliminate the

Truths Laid Bare by Technology

Many now work in a totally filmless environment; all imaging is displayed only on computer displays. This new workflow has many advantages. Today, we can interactively adjust the contrast of the image and magnify areas of interest at will. These new tools open our eyes to yet unseen parts of the clinical images we review on a daily basis.

In years past, MRI images were printed on photographic film by the MRI technologist. The printing of images on film was truly an art form, as the technologist would carefully adjust image contrast and brightness. In addition, the technologist was expected to magnify and crop the image to show the area of interest to best advantage.

possibility of aliasing. The downside is that, because the same number of voxels is now spread across a larger FOV, our image will now have lower in-plane spatial resolution. To preserve voxel size, we can divide our large FOV into a larger number of voxels but at the expense of increased imaging time for each of those additional phase-encoding steps.

Options are available that, at the click of a mouse, seem to magically eliminate aliasing without any increase in

Axial images of the spine (Fig. 10-3), for example, had always appeared on film showing a very limited "FOV": only the vertebra was included, leaving out almost all of the paraspinal tissue. As it turns out, these "small FOV" images were extensively affected by wraparound artifact. We never saw the artifact because the technologist excluded it when cropping the images for display on film. It is not at all important, of course, to know that this wraparound is in fact there. Nonetheless, it is instructive to see that in many cases, we can actually live with wraparound artifact.

imaging time or loss of spatial resolution. By this point, we see that this is physically impossible. In reality, these options do eliminate aliasing by oversampling—the FOV is increased—and they do maintain spatial resolution by increasing the number of phase-encoding steps. The "smoke and mirrors" are revealed when we examine the way in which imaging time

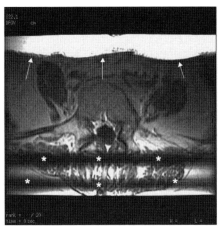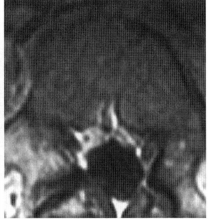

FIGURE 10-3. "Fixing" wraparound artifact. The buttocks are superimposed on the abdomen (arrows) due to the too-small field of view in this image (left). Because this is a spine examination, however, artifacts affecting the abdomen are inconsequential and can even be masked when the region of interest is displayed (right). Notice that artifact due to cross talk (left; asterisks) is also excluded by this display.

is maintained without change. These options cut the number of signal averages by the same proportion at which they increase the number of phase-encoding steps. Thus, while we do eliminate aliasing and maintain spatial resolution and imaging time, we pay the price in a reduction in SNR. Again, there is no free lunch.

Susceptibility Effects: Signal Loss and Geometric Distortion

The details of magnetic susceptibility will be covered in Chapter 18, but we will highlight here the basics required for understanding the artifacts produced by magnetic susceptibility effects. Magnetic susceptibility gradients occur

Minimizing Signal Loss and Distortion

- Remove the offending object
- Spin echo
- Short TE
- Long ETL

in the presence of materials such as metals and tissues such as bone, and in the presence of air, calcification, and certain blood products. The effects that underlie the artifacts we will observe are due to variability in the static magnetic field strength. As a result, we have a point-to-point variability in magnetic field strength, and, it follows, spins will precess at a range of frequencies, not simply at ω_0.

Signal Loss

When field strength varies enough that spins within a single voxel precess at significantly different frequencies, dephasing will occur. Dephasing leads to a rapid decline in net M_t: this is the concept of T2′ relaxation introduced in Chapter 3. Thus, spins in the vicinity of magnetic susceptibility gradients will demonstrate less signal (M_t) when we measure signal at TE. The degree to which signal loss due to magnetic susceptibility effect will manifest is dependent on the severity of the magnetic susceptibility gradient and the sensitivity of the imaging protocol to these effects (Fig. 10-4). The box in this section shows options for making an image less sensitive to magnetic susceptibility effects.

Geometric Distortion

As a clinician, I rely on the image as a true representation of the normal anatomy and pathology I am evaluating. The surgeons I work with rely on

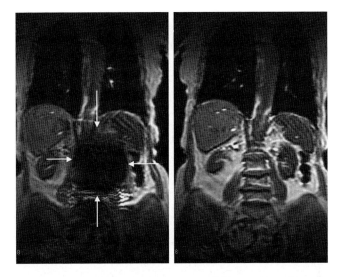

FIGURE 10-4. Signal loss due to magnetic susceptibility artifact. The area of signal loss (left; arrows) is due to a metallic component of the patient's clothing. After the article is removed, the artifact is resolved (right).

the shape and position of a tumor in planning its resection. In functional MRI (fMRI), we rely on the accurate location of regional brain activity in planning the safe extent of surgery. All of these assumptions may not hold up in the presence of magnetic susceptibility gradients. The variability in magnetic field strength and precessional frequency destroy the reliability of our spatial localization techniques. In spatial localization (see Chapter 6), we expect frequency of precession to vary in a precise linear fashion because of application of linear gradient magnetic fields. When spins actually precess at different frequencies that we cannot predict—the variability of frequency due to susceptibility effects is random—the signal will be written to the wrong location in the image. Because the effects are not linear or directionally specific, we will see misplacement of signal in all directions. The result is distortion of the expected geometry of the image. Keep in mind that because these susceptibility effects alter precessional frequency, they also corrupt slice selection. Thus, we may see signal within an image that does not belong there (Fig. 10-5). This is because, due to susceptibility gradients, frequency no longer varies in a linear fashion along the slice dimension. When we apply our RF pulse in the presence of the slice select gradient, spins at varying locations along the slice dimension will be excited, depending on the frequency of precession conferred by the combination of B_0, the slice select gradient, *and* the magnetic susceptibility effect.

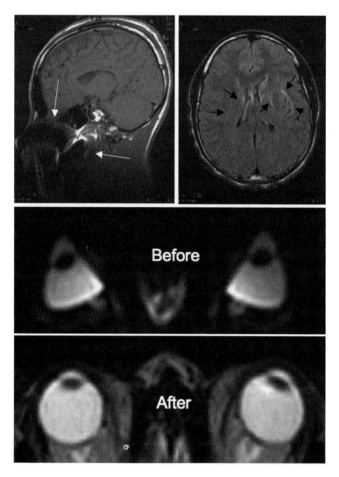

FIGURE 10-5. Geometric distortion due to magnetic susceptibility artifact. The subject's braces (top row) lead to signal loss but also distortion. Signal (arrows at top right) "abnormality" within the brain actually arises near the braces, but alteration of B_{net} makes this signal behave as if it arises in the brain. Eye makeup ("Before") containing paramagnetic components leads to bizarre appearance of the eyes that resolves with removal of the makeup ("After").

Truncation (Gibbs Artifact)

How do the spatial localization techniques we described in Chapter 6 allow us to precisely define an edge? If we have a phantom image, for example,

Minimizing Truncation (Gibbs) Artifact

- Increase resolution in the affected dimension (usually phase).

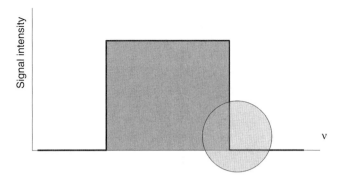

Signal intensity

v

FIGURE 10-6. Truncation artifact. In order to accurately locate the sharp edge, measures of signal intensity must be available at an infinite number of frequencies (v) in the region of the edge (gray circle). If not, we will inevitably undersample signal at the edge, aliasing it to an incorrect location.

there is an abrupt interface between the outer edge of the phantom and the surrounding air. Frequency is location, of course! In order to accurately depict the edge, we should have a range of frequencies at which we detect signal from the phantom with an *abrupt* transition to no signal (air) (Fig. 10-6). The degree to which this transition is truly abrupt is the determinant of the sharpness of the edge. In order to accurately localize the edge, we need to know the signal amplitude at an infinite number of frequencies. Because we can never have information about so many frequencies, we end up interpolating signal amplitude at the "missing" frequencies. Notice that we are not accurately sampling all of the frequencies contributing signal to the image. It follows that we will incorrectly sample some of those frequencies, assigning the incorrect frequency to some portions of the signal. This incorrect sampling results in the truncation artifact where signal from abrupt tissue interfaces is misplaced in the image along the phase-encoding dimension.

When tissue interfaces are oriented perpendicular to the phase-encoding dimension, we will see a series of parallel lines of misplaced signal. A common manifestation of truncation occurs when we image the spine in the sagittal plane and phase encode anterior to posterior. Multiple alternating bright and dark lines will appear parallel to the edges of the spinal cord and spinal canal (Fig. 10-7). The bright lines represent the misplaced signal, and the dark lines represent intervening areas. Looking at an image with high signal arising from CSF, it is possible for the bright lines to end up running down the center of the spinal cord. It is obviously important not to mistake this bright line for either the central canal of the cord (which is much too small to see on typical MR images) or a syrinx within the cord.

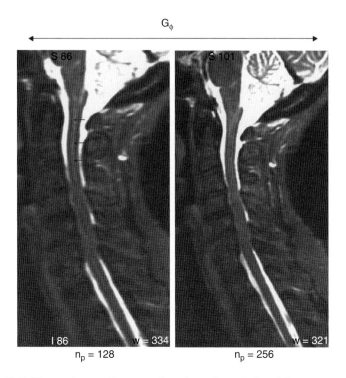

FIGURE 10-7. Truncation artifact as a function of resolution. Numerous vertically oriented striations are present parallel to the spinal column and cord, that is, propagating along the phase encoding dimension (G_ϕ). The most prominent of these lines is positioned in the center of the cord (arrows). This is misplaced signal due to truncation and does *not* represent a syrinx or the central canal of the spinal cord. The artifact is much less noticeable when resolution (N_p) is increased along the phase encoding dimension (right).

If this discussion sounds similar to aliasing because of undersampling along the phase dimension, it is in fact very much the same thing. Truncation is essentially aliasing because of undersampling along the phase dimension. The artifact tends to occur predominately along the phase-encoding dimension because we generally have a smaller number of voxels along the phase dimension. Increasing the number of voxels will diminish or resolve the artifact altogether (Fig. 10-7). Truncation can, of course, occur in the frequency dimension if we have an insufficient number of voxels. As we discussed, however, most scanners oversample along the frequency dimension by default, making truncation uncommon along this dimension of the image.

Radiofrequency Leak (Zipper Artifact)

A fact of life in MRI is that the receiver coils detect any signal present in the scanner room as long as it is in a frequency range to which the coil is sensitive. We have no means for making coils selective for signal arising from

Minimizing RF Leak Artifacts

- Close the door
- Clear all waveguides
- Check penetration panel connections
- Have the RF shield serviced

the patient. For this reason, the MRI scanner room is shielded to prevent any unwanted signal from reaching the coil (see Chapter 5). If it happens, as it certainly will in real life, that unwanted signal enters the room, we may see artifacts in our images. Entry of unwanted signal is usually due to either a breach in the RF shield or a malfunction of the MR hardware. Leaving the door to the scanner room open or having unfiltered electrical signals entering the room through the penetration panel. Both are common causes that are also easy to remedy. Actual failure of the shield can also occur—consider this after any structural work has been done on the room—and may be much more difficult to fix.

Excess signal at a specific frequency will appear as a straight line across the image perpendicular to the frequency-encoding dimension (Fig. 10-8), that is, at a single frequency. Multiple lines might appear if multiple frequencies are present. In the case where broadband noise is present, the entire image might be degraded with no recognizable representation of the subject.

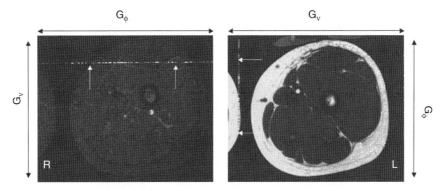

FIGURE 10-8. RF leak. Lines of signal intensity (arrows) are present perpendicular to the frequency-encoding dimension (G_v), each representing a single RF frequency that has contaminated the signal. Notice that when phase (G_Ω) and frequency (G_v) directions are swapped (right), the artifact is transposed accordingly.

Most commonly, such RF noise will be present at one or a few frequencies. For example, a truck driver's CB radio might be transmitting at a frequency in the megahertz range while his truck is passing by the MRI facility. If the shield is not intact, signal at that specific frequency will enter the room and be detected by the coil. This scenario, by the way, is one that actually happened at a facility that I was supervising. It was due to some shoddy work that had been done on the RF shield.

k-Space Corruption: (Corduroy, Herringbone, and Spike Artifacts)

This uncommon artifact is most important because it reinforces our understanding of k-space (see Chapter 6). We will see a repetitive pattern across the *entire* image (Fig. 10-9).

The zigzag appearance of the artifact gives it its name. This problem occurs because of aber-

Dealing with the Corduroy Artifact

- Rescan the patient
- If your scanner and technologist have the ability:
  - Edit the raw data
  - Reconstruct the image again

rant signal amplitude at even one single location in the raw data. This is typically referred to as a spike in the raw data because the abnormality is one of very high signal. Notice that although the problem with the data is at a single point in k-space, the artifact propagates throughout *all*

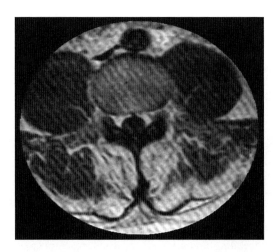

FIGURE 10-9. *k*-space corruption. This artifact manifests as uniform disturbance of *the entire image*, driving home the point that data from each point in k-space contribute to signal at every point in the image.

locations in the image. This, of course, is because the location of signal in *k*-space has no direct correlation with a specific spatial location in the image; each and every location in our raw data contributes to the signal at each and every location in the image.

The data spikes leading to the corduroy artifact are generally random and infrequent. For this reason, it is not usually fruitful or worthwhile to pursue the source of the artifact. Most often, it is actually best to just repeat the scan. In the event that such an artifact occurs frequently, a search for problems would be indicated. With special software tools, the spikes can be identified and edited out of the raw data. Reconstructing the image again after such editing will generally resolve the artifact. The absent data point, by the way, will likely not be noticeable in the reconstructed image.

Chemical Shift Artifact

The concept of chemical shift will be discussed in detail in Chapter 12. The chemical shift is the difference in precessional frequency (relative to that of pure water) conferred by the electron clouds present in the molecular envi-

Minimizing Chemical Shift Artifacts

- Increase receiver bandwidth
- Decrease spatial resolution
- Fat suppression

ronment within tissue. A chemical shift will be present in any tissue. However, the chemical shift of most tissues is so small that they behave, for purposes of practical imaging—spectroscopy is another story as we will see in Chapter 19—just like water. Fat, on the other hand, has a large chemical shift relative to water. Because fat occurs as an abundant homogeneous tissue, the chemical shift of fat relative to that of tissue is quite relevant. We exploit it for fat saturation and must be aware of the artifacts it can cause.

Consider a common scenario: in an axial image of the abdomen, we will view the kidneys—tissue, including the kidneys precess at a frequency similar to that of water—surrounded by perinephric fat. Along the frequency-encoding direction, we rely on the precessional frequency of spins as modified by a linear gradient magnetic field to correctly localize the signal. This scenario works out fine when we deal only with tissue (water) spins. Signal arising from fat, however, comes with a substantial frequency shift. As a result, we will misplace signal arising from fat along the frequency-encoding dimension. Within a large area containing fat, all of the signal arising from fat will be displaced, and, so to speak, voxels vacated by displaced fat signal will be reoccupied by signal displaced from other voxels. It is only at an interface between fat and water that we will detect this effect. The type of effect depends on the direction of the chemical shift relative to the tissue interface. As shown in Figure 10-10, when the displacement of fat is away from the water signal, we will see a black line

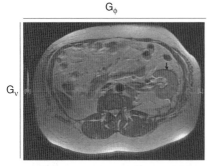

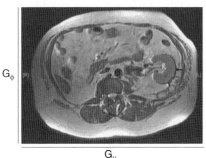

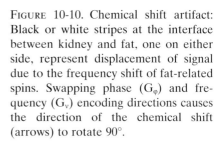

FIGURE 10-10. Chemical shift artifact: Black or white stripes at the interface between kidney and fat, one on either side, represent displacement of signal due to the frequency shift of fat-related spins. Swapping phase (G_φ) and frequency (G_v) encoding directions causes the direction of the chemical shift (arrows) to rotate 90°.

separating the water signal and fat. This line represents locations from which fat was displaced. On the other hand, if the fat signal is displaced toward the water signal, we will see a bright line at the interface. This is because fat signal is displaced into voxels containing water signal. Because the water signal is not displaced, we have a region where signal from *both* the resident water and displaced fat is detected as arising from the same voxel and summed. No black line is present because the voxels on the fat side of the interface that are "vacated" due to the chemical shift effect are "reoccupied" by fat signal next door.

The chemical shift artifact can sometimes be problematic, but it also has diagnostic utility. When there is question, for example, whether high signal on a T1-sensitive image represents fat or not, the presence of a chemical shift artifact may answer the question. In cases in which it is not clear whether a signal aberration is due to chemical shift, a simple way to verify the effect is to repeat the pulse sequence but swap the phase and frequency dimensions. The chemical shift artifact will follow the direction of frequency encoding. The likelihood that the chemical shift artifact will be seen is related to resolution along the frequency-encoding dimension. With larger voxels, the frequency range within a voxel may be larger than the magnitude of the chemical shift. As a result, displacement due to chemical shift will occur mostly within the voxel, and the chemical shift artifact will not be seen. Finally, receiver bandwidth modulates the magnitude of the chemical shift artifact. Similar to a decrease in resolution, increasing the bandwidth will lead to a greater range of frequencies per voxel, and any displacement of signal due to the chemical shift effect will be confined to the voxel and not manifest as a shift in signal within the image.

Slice Profile Interactions (Cross-Talk Artifact)

We learned in Chapter 6 that, whereas we might think that our images derive from perfectly even slices of tissue with perfectly parallel edges, this is clearly not the case. The edges of real-world slices have decidedly nonparallel edges; they are thicker at one edge and narrower at the opposing edge. Thus,

Minimizing Cross Talk

- Use an interslice gap
- Interleave slice acquisition
- Avoid multislice imaging
- Use a 3DFT pulse sequence

whereas our idealized even slices would stack up one next to the other, real slices will have some overlap. Tissue in the region of the overlap will be excited during acquisition of both of these adjacent slices. If we excite the two slices one after the other, as in multislice imaging (see Chapter 8), signal arising from the region of overlap will end up receiving multiple RF pulses in rapid succession, and this signal will be saturated. This is the major manifestation of slice interaction: saturation in the region of overlap. To minimize this problem, we can space our slices at a distance sufficient to make the real slice profiles truly separate, or we can just increase the time interval between excitation of adjacent slices. This is the reason for interleaving of our multislice acquisition where we excite slices out of order (e.g., slices 1, 3, 5, 7, 9 during one TR and slices 2, 4, 6, 8, 10 during a second TR). Figure 10-11 shows a unique case of cross-talk resulting from slice positioning.

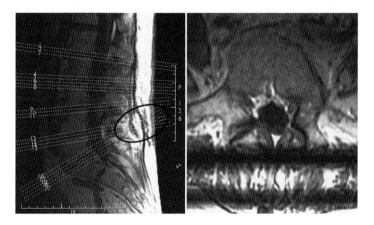

FIGURE 10-11. Cross talk. Horizontal black lines (right) are due to saturation where slice profiles intersect (black circle in the plane scan at left). In this case, the intersection was necessary to achieve appropriate slice position and did not degrade the essential portion of the image for the study being conducted.

11
Safety: First, Do No Harm

Who Cares?

If you plan on having anything to do with MRI, you had better care about safety. Whereas MRI is a powerful diagnostic tool that has become indispensable in health care delivery, it is potentially a double-edged sword. Patients have literally lost their lives due to errors in the use of clinical MRI scanners, and others have been seriously injured. Although the safety issues surrounding MRI have been know since its inception, renewed interest and serious attention to MRI safety dates from summer 2001. In July of that year, a 6-year-old boy who had just recovered from curative surgery for a brain tumor was killed during a follow-up MRI scan. During the scan, a ferromagnetic oxygen tank was brought into the scanner room and it launched into the bore crushing the little boy's head. This event received international media attention and instigated the American College of Radiology (ACR) to convene a Blue Ribbon Commission to assess the state of MR Safety and the scope of safe MRI practice. The commission published a White Paper on MRI Safety, which has been updated since its initial release (see Appendix 4 for the complete citations), delineating, in considerable detail, the parameters of safe MRI practice. The ACR White Papers are required reading for anyone involved in MRI and especially for physicians responsible for the safe operation of an MRI facility. If the urge to do good by patients does not suffice to encourage compliance and attention to detail, the fact that such policy papers are likely to form *de facto* standards used in litigation should help us all wake up and pay attention.

The Safety of MRI Versus Iatrogenic Injury

One of the major selling points in favor of MRI as a first-line diagnostic modality is its safety. The bioeffects of MRI are generally harmless. There is, to date, no evidence of any immediate or long-term adverse effect of

MRI on human subjects (the scanning itself; that is, this does not address the safety issues related to contrast agents and other "accessories"). This contrasts starkly with imaging modalities that employ ionizing radiation and carry well-documented risks of carcinogenesis, cataract formation, and harm to the developing fetus. The only caution we must keep in mind is that clinical MRI has been around only for a bit more than two decades. Long-term ill effects might not yet be known. To put this into perspective, however, the danger of ionizing radiation was quite evident in the first years of its development. NMR methods have been in use for decades without evidence of ill effects on humans.

If MRI is so safe, what's the danger? The problem with MRI is not so much the procedure itself, but rather when things go wrong or when humans interact with the magnetic field or the MR scanner in an unsafe manner. MRI risks are essentially risks of injury due to human error. Finally, we must realize that definitions and requirements of MRI safety change rapidly because of changes in the MRI equipment as well as other medical and nonmedical equipment that, for one reason or another, comes to interact with MRI.

Types of MRI Risk

There are many ways to break down the potential risks, and this chapter, because of space constraints, will necessarily provide only a summary overview. The safety of specific devices and implants is beyond our scope. For more detailed information, I refer you to the sources in Appendix 4. To keep things simple and clinically relevant, I will categorize the safety issues based on the type of adverse outcome.

Projectiles

The B_0 magnetic field is many-fold stronger than the powerful crane-mounted electromagnets used to move junk cars around a dump. *Anything* ferromagnetic will be pulled toward the bore of the MRI scanner with dramatic acceleration. If, for example, a pen or screwdriver is released opposite the bore of a 1.5-Tesla MRI scanner, it will be traveling at, perhaps, 65 miles per hour when it enters the bore. Were this to happen while a patient was lying in the scanner, serious injury could result. I once had the misfortune to witness the untimely demise of a rat (fortunately under anesthesia) when just such a flying screwdriver impaled it at a high rate of speed in the MRI scanner. The course such a projectile will take is random and unpredictable. The bottom line is that *all* ferromagnetic objects must be kept out of the MRI scanner room, whether oxygen tanks, hairpins, or hypodermic needles. For service work, by the way, special nonferromagnetic (usually beryllium alloy) tools are kept at the ready.

Projectiles Inside the Patient

Although we may not think of these as projectiles, bioimplants and foreign bodies containing ferromagnetic components also will be displaced by the B_0 field. Metallic fragments in the eye can lead to vitreous hemorrhage and blindness, and bullet fragments, if ferromagnetic, could be displaced and lead to injury. A major concern in this category is the ferromagnetic aneurysm clip. These are metallic objects with a high length-to-girth ratio, kind of like a compass needle. During surgery to repair an intracranial aneurysm, the clip is attached to an intracranial artery. If the clip is ferromagnetic, it will tend to line up with B_0, just like a compass needle will align with the earth's magnetic field. The force of this torque (as well, of course, as translational force) may (and has in at least one reported case) cause laceration of the artery, hemorrhage, and death. Other devices, although somewhat ferromagnetic, may not present a hazard because they are firmly attached to tissue in a way that sufficient movement to cause injury cannot occur. Heart valve prostheses, for example, although they might be somewhat ferromagnetic, are subject to greater force from the beating heart than due to interaction with the magnetic field B_0 and do not present a hazard once biointegration of the prosthesis has occurred several weeks after implantation. Orthopedic devices are generally so securely bolted in place that, even if ferromagnetic, would not pose a hazard related to displacement.

Bioimplant Malfunction

Patients may present for MRI with many different types of electronic implants. Even if these devices present no concern with regard to projectile hazards (e.g., they are made with only nonferromagnetic components), the MRI scanner or one of its components may cause malfunction of the device. In the best-case scenario, such device failure will damage the device without causing harm to the patient. In other cases, serious harm or death can result. We will consider each case separately.

Risk to the Patient

The device subject to greatest concern (and controversy) is the cardiac pacemaker/defibrillator. Although the medical literature has seen debate regarding the safety of pacemakers in the MRI environment, numerous cases of sudden cardiac death have been reported in which patients with pacemakers expired during an MRI scan. There are several potential mechanisms by which pacemakers may pose such risk. At the same time, there may be some patients that can, under specific conditions, survive MRI without ill effects. The problem is that it is not necessarily possible to accurately identify such patients in advance. In fact, risk may depend on the nature and timing of the patient's heart rhythm at the time of the scan. At this time, it should not be considered safe to subject a patient with a pacemaker to MRI unless a specially trained team is present and is intimately familiar with both the MRI and cardiac/pacemaker issues involved. For almost all MRI sites, excluding pacemakers without exception remains prudent practice.

Other devices, such as nerve and spinal cord stimulators, also may pose hazards because of unintended discharge of the device during MRI. A major concern for these devices also will be addressed below in our discussion of MRI-related burns.

Risk to the Device

Many types of devices, such as the cochlear implant, may be irreparably damaged by exposure to the MRI environment. Others, such as pumps and programmable CSF shunt valves, may require reprogramming or testing after the patient leaves the MRI scanner.

Burns

The RF pulses that generate the MR signal deposit relatively large wavelength energy in the patient. The energy deposition leads to heating, which is an inevitable consequence of MRI. Power deposition increases in proportion to the magnitude and duration of the RF pulses and also rises with the strength of B_0. For example, a turbo spin echo (TSE) pulse sequence that applies a series of $180°$ RF pulses delivers more energy than the single $180°$ RF pulse of a spin echo pulse sequence or the series of $15°$ RF pulses that might be used in a fast GRE acquisition. Excess RF power can lead to burns that can be quite serious. The FDA recognizes this hazard and has set strict guidelines for acceptable RF deposition, based on body size. The limits are expressed as either the specific absorption rate (SAR) or as an absolute temperature increase. Separate limits are set for the entire body and for specific body parts. MRI scanner manufacturers determine the SAR for each pulse sequence and coil and set limits within the system to prevent the limits from being exceeded. Additionally, all human MR scanners must be equipped with a real-time SAR monitor. Because the size of the patient affects SAR (larger patients can receive more energy without incurring as much heating as smaller patients), this system measures SAR for each pulse sequence performed on each patient and prevents the operator from exceeding SAR limits. For example, you might be prevented from further increasing the echo train length in a TSE pulse sequence due to the SAR monitor.

Beware Conductive Materials and Loops

The SAR limits described above are calculated based on the efficiency of energy transfer to tissue. Other materials, specifically electrical conductors, will absorb RF energy even more efficiently. If, for example, a conductive cable such as the one connecting the coil to the scanner is in contact with the patient during the scan, it may, despite a "safe" level of SAR, be heated to the point that a full-thickness burn occurs at the point where the patient's skin touches the cable. Insulating material (foam pads, blankets, etc.) should always be placed between the patient's skin and any conductive surface including the coil, cables, and the scanner bore. Because current will be more readily induced in looped conductors, it is essential to avoid all conductive loops; cables should be straight and the patient's arms and legs should not be crossed (forming a conductive tissue loop).

Nerve Stimulation

The RF and gradient magnetic fields applied during the MRI pulse sequence will induce current in conductors according to Faraday's law of induction. One potential consequence of this effect is direct stimulation of peripheral nerves by these time-varying magnetic fields. The patient may experience effects such as twitching and tingling, especially during high-duty-cycle pulse sequences (especially EPI [echoplanar imaging]) performed at high field strength. There is, however, no evidence of an enduring adverse effect of this type of nerve stimulation. For this reason, the FDA guidelines state that the threshold above which nerve stimulation must be avoided is pain.

Additional concern exists that current induced in implanted conductors such as pacemakers or nerve stimulators could lead to unwanted electrical stimulation of the heart or nerve. This effect is in addition to those discussed above regarding heating and burns and would apply in the presence of such wires even if no pulse generator is present. For this reason, it may be prudent to avoid high-duty-cycle acquisitions in the presence of such abandoned leads.

Hearing

The time-varying magnetic fields generate substantial acoustic noise and can potentially have an adverse effect on hearing. However, risk is proportional not just to amplitude, but also to duration of exposure. Thus, noise risk is especially concerning for those with repeated occupational exposure to the scanner room (as in MRI research environments). It is advisable that patients and workers always wear hearing protection when inside the scanner room during active scanning.

Psychological Distress

Claustrophobia, anxiety, and restlessness are relatively common among MRI patients. Although there have been individual reports of "permanent" psychopathology after the stress of an MRI procedure, there is no clear evidence that real risk exists. In the interest of maximizing the diagnostic yield from MRI, many steps can be taken to put patients at ease, including providing information about MRI and visits to the scanner in advance, playing music or a video for the patient during the scan, providing blind-folds, placing mirrors that allow the patient to see out of the scanner, and providing ongoing two-way verbal contact between the patient and scan operator. When appropriate and not medically contraindicated, oral anxio-lytic medications may be helpful. For extreme cases and in young children, scans may be performed under sedation or anesthesia. In such cases, skilled staff, resuscitation equipment, and MRI-compatible monitoring equipment must be readily available.

Pregnancy

To date, there is no evidence that exposure to MRI during pregnancy has an adverse effect on fetal outcome. *In vitro* and animal studies from which risk might be implied employed extreme levels of RF power and duty cycle making translation to human clinical MRI questionable. In fact, MRI has evolved into a favored modality for fetal imaging. Nonetheless, our experi-ence with MRI in pregnancy is limited to little more than two decades. As such, it is prudent to avoid MRI during vulnerable periods of fetal develop-ment (the first and, to a lesser extent, the second trimesters) unless there is a clear medical indication and no other nonionizing imaging modality can be used to answer the clinical question.

Gadolinium contrast agents should be avoided during pregnancy if at all possible. Because these agents cross the placenta and are excreted into amniotic fluid via the fetal urinary system, they may persist in the fetal cir-culation long enough for the chelate to dissociate, leading to exposure of the fetus to toxic free gadolinium ion.

Keeping It Safe: S⁴

After becoming familiar with the potential adverse effects related to MRI that we outlined above, a clear approach must be implemented to manage risk in the MRI facility. This can be remembered as the four "S's" of MRI safe practice.

Safety

Safety implies being cognizant of the potential risks and taking steps to minimize them through policy and, especially, training. Chief among these steps is the adoption and enforcement of a strict MRI safety policy. Such a policy is suggested in the ACR White Papers (see previous discussion in this chapter and Appendix 4) and should codify means to address each of the hazards discussed in this chapter. This policy largely relies on training of individuals involved in MRI. Annual formal in-service training and rec-redentialing of MRI staff is essential.

TABLE 11-1. MRI security zones.

Zone title	Area encompassed	Who gets access	What is allowed
Zone 0	Outside the MRI scanner facility including waiting areas, offices, etc.	No restriction	No restriction
Zone I	Areas with immediate access to the MRI scanner room door	All trained MRI personnel	Unsafe objects must be labeled
Zone II	The scanner room	MRI operators	Safe objects

Table based on concepts from Lipton ML. Keeping it safe: MRI site design, operations, and surveillance at an extended university health system. *Journal of the American College of Radiology* 2004;1(10):749–754; Kanal E, Borgstede JP, et al. American College of Radiology White Paper on MR Safety: 2004 update and revisions. *American Journal of Roentgenology* 2004;182(5):1111–1114; and Kanal E, Borgstede JP, et al. American College of Radiology White Paper on MR Safety. *American Journal of Roentgenology* 2002;178(6):1335–1347.

Security

Because of the projectile risk in the MRI scanner room, it is essential that the MRI facility be effectively locked down so that only individuals with appropriate training have access. Effective security can obviate major mishaps, such as the eager cleaning staff who decide to polish the MRI scanner room floor after hours and find their machines fly into the scanner bore, causing severe damage and perhaps, injury. We have implemented a scheme of secure zones that, in the interest of simplicity and compliance, is modified from that suggested in the ACR White Paper (Table 11-1). The essence of these restrictions is that, although unsafe objects might be necessary in the areas outside the scanner room (Zone I), they must be clearly identified with a conspicuous label so that they are not inadvertently brought into the scanner room (Zone II). All secure zones must be physically locked and only appropriately trained personnel (Table 11-1) may have unsupervised access.

Screening

It is imperative that *everyone* who enters the MRI scanner room (Zone II) is carefully screened to be sure he or she does not harbor an implant that might endanger him or her in the MRI environment. This applies to staff and visitors as well as patients. Trained MRI personnel should accomplish screening using a standardized form as well as at least two face-to-face screenings. A sample screening form is shown in Figure 11-1.

Surveillance

Any safety policy is only as good as its implementation. It is essential to establish a program for ongoing monitoring of the safety policy's adequacy

* RADSCR *

MONTEFIORE MEDICAL CENTER
The University Hospital
for the Albert Einstein
College of Medicine

MAGNETIC RESONANCE IMAGING
SAFETY SCREENING FORM

ADDRESSOGRAPH

NAME: _____

DATE: _____   WEIGHT: _____

YES	NO	PLEASE CHECK. ALL QUESTIONS MUST BE ANSWERED.
☐	☐	**Have you EVER had a pacemaker/defibrillator/ ICD/AICD?**
		(Implantable Cardioverter Defibrillator / Automatic Implantable Cardioverter Defibrillator)
☐	☐	**Have you EVER had an Electrical/Nerve/Spinal/Bone Stimulator?**
☐	☐	**Do you use hearing aids?**
☐	☐	**Have you EVER had a cochlear implant?**
☐	☐	Have you ever been told you have kidney disease? If yes, please specify: _____
☐	☐	Are you currently receiving dialysis?
☐	☐	Have you ever been a machinist, welder or metal worker?
☐	☐	Have you had metal removed from your eyes?
☐	☐	Have you been shot with bullets, BBs, or shrapnel?
☐	☐	Any surgery? If yes, please specify:
		OPERATION: DATE:

YES	NO	
☐	☐	Brain/Aneurysm clips
☐	☐	Ear Implants
☐	☐	Infusion pumps
☐	☐	Coils, catheters, filters or wires in blood vessels
☐	☐	Artificial heart valves
☐	☐	Magnetic dental implants
☐	☐	IUD
☐	☐	Tissue expander for future implants
☐	☐	Body piercing
☐	☐	Stents, filters, coils, shunts
☐	☐	Removable dental work such as bridges or dentures
☐	☐	Transdermal patches
☐	☐	Are you pregnant? - Obtain informed consent
☐	☐	Artificial limbs or joint replacement
☐	☐	Tattooed eyeliner/Permanent makeup
☐	☐	Any type of metal: rods, pins, screws, nails, plates, wires, mesh, or other

PATIENT SIGNATURE _____

PRINT NAME _____

TECHNOLOGIST'S USE ONLY

- I have reviewed the above form with the patient. The patient and/or guardian appear competent to respond.
- **Based on my review, I have made the following determination**
☐ No safety contraindication for MRI
☐ **MRI contraindicated (exam canceled)**
☐ Further clarification by the Radiologist: ☐ Approved   ☐ Exam canceled

_____
Radiologist Name   Date   Time

☐ Specific Precautions Will be Taken

TECHNOLOGIST SIGNATURE: _____

PRINT NAME: _____

XR9033M (06/07)

FIGURE 11-1. MRI screening form. This version of the MRI screening form is specifically designed to ensure the safety of MRI personnel. (Reprinted with permission of Montefiore Medical Center, The University Hospital for the Albert Einstein College of Medicine, Department of Radiology, New York, NY.)

and implementation. Changes will inevitably be required to address issues unique to each site. The surveillance process should include, but not be limited to, adverse event monitoring. The goal should be to identify policy breaches before they manifest as an adverse event. Many approaches such as electronic security systems that monitor door access and periodic "environmental rounds" to inventory and check labeling of safe and unsafe equipment can be used. It is, however, the responsibility, knowledge, and, above all, vigilance of MRI personnel that make any safety program a success.

Part III
To the Limit: Advanced MRI Applications

12
Preparatory Modules: Saturation Techniques

As mentioned in Chapter 8, the basic pulse sequence requires both an excitation module and a readout module. These pulse sequences can be modified, however, by adding preparatory modules (appetizers in the "pulse sequence menu" of Fig. 8-2). These preparatory modules are essentially different types of saturation techniques. In Chapter 8, we introduced the idea of saturation as a consequence of applying multiple RF pulses. In this chapter, we will apply additional RF pulses to deliberately cause specialized types of saturation in an effort to modulate image contrast in unique ways.

It is important to keep in mind that these preparatory modules are merely added to the front end of another pulse sequence. The core pulse sequence (excitation and readout modules) to which the preparatory module is added can be of virtually any type.

Inversion-Recovery Imaging

Inversion recovery (IR) simply implies adding a 180° RF pulse to the *beginning* of the core pulse sequence (Fig. 12-1). Yes, *before* the 90° RF pulse.

Immediately after the 180° RF pulse, the NMV is oriented at 180° relative to M_0; the magnitude of M_z is equal to M_0 and net M_t is zero. As we observe the behavior of M_z after the 180° RF pulse (Fig. 12-2), note that the magnitude of M_z gradually shrinks to zero and then grows back to M_0. Importantly, during recovery of M_0, *no net M_t is achieved*. This is because we are observing relaxation; no energy is being added to the system. Because the phase coherence required to achieve net M_t implies a higher energy configuration relative to phase dispersion, M_t cannot develop without addition of energy. Thus, during recovery of M_z, the NMV does not rotate through 90° but rather shrinks to 0 and grows back to M_0.

How is this phenomenon useful? After a delay following the 180° RF pulse, we begin our core pulse sequence starting with, for example, the 90° RF pulse of a SE pulse sequence. The time between the initial 180° RF pulse

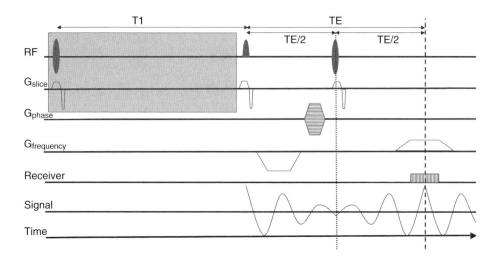

FIGURE 12-1. IR spin echo pulse sequence. An IR preparatory module (shaded box) is added to the front end of a standard spin echo pulse sequence. The time between the 180° and 90° RF pulses is termed TI. (For an explanation of the striped and solid symbols, see Figure 8-1.)

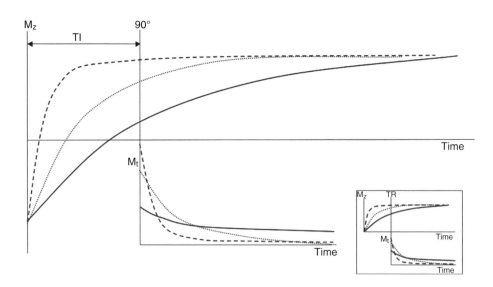

FIGURE 12-2. IR mechanisms. The 90° RF pulse that generates signal (M_t) is applied during recovery of M_z. T1 contrast (differences in signal immediately after the 90° RF pulse) differs from the standard pulse sequence (inset) based on the time TI.

and the subsequent 90° pulse is denoted by the Greek letter τ or the abbreviation TI. Looking at the broken lines in Figure 12-2, we can see that in the case of two tissues with similar proton density (similar M_0) and only slightly different T1, the steady state M_z will not be very different even when TR is short. However, when we precede the 90° RF pulse with an IR (180° RF pulse) preparatory module, the steady-state difference in M_z is greater. Thus, IR is a means for imparting T1 contrast. Every IR-prepared pulse sequence contains a significant component of T1 contrast; no matter how long the TR or how narrow the flip angle. As a clinical example, the greatest gray matter/white matter contrast is achieved with the use of IR. Magnetization-prepared rapidly acquired gradient echo (MP-RAGE) pulse sequences employ an IR preparatory module at the front end of a fast gradient echo pulse sequence. To achieve high grey/white contrast.

IR-prepared pulse sequences are perhaps most commonly used as tissue suppression techniques such as the fat-suppressed short τ inversion-recovery (STIR) pulse sequence. Notice in Figure 12-2 that the curves representing recovery of M_z cross the x axis. At the moment the curve crosses, the tissue has no net M_z (and also no net M_t as explained earlier). This point in time is termed the *null point* for the tissue. Remember that the RF is oriented perpendicular to B_0 and can only flip magnetization perpendicular to its plane of rotation. If the 90° RF pulse is applied at the null point when tissue magnetization has no net M_z, no M_t (i.e., no signal) will be generated from that tissue's magnetization. Other tissues with even slightly different T1 will generate signal after the 90° RF pulse, as they will be on one side of their null point or the other (Fig. 12-3).

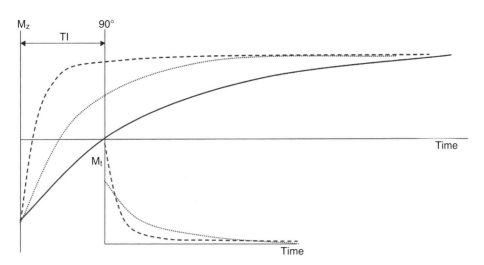

FIGURE 12-3. Tissue suppression with IR. TI is set so the tissue depicted by the solid black line has no net M_z at the time the 90° RF is applied. Thus, no signal is generated from this tissue; it is absent from the graph of M_t.

Creating a tissue suppression image requires knowing the time after an 180° pulse at which M_z of the tissue will be zero and applying the 90° RF pulse at exactly that time. The time interval between the 180° and 90° RF pulses is designated by the symbol τ or by TI. For tissues with a short T1 such as fat, a short TI will be required yielding a pulse sequence such as STIR (described earlier). To suppress signal with a very long T1 such as CSF, a long TI will be required, yielding a pulse sequence such as fluid attenuated inversion recovery (FLAIR). Modifying TI can also be employed to suppress signal from other tissues such as myelin. Figure 12-4 shows how tissue suppression and contrast is determined by TI.

While STIR is commonly touted as a "fat-suppression" technique, keep in mind that the tissue suppression is in no way specific for fat, only for tissues with short T1. Caution is especially in order when performing STIR in conjunction with contrast agents. As a practical example, consider the case of a tumor within the subcutaneous fat of the arm. STIR can quite nicely show the tumor. Fat is suppressed, but not the tumor tissue, which

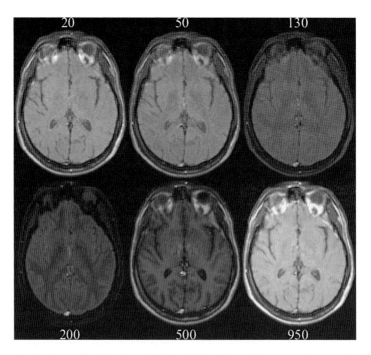

FIGURE 12-4. Contrast variation with TI. TI (indicated above or below the image) was varied as indicated; no other parameters differ between images. Notice that fat suppression is maximal at TI = 200 milliseconds, approximately the TI that would be chosen to create a STIR image. Contrast between gray and white matter reverses between TI = 200 and TI = 500 milliseconds due to modulation of T1 contrast by the IR preparatory pulse.

has longer T1 and T2 than fat. What happens on the postcontrast images? Fat is again nicely suppressed. The tumor, however, will have a much shorter T1 because of the presence of the contrast agent (see Chapter 4), and, as a result, the null point of the contrast-enhancing tumor may coincide with that of fat, and both fat *and* tumor will be suppressed, making the tumor *less* conspicuous than on the precontrast images. Watch out!

Spectral Saturation Techniques

Because IR is not a tissue-specific signal suppression technique, it will not be effective in all applications that require tissue suppression. How then can we do the job?

Chemical Shift

In Chapter 1, we explained that the frequency at which spins precess in the MR scanner's magnetic field (B_0) is determined by the strength of the *net* magnetic field (B_{net}) to which the spins are subjected. One component of B_{net} of course is B_0. ω_0 is the precessional frequency of pure water spins at the field strength B_0. Spins within soft tissue are often called *water spins* because the frequency of precession within most tissues is extremely close to that of pure water.

The tissue itself may also contribute to B_{net}. Electron clouds of molecules within tissue generate local magnetic fields that sum with B_0 yielding B_{net}. As a result, ω_{net} will vary, albeit to a miniscule degree, with the tissue the spins reside in. For example, when B_0 is 1.5 Tesla, the additional field generated by the electron clouds of fat molecules (specifically the numerous methylene groups on fatty acids) causes spins within fat to precess 224 Hz faster than those within soft tissue.

The change in precessional frequency conferred by the environment (in this case fat) is termed the *chemical shift*. Note that the chemical shift is a shift in the precessional frequency

> Chemical shift is the change in ω relative to ω_0 due to slight variations in B_0. It does *not* refer to spatial displacement of signal, that is, the *chemical shift artifact*.

and does not necessarily imply an alteration in signal within the image. The chemical shift artifact was addressed in Chapter 10; this artifact is a consequence of the chemical (frequency) shift described here.

Chemical shift is a function of field strength, and the absolute magnitude of the chemical shift will increase as field strength increases. The chemical shift of fat relative to water is 224 Hz at 1.5 Tesla, 447 Hz at 3 Tesla, but only 45 Hz at 0.3 Tesla. Rather than recalling or needing to look up the chemical shift for a specific field strength, it can be expressed as a fraction of the precessional frequency in parts per million (ppm), a field strength–independent parameter. The chemical shift of fat relative to water is 3.5 ppm regardless of field strength; multiplying ω_0 by the chemical shift in parts per million yields absolute chemical shift in hertz.

Note that since chemical shift becomes smaller as the strength of B_0 declines, lower field strength scanners will demonstrate much smaller chemical shift than at higher field strength. This, of course, means that artifacts due to chemical shift (see Chapter 10) will be much less troublesome at lower field strength. In addition, however, techniques that manipulate image contrast based on chemical shift, such as spectral fat saturation described in the next section, will be much less effective or impossible at low field strength.

Exploiting Chemical Shift to Saturate Tissue

From the preceding section, we see that a clear distinction can be made between the precessional frequency of fat and tissue (AKA water). We can thus design an RF pulse that is precisely tuned to excite spins precessing with ω_{fat}, but not with ω_0. If we apply several such fat-specific RF pulses in rapid succession (very short TR), the M_z of fat will be saturated, but tissue (water) will be unaffected. When we immediately apply the 90° RF pulse (not specific for fat) of our core pulse sequence, only the tissue in the slice that has net M_z will be excited. Because of the preceding fat-specific RF pulses, fat will have no net M_z, and no signal will be generated from fat. The image will indeed be fat suppressed. Unlike inversion recovery, however, the suppression in this case is quite specific to fat; it is termed *chemical shift selective* (CHESS) and commonly referred to as *fat sat* or just *fat suppression*.

Just as we can tune our CHESS RF pulses to be specific to fat, they can be tuned to be specific to other "tissues" as well. Water suppression is one example and is extensively used in MR spectroscopy.

Hybrid Techniques

Toward optimizing tissue, suppression techniques have been developed that combine aspects of both CHESS and IR. Spectral presaturation with inversion recovery (SPIR), for example, applies an IR preparatory module where the 180° RF pulse is tuned to ω_{fat}. Thus, only the M_z of fat is inverted. The 90° RF of the core pulse sequence is then applied when M_z of fat is zero. In this technique, two methods of fat suppression are combined.

Selective Excitation

Recently, precisely tuned RF pulses that excite tissue spins, but *not* fat spins, have been used to generate images with excellent "suppression" of fat or water. No signal is in fact suppressed in these images: the undesirable tissue is just never excited.

Spatial Saturation

We learned in Chapter 7 that aliasing will occur if the field of view is small relative to the true size of the body part being imaged. One approach to minimize aliasing is to oversample; but oversampling entails additional imaging time (at least when done in the phase direction). Another approach is to eliminate the signal outside of the field of view of interest using spatial presaturation pulses. This approach is essentially the same as spectral presaturation except that instead of applying saturation pulses tuned to a specific tissue's precessional frequency, we employ pulses that are slice selective for the region of the unwanted tissue. If we wish to image only a short segment of the leg in the sagittal plane, RF can be applied in the presence of a gradient magnetic field along z with the RF tuned to excite a thick axial slice on either side of the region of interest. When the core pulse sequence begins immediately after the saturation pulses, tissue outside of the field of view will have no net M_z and will contribute no signal (net M_t) to the image.

The application of spatial presaturation is also termed *outer volume suppression*. Another, even more common use of spatial presaturation is in the suppression of motion artifacts. In cervical spine imaging, for example, pulsation of the cervical carotids as well as swallowing lead to motion artifacts that extend across the entire image in the phase-encoding direction (see Chapter 10). By applying spatial presaturation to the soft tissues anterior to the spine, these structures, while still moving, have no net M_z and contribute no signal (net M_t) to the image (Fig. 12-5).

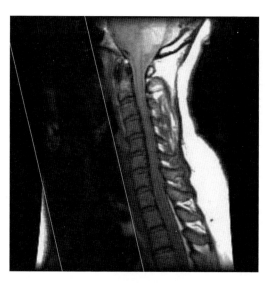

FIGURE 12-5. Spatial presaturation: Absent signal between the white lines anterior to the cervical spine is due to a presaturation pulse used to suppress motion from blood vessels and swallowing.

Spatial presaturation is also a key component of time-of-flight MR angiography (MRA). This will be discussed in Chapter 16.

Magnetization Transfer Contrast

Magnetization transfer contrast (MTC) is a special case of spectral saturation in which the suppressive effect of the saturation pulses indirectly decreases signal from tissue.

Just as the environment within fat modifies the precessional frequency of spins, other large molecules can have a similar effect. In fact, the frequency of precession conferred by this macromolecular pool is several hundred hertz different (termed *off resonance*) from that of water. This macromolecular pool has relatively low abundance; but when an RF pulse is applied tuned to its frequency range, energy conferred on the macromolecular pool will ultimately transfer to adjacent water spins. As a result, the nearby water spins will become partially excited (saturated) and have reduced M_z when the RF excitation of the core pulse sequence is applied. If we compare two images, one with the MTC presaturation pulse and one without it, signal will be lower overall on the MTC-prepared image but will vary spatially in inverse proportion to the macromolecular concentration.

MTC has limited clinical utility but is used as a tissue-suppression technique in MRA and can be used to improve the apparent intensity of contrast enhancement on gadolinium-enhanced images (Fig. 12-6). Important

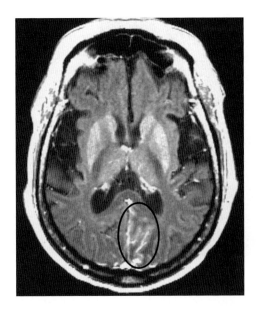

FIGURE 12-6. Magnetization transfer contrast. MTC was used to make contrast enhancement more obvious in this occipital infarct (black oval).

research applications of MTC employ quantitative measurement of the MTC ratio (comparing two identical images, one with and one without MTC preparation) in diseases such as multiple sclerosis. Although these quantitative measures are not in clinical use today, they may well be in the future.

13
Readout Modules: Fast Imaging

Whereas the preparatory modules discussed in the previous chapter were added to the front end of a core pulse sequence to further modify its contrast, this chapter will explore modification of the readout module of the core pulse sequence, principally in order to accelerate the speed of imaging. We learned earlier that the pulse sequence (time period = TR) must be repeated once for each line of k-space (which, of course, determines the number of voxels in the phase-encoding direction). Thus, TR and the number of phase-encoding steps (lines in k-space) are the factors that determine imaging time:

$$\text{Imaging time} = \text{TR} \times \text{N}_p$$

Faster imaging can be accomplished by shortening TR, as in fast gradient echo imaging. However, fast imaging is even more efficient when we actually fill more than one line of k-space during each TR. This central concept, filling multiple lines of k-space (or even all of it) during a single TR, is the foundation of many newer fast-imaging techniques. Be advised that this is the point at which your understanding of k-space (see Chapter 6) will come to real-world clinical application.

Gradient Echo Approaches: Turbo-Fast Low Angle Shot, Fast Gradient Recalled Echo, Turbo Field Echo

In Chapter 8, we pointed out that because the GRE pulse sequence does not include a spin echo (180° RF pulse with delays before and after for dephasing and rephasing), it can be accomplished faster than a SE pulse sequence. Additionally, we learned that while a short TR generally confers a large degree of T1 contrast, T1 contrast is also controlled quite nicely by modifying the flip angle of the RF pulse. Thus, we can image rapidly using GRE by simply shortening the TR. In fact, such fast gradient echo (FGRE) techniques often employ a TR of only a few milliseconds duration.

Because T1 contrast is controlled with the flip angle, the only limitation on shortening TR is the time required to switch the gradients on and off and to sample the signal at TE (dependent on receiver bandwidth as discussed in Chapter 7). Flip angle is also modified in an effort to maximize signal. At very short TR, saturation becomes problematic if the flip angle is too large: recall and be mindful of the Ernst angle (see Chapter 8).

Residual Transverse Magnetization and Spoiling

Another problem arises in FGRE where the TR may be only slightly longer than TE. Let us consider two successive RF pulses (RF_1 and RF_2) separated in time by TR and each followed by signal sampling at TE (TE_1 and TE_2) (Fig. 13-1). To this point, we have correctly assumed that the signal

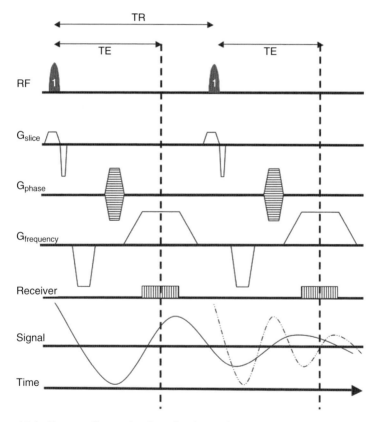

FIGURE 13-1. Fast gradient echo. Imaging is accelerated by simply making TR very short. As a result, signal generated by the initial RF pulse has not fully decayed when subsequent echoes are sampled. This signal will be detected in summation with signal from subsequent echoes unless it is spoiled. (For an explanation of the striped and solid symbols, see Figure 8-1.)

generated by RF_1 has completely relaxed by the time TE_2 arrives. As a result, we sample *only* signal generated by RF_1 at TE_1 and only signal generated by RF_2 at TE_2. This is because in previous chapters, we always employed a TR that was much longer than T2* of the tissue being imaged. However, when TR is very short, signal generated by RF_1 may still exist when signal is sampled at TE_2. This persistent or residual signal has continued to relax (according to T2*) from the time the spins were excited by RF_1; these spins will demonstrate greater T2* contrast than spins excited by RF_2. Furthermore, because the receiver coil detects all signal emanating from the tissue and cannot separate the component due to RF_1 from the component generated by RF_2, the image will demonstrate contrast that is a composite of signal acquired at two different TEs. Such residual transverse magnetization will be a particular problem if we are attempting to minimize T2* contrast and generate an image where T1 contrast predominates.

To minimize this problem, spoiling techniques are employed that either destroy or preempt the buildup of residual transverse magnetization. Gradient spoiling employs brief application of a strong gradient magnetic field after signal sampling is complete for each TR. As a result, all residual signal is dephased so that no coherent transverse magnetization (i.e., signal) persists.

A more sophisticated and effective approach is RF spoiling. Recall that the RF is a rotating magnetic field B_1. Just as we prescribe the frequency of the RF to accomplish slice selection, we can also prescribe the phase of the RF. It turns out that the phase of the RF determines the phase of the coherent transverse magnetization (signal) that is produced. If the phase of the RF is varied such that it is different for each TR, residual coherent transverse magnetization may persist after each TR, but net residual coherent transverse magnetization from multiple successive RF pulses will cancel to zero (Fig. 13-2).

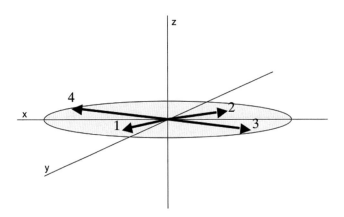

FIGURE 13-2. RF spoiling. Signal from four successive RF pulses (1 to 4) was applied with progressive change in phase to minimize net accumulated M_t (from prior TRs). The signals continue to decay with T2*, hence their different magnitudes, but basically sum to zero.

A footnote to our discussion of spoiling relates to the etymology of a venerable MR pulse sequence acronym: SPOILED-GRASS. This is an early, although still useful, implementation of gradient echo designed to generate images that demonstrate T1 contrast. The core of this pulse sequence is a gradient echo acquisition: GRA is gradient recalled acquisition. As with almost all MR pulse sequences, we discard data from the first few TRs in order to image in the steady state: GRASS is Gradient Recalled Acquisition in the steady state. Because we are interested in T1 contrast to the exclusion of T2* contrast, we will invoke spoiling to eliminate residual transverse magnetization: hence, SPOILED-GRASS is spoiled gradient recalled acquisition in the steady state.

Steady-State Free Precession: Balanced Turbo Field Echo, True-Fast Imaging with Steady-State Precession, Fast Imaging Employing Steady-State Acquisition

What happens if we do not spoil the residual transverse magnetization during a fast gradient echo pulse sequence? With a fast sequence that employs a TR that is shorter than T2*, when each RF pulse is delivered, magnetization, both M_t and M_z, from the preceding RF pulses will not have fully relaxed; both transverse and longitudinal magnetization will be present. By applying a closely spaced series of RF pulses, we will produce a series of gradient echoes and spin echoes (see Chapter 3) that merge one into the next. Because signal appears to never decay between RF pulses, we essentially have a perpetual signal to sample. This is called a steady-state free precession (SSFP) where the NMV is maintained at a fixed angle (β) relative to B_0, precessing around it. This approach is used to generate fast T2-weighted images, but note that, because M_z never relaxes completely, substantial T1 information is present in the images. Also note that, whereas this may seem like a gradient echo technique (no 180° RF pulses), the series of RF pulses does in fact generate spin echoes (see Chapter 3). Thus, we have less sensitivity to T2* than with typical gradient echo imaging. A major advantage of SSFP is its speed. Because of the extremely short TR, the images can be quite motion insensitive and useful for abdominal and cardiac imaging where fluid-sensitive images (heavily "T2 weighted") must be obtained faster than physiologic motion such as breathing.

Manipulating *k*-Space: Rapid Acquisition with Relaxation Enhancement, Turbo Spin Echo, Fast Spin Echo

Jürgen Hennig and colleagues at the University of Freiburg developed the concept of acquiring multiple lines of *k*-space after a single RF pulse in 1986. Implemented as rapid acquisition with relaxation enhancement

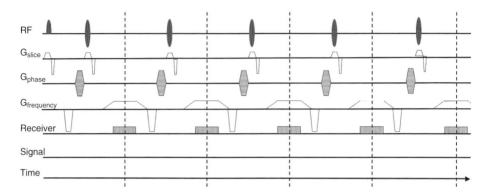

FIGURE 13-3. Turbo spin echo pulse sequence. All signals are acquired after a single 90° RF pulse. Additional phase-encoding gradient is applied before each subsequent 180° RF pulse. Thus, each time we record signal, it has unique phase encoding and can be written into a new line of k-space. In this example, five lines of k-space are filled after a single RF excitation (during one TR), shortening imaging time by a factor of five. (For an explanation of the striped and solid symbols, see Figure 8-1.)

(RARE), this technique is better known by the trade terms fast and turbo spin echo (FSE and TSE) used by the major commercial MRI equipment manufacturers.

Looking at Figure 13-3, we see that TSE begins as a typical SE pulse sequence. After the spin echo is sampled (at, let's say, TE_1) and written into the first line of k-space, however, a second 180° RF pulse is applied. This RF pulse is selective to the same slice as the original 90° and 180° RF pulses. Applying the additional 180° RF pulse causes the remaining transverse magnetization to be refocused with maximum signal occurring at a point equal to twice the interval between TE_1 and the second 180° RF pulse. A second echo is thus created and sampled (at, let's say TE_2). At this point, things seem very similar to the multiecho pulse sequence. The only difference is that we apply the phase-encoding gradient *again* before the second 180° RF pulse. This allows us to write the signal acquired after the second 180° RF pulse into a separate line of k-space *for the same image*. Additional 180° RF pulses can then be applied, each preceded by additional phase encoding followed by signal sampling. In each case, signal will be sampled at twice the interval between the preceding TE and the 180° RF pulse, and the data are written into the next line in k-space. Let's say, for example, that we generate eight spin echoes in this manner, filling eight lines of k-space. After we finish collecting the eight echoes, we must wait until the end of TR and begin again. As eight lines in k-space are filled within each TR, it follows that total imaging time will no longer be a simple function of TR and N_p but will be reduced by a factor equal to the number of echoes sampled during each TR. The number of echoes is termed the *echo train length* (ETL, or turbo factor). In our eight-echo example, imaging time will be one eighth as long as the equivalent SE pulse sequence!

During the time that we continue to apply the series of 180° pulses, the signal is, of course, decaying with the time constant T2 (each 180° RF pulse recovers signal lost due to T2′). The only limitation on the number of echoes we can create during a single TR (and as a result further accelerate the imaging time) is the longevity of the signal; we need to finish sampling before the signal has vanished completely. It follows that the closer we can space the 180° RF pulses together, the more echoes we can sample and the more lines of *k*-space we can fill after the single 90° RF pulse that started the pulse sequence. *Echo spacing* is determined by hardware performance including RF power, gradient speed, and receiver bandwidth. Very close echo spacing is a feature of newer and more expensive scanners. Once again, you get what you pay for when it comes to hardware: dollars invested in higher-performance hardware and the ability to space TSE echoes close together pays off in reduced imaging time and improved SNR.

Fast Spin Echo Contrast

Notice that each line of *k*-space was not acquired at the same time after the 90° RF pulse; each line, so to speak, has a different TE. Thus, we cannot say that the image created in this manner was acquired with a specific TE (Fig. 13-4). Rather, we speak of the effective TE (TE_{eff}) that indicates the dominant contribution to image contrast. What then determines TE_{eff}? It turns out that it is not merely a composite or average of the various TEs at which signal was sampled.

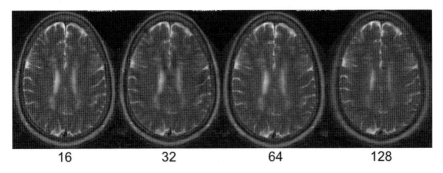

| 16 | 32 | 64 | 128 |

Figure 13-4. Echo train length. Image contrast is similar at these different ETL (below each image) settings, but speed varies dramatically. In addition, with increasing ETL, edges become blurred because very little signal amplitude is available in the periphery of *k*-space. The image on the far right is from a half Fourier single-shot TSE acquisition.

Recalling our discussions of k-space, remember that it is the central lines of k-space, those with the greatest signal amplitude, that govern image contrast. The peripheral lines of k-space, of course, have lower signal but higher frequency and govern spatial resolution in the final image. What determines TE_{eff} is the TE of the echoes *you choose* to place in the center of k-space. The signal acquired at each TE does *not* have to be entered into k-space in the order in which the TEs occurred in the pulse sequence. If signal acquired during the earlier echoes in the echo train are written to the center of k-space, TE_{eff} will correspond with a relatively short TE, and placement of later echoes in the center of k-space will confer an image contrast that reflects a longer TE_{eff}.

In our discussion of spatial localization, signal acquired using the lowest amplitude of the phase-encoding gradient (and therefore with the highest signal amplitude) was written to the central lines of k-space, and signal acquired with increasing strength of the phase-encoding gradient were entered more peripherally in k-space such that the signal was listed in order of the phase-encoding gradient strength. In TSE, notice that each successive echo in the echo train is encoded with the cumulative effect of *all* previous applications of the phase-encoding gradient during that TR. Thus, in general, earlier echoes have "seen" lower phase-encoding gradient strength, have higher signal, and are indeed written to the center of k-space. Subsequent echoes have "seen" higher phase-encoding gradient strength, have lower signal, and are written to increasingly peripheral locations in k-space. This results in a TE_{eff} that is in the range of the TE at which the earliest echoes were acquired. Modifying T2 contrast entails adjusting the amount of time between the initial $90°$ RF pulse and the beginning of the echo train, which modifies TE_{eff}.

Extreme Speed: Single-Shot Turbo Spin Echo, Single-Shot Fast Spin Echo, Half Fourier Acquisition Single-Shot Turbo Spin Echo

Assuming our hardware is fast enough, it may actually be possible to acquire enough echoes (maybe 128 or more) after a single RF excitation to fill all of k-space. Thus, the entire image is acquired within a single TR or in a "single shot." Such single-shot techniques (also called SSFSE, single-shot TSE, etc.) can acquire images in much less than one second—motion stopping speed—and are central to high-speed imaging such as breath-hold imaging of the abdomen.

The major limitation of single-shot techniques centers on the need to finish sampling and record all of the lines of k-space before the signal has vanished. If not, SNR will suffer in proportion to the portion of k-space that contains less than adequate signal amplitude. Because the central lines of k-space are generally filled from the earliest echoes, overall image intensity and contrast are quite robust, even with the most aggressive single-shot approaches. The area of concern is the periphery of *k*-space. With a very long echo train, especially with a long TE_{eff}, the most peripheral lines of *k*-space that contribute most to spatial resolution will have very low signal amplitude. As a result, long echo train techniques such as single-shot TSE will suffer some loss of spatial resolution and blurring of fine detail (Fig. 13-4). This occurs despite the actual spatial resolution of the image dictated by the number of lines in *k*-space; if the most peripheral lines in *k*-space have no signal, not only the periphery of the image but the entire image will have poor edge definition.

From the preceding section, it is apparent that it will be difficult to generate very high resolution single-shot images because of the limited signal available for sampling at the latest echoes. The conjugate symmetry of *k*-space (see Chapter 6) can be used in conjunction with a single-shot acquisition to permit very high speed, high-resolution imaging. These partial Fourier techniques often go by the acronym HASTE (HAlf Fourier single-shot TUrbo spin ECho) and entail using a single-shot TSE pulse sequence to acquire, for example, 129 echoes that are written into the first 129 lines of a 256×256 *k*-space grid. The remaining 127 lines are constructed from the acquired data based on the principle of conjugate (diagonal) symmetry. The result is a high-resolution image acquired in a very short time frame. The price: a small loss in SNR relative to a full *k*-space acquisition.

T1 Contrast in Single-Shot FSE

What is the TR of such a single-shot image? TR is the time interval between one RF excitation and the next, but during single-shot acquisitions, all of *k*-space for an entire slice is filled after each TR. The next RF pulse excites an entirely different slice. We do not, by definition, repeat the same RF excitation during a single-shot acquisition, and there is, in effect, *no* TR. If we use the term TR in describing a single-shot acquisition, it refers to the time between acquisitions of individual slices, not the time between multiple excitations of the same slice. Because all spins are fully relaxed at the time of the initial RF excitation, the rate at which their M_z recovers (their T1) has no bearing on the signal we sample. It follows that single-shot images cannot have T1 contrast. The only means for generating a single-shot image with any T1 contrast will be to apply an IR preparatory module. See Chapter 12 if it is unclear why IR will confer T1 contrast on the image.

Contrast Inversion: MR Hydrography

What happens if we write the latest echoes into the central lines of *k*-space and put the earliest echoes in the periphery? TE_{eff} is very long, and contrast will be strongly dominated by T2. On the other hand, significant signal (earlier echoes) will be placed in the periphery of k-space, ensuring adequate spatial resolution. This approach is one used to generate images showing fluid to the exclusion of all else, such as MR urography, myelography, cholangiopancreatography (MRCP), and so forth.

Gradient and Spin Echo

A variant of FSE is GRADIENT AND spin ECHO (GRASE) imaging. In this technique, some of the 180° RF pulses in the echo train are removed. As a result, signal sampled at these time points is due to the gradient echo phenomenon only. Our echo train thus contains some spin echoes and some gradient echoes. This approach can save some time because the time required to elicit a gradient echo is significantly shorter than that required to elicit a spin echo. The main use of the technique is to confer T2* contrast on the image.

Hyperspace: Echoplanar Imaging

Sir Peter Mansfield developed the concept of echoplanar imaging (EPI) in 1977, although it would be another 20 years before the necessary MRI hardware would be available to make the technique usable in practice. As we will see, gradient speed and strength are essential requirements of EPI.

Like the TSE techniques, EPI employs a unique readout module to dramatically accelerate imaging speed (Fig. 13-5). It will be useful to first examine an older implementation of EPI in order to understand the technique. Be advised, however, that this first approach is no longer widely used. After the initial 90° RF excitation, the phase-encoding gradient is turned on and *left on* at a fixed strength throughout the readout period. As a result, spins will experience a progressively increasing degree of phase encoding as the readout period progresses. Simultaneous with the phase-encoding gradient application, the frequency-encoding gradient is set to oscillate between two settings that have equal magnitude but opposite polarity (Fig. 13-5). The signal continues to decay with T2* as the gradients switch polarity back and forth, generating multiple gradient echoes. Each of these gradient echoes is sampled, and signal acquired during each echo is written into a new line in k-space. Using this approach, many lines of k-space can be filled after a single RF excitation. In practice, EPI is most commonly implemented as a single-shot technique where all of k-space is filled after a single RF excitation. Note that, in this implementation of EPI, the degree of phase encoding changes continuously throughout the readout period. Because the phase-encoding gradient is left on throughout the readout period, each time point within each line of k-space is acquired with

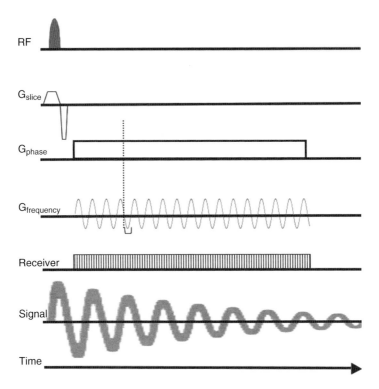

RF

G_{slice}

G_{phase}

G_{frequency}

Receiver

Signal

Time

FIGURE 13-5. Original EPI pulse sequence. The phase-encoding gradient is on at constant low amplitude, whereas the frequency-encoding (readout) gradient is oscillated such that a full line of k-space is sampled during each half cycle of the frequency-encoding gradient oscillation, indicated by the bracket. (For an explanation of the striped and solid symbols, see Figure 8-1.)

a different degree of phase encoding. This means that we fill k-space diagonally, resulting in phase artifacts that must be corrected in order to generate a coherent image.

To create a modern EPI pulse sequence, such as you will find in use on many commercial MRI scanners, we will significantly modify the phase-encoding gradient application. Rather than maintaining a continuous and constant strength, the phase-encoding gradient will instead be turned on very briefly each time the amplitude of the frequency-encoding gradient traverses zero (Fig. 13-6). These brief "blips" of the phase-encoding gradient give this form of EPI its name: *blipped EPI*. Another modification that improves the efficiency of EPI is sinusoidal oscillation of the frequency encoding gradient.

Notice that during the EPI readout, signal is sampled during periods of opposite frequency-encoding gradient polarity. This characteristic of

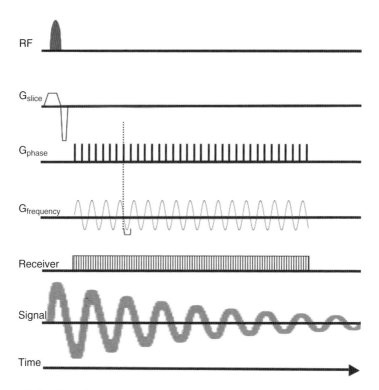

FIGURE 13-6. Blipped EPI pulse sequence. The phase-encoding gradient is only applied briefly each time the frequency-encoding gradient reaches zero amplitude between sampling periods. (For an explanation of the striped and solid symbols, see Figure 8-1.)

the EPI readout has specific implications for the filling of k-space. The right-to-left filling of k-space is ordered based on the polarity of the frequency-encoding gradient. Because the polarity of the gradient inverts for each successive gradient echo, we alternately fill k-space from right to left and then from left to right. Filling of k-space is thus rectilinear (Fig. 13-7).

As EPI, by definition, employs a long train of gradient echoes, it exhibits many characteristics of the GRE pulse sequence. Contrast in any EPI image is heavily dependent on T2*. Whereas spin echo EPI is accomplished by placing a 180° refocusing pulse between the RF excitation and the EPI readout module, because of the numerous gradient echoes, there can be no such thing as a truly T2-weighted EPI image. Despite the name *spin echo EPI*, the large number of gradient echoes confers image contrast that is more typical of a GRE image, dependent on T2* rather than T2 alone. As we will discuss in Chapter 18, the combination of speed and sensitivity to T2* make EPI an ideal technique for perfusion imaging and functional MRI (fMRI).

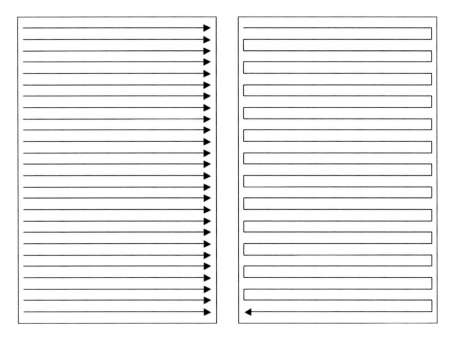

FIGURE 13-7. k-space filling. The diagram on the left shows standard left-to-right filling of k-space, and rectilinear filling as employed in EPI is shown on the right.

Further Exploits in k-Space

As discussed in Chapter 6, the phase-encoding gradient strength determines the location in k-space where a specific component of the MR signal will be written. Furthermore, within a given line of k-space, the time during readout at which a sample of the signal was acquired determines the location into which that sample will be recorded along that line of k-space. Each sample of the signal must occupy a specific location within k-space that is determined by the pulse sequence parameters, not necessarily the order in which the signal was sampled. We could, for example, record the samples "out of order." As long as we record them in the correct locations in k-space, the image will reconstruct correctly.

Applying this principle, we can develop unique approaches for the filling of k-space that may confer advantages, such as reduction of imaging time and decreased sensitivity to motion artifacts. In the constant phase-encoding gradient implementation of EPI discussed above, for example, phase changes throughout the readout period of a given line of k-space. This means that samples acquired in sequence will actually reside in different lines of k-space leading to a diagonal trajectory for k-space filling. Similarly, whereas typical pulse sequences fill each line of k-space from left to right, the oscillating readout gradient employed in EPI leads us to fill in a rectilinear fashion as described above.

SPIRAL imaging is essentially an EPI technique, but the readout and phase gradients are *both* oscillated so that *k*-space is filled in a spiral fashion. SPIRAL is also a fast-imaging technique, but its main advantage lies in the order in which *k*-space is filled. Because the center of *k*-space is filled first (recall that the center of *k*-space controls image contrast and intensity), before phase errors have developed, the resultant image will be relatively insensitive to the phase errors that plague standard EPI.

Although these varied approaches employ different methods for *filling* *k*-space, all techniques must ultimately convert the *k*-space data to a linear grid-like array in order for the Fourier transform to perform correctly. This regridding is one of the most challenging aspects of techniques such as SPIRAL that fill *k*-space through unconventional trajectories.

14
Volumetric Imaging: The Three-dimensional Fourier Transform

Multislice Versus Volumetric Imaging: Three-dimensional Versus Two-dimensional

In almost all imaging applications, we are in fact interested in viewing a volume of tissue; a single slice just does not convey sufficient clinical information to be useful. How then do we do it? In many, perhaps most, cases, we acquire a set of separate images, each representing a slice of tissue. If we set up the scan so that the slices are adjacent to each other, we will represent the volume of interest as a set of contiguous slices. However, it is important to recognize that these slices are in fact independently acquired images. We will now discuss an alternative approach. In three-dimensional imaging, the entire volume of tissue is imaged at once and, so to speak, chopped up after the fact into a group of slices.

Notice that the terms two-dimensional (2D) and three-dimensional (3D) do not describe the *display* of the imaging data, but how it is *acquired*. We can feed a set of 2D slices into a software program that creates a 3D rendering of those slices. On the other hand, even when we employ 3D imaging, the data are commonly viewed as a set of 2D slices.

Two-dimensional Imaging: How Do We Do It?

The answer to this question is quite simple: we perform some form of multislice imaging as described in detail in Chapter 8. The extent of the volume of tissue we will cover is determined by the number of slices, the slice thickness, and the gap between slices, if any. Remember that cross talk between the slices is an issue, and, for this reason, we generally interleave the order in which we acquire the slices.

Three-dimensional Imaging: How Do We Do It?

In contrast with the multislice approach, 3D Fourier transform (3DFT) imaging acquires signal from an entire volume of tissue at once. Just as we employ phase encoding to separate signal across the width of a 2D slice, the same concept of phase encoding is used in the "slice" direction to separate signal across the thickness of the volume.

Slab Selection

In 3DFT, we do not select an individual slice but rather a thick slab of tissue. Whereas in 2DFT the RF pulse might excite 20 separate adjacent slices to image a volume of tissue, in 3DFT we design our pulse sequence so that the RF pulse excites the entire volume of tissue (the slab) at once. The *entire* volume of tissue will be excited during *each* iteration (i.e., each TR) of the pulse sequence.

A Variation on Phase Encoding

Our first step in a 3DFT pulse sequence is exactly the same as the 2DFT pulse sequence we learned about in Chapter 8. After each RF excitation, we acquire a series of samples of signal and record them into one row of k-space. We then repeat the entire procedure once more for each additional line of k-space. The number of samples we record in each row, of course, determines the number of pixels we will have along the frequency-encoding direction of our image. The number of rows we fill determines the number of pixels we will have along the phase-encoding direction of the image. Once we have filled all the lines of k-space, executing the Fourier transform, first across the frequency-encoding dimension and then along the phase-encoding dimension, will yield a 2D image of our entire slab (Fig. 14-1). The thickness of this "slice," of course, is the thickness of the volume of the tissue (the slab) that we excite. We now have an image of a single thick slice to show for our efforts.

Once we have completely filled k-space, we will acquire a second image of this same thick slice, repeating the entire process with only one alteration. During acquisition of this second image, we will turn on the slice select gradient (Fig. 14-2) for an additional brief period of time after slice selection is complete and the RF has been turned off. This additional gradient will be applied at exactly the same time and with exactly the same strength during each repetition of the pulse sequence used to generate the second thick slice image. The signal acquired during each repetition will be written to a separate "page" of k-space. At the end of the process, we will have a spreadsheet file with two pages. Each page contains complete information for a 2D image of the same thick slice. If we apply the

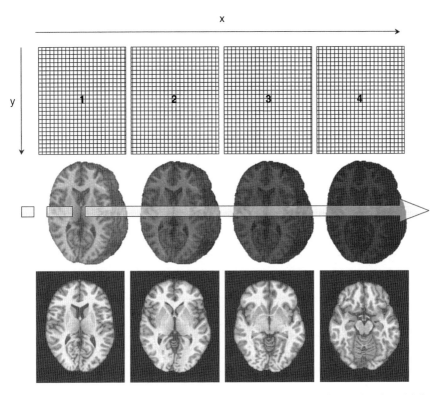

FIGURE 14-1. Schematic of 3DFT. A 2D matrix of raw data is obtained multiple times from a single thick slice. Each data set is written into a separate 2D k-space (1 to 4). The four data sets differ in that each was subjected to an additional application of G_{slice} (see Fig. 14-2). When we reconstruct each data set, we generate an image of the thick slice with overall signal altered based on the magnitude of the extra G_{slice} (middle row). In the final step, we perform a Fourier transform on the signal found at the same xy location in each thick slice image. This process is repeated for each and every xy location, yielding four separate partitions (bottom row).

2D Fourier transform separately to each of the pages, we will have two images of the entire thick slice. Will these two images be identical? Not really. Remember the extra gradient. The second image will have lower signal amplitude due to the extra dephasing induced by the extra application of the slice select gradient. Notice that the magnitude of this extra dephasing and signal loss will be the same everywhere along the phase- and frequency-encoding dimensions of the slice; because we are using the slice select gradient, phase changes are only induced along the slice dimension.

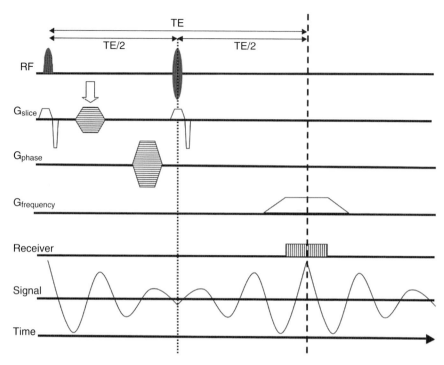

FIGURE 14-2. 3DFT pulse sequence. This standard spin echo pulse sequence has been transformed into a 3D acquisition simply by adding a *second* application of G_{slice} (open arrow) that will be set to a different amplitude during acquisition of each "page" of k-space (one for each partition we wish to generate, of course). (For an explanation of the striped and solid symbols, see Figure 8-1.)

The next step is to collect additional thick slab images, one acquisition entered into its own separate k-space "page," for each slice we wish to divide our thick slab into. As a simple example, let's assume we wish to divide our slab into four slices. We will need to acquire four thick slab images where the extra slice select gradient is applied at a different strength during acquisition of each image. What does k-space look like at this point? We have four separate "pages," each containing enough information to produce an entire 2D image of the entire thick slice (Fig. 14-1). The *only* way in which the values written into each "page" of k-space differ from those at corresponding xy locations in the other pages is due to the effect of the additional slice select gradient. This difference, of course, is due to dephasing and resultant signal loss induced by the extra application of the slice select gradient. If this is beginning to sound somewhat familiar, it is because we are setting up a scenario just like the phase encoding used to localize signal along the phase-encoding dimension of the slice.

Once we have filled all four pages of k-space, we can proceed to reconstruct the final image. The first step is identical to the procedure we discussed in Chapter 6: each of the four pages of k-space is subjected to the two steps of the 2D Fourier transform. Once complete, we have our four images, each of the entire slab. Now examine the signal located at a single xy location in each of the four slices. This signal in each and every one of the images is correctly localized along both the phase and frequency dimensions. If we ask where signal from this location in each of the thick slices comes from along the thickness of the 3D slab, we cannot localize it; it comes from *everywhere* along the slice direction, but only at that xy dimension. Signal from this location in each thick slice contains different overall signal intensity due to dephasing caused by the extra slice select gradient application. Just as with the phase encoding we discussed in Chapter 6, when we compare the four images, the degree of dephasing and therefore signal loss is greater for spins located farther from isocenter. If we now subject the values from this one xy location to the Fourier transform, we can separate the acquired signal into four locations along the slice select dimension. This is the third dimension of the 3DFT. After we perform the 3DFT, we will no longer have four images of the same thick slice, but four adjacent slices, each with its thickness one fourth of the thickness of the thick slab. To divide our slab into more and thinner slices, we need only acquire additional thick-slice images, applying a unique strength of the phase-encoding gradient during acquisition of each. The third application of the FT will then separate our slab into a number of partitions equal to the number of thick slice images (again, each acquired with a unique strength of the additional slice gradient) supplied to the FT.

The Price: Imaging Time

Because we must acquire a complete thick slice image for each slice we wish to divide our volume into, the number of slices now becomes a direct determinant of imaging time. In 2D multislice imaging, we could excite multiple slices within a single TR, significantly enhancing the efficiency of the overall acquisition sequence. In 3DFT imaging, because we excite the entire slab every time we apply an RF excitation pulse, a multislice approach would effectively alter the TR of our acquisition and lead to saturation. In the end, the total time to acquire our four slices will be four times as long as if we used a 2DFT multislice approach. In 3DFT imaging, total imaging time is determined as follows:

$$T = TR \times N_p \times N_{sl}$$

where N_p is the number of in-plane phase encoding steps and N_{sl} is the number of slices.

The Payoff: Spatial Resolution and Signal to Noise

Because it costs so much in terms of time to complete a 3DFT acquisition, why do it? There are two very good answers to this question. First, spatial resolution can be dramatically improved using 3DFT. Second, signal to noise will always be much better for a given voxel size when we use 3DFT.

The key to spatial resolution improvement is the thickness of the slice. In 3DFT, we are able to generate a much thinner slice than with 2DFT. Remember in Chapter 5 that we discussed limitations on the precision of RF slice selection profiles. Because of physical limitations on how narrowly and precisely we can tune our RF pulse, selection of very thin (approaching 1 mm) slices is not reliable. The outer edges of our slice will simply not be as straight and parallel as we expect. The 3DFT approach, on the other hand, selects a thick slice and divides it into thinner slices using the concept of phase encoding. Just as the voxels delineated within the plane of a 2D slice will be perfectly regular and square, 3D slices delineated using phase encoding will be extremely precise and regular. We can achieve a set of perfectly parallel and regular submillimeter slices. A 3DFT acquisition designed using small isotropic (cubic) voxels can be reformatted into 2D images in multiple planes (Fig. 14-3) that are indistinguishable from the images initially acquired. 3DFT using isotropic voxels also facilitates true 3D volume rendering (Fig. 14-4).

Improvements in signal to noise actually facilitate the high-resolution capabilities of 3DFT. When we perform 2DFT, each RF pulse generates

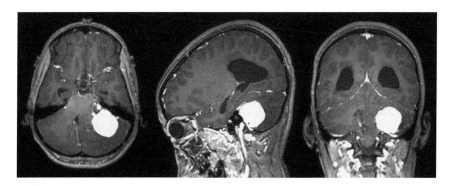

FIGURE 14-3. High-resolution 3DFT imaging. These three images, each in an orthogonal plane, were generated from a single 3DFT acquisition. Slice selection was performed in the sagittal plane, and parameters were set to generate voxels that are 0.6 mm on each side. Because of the high resolution and cubic voxel shape, you probably cannot tell that the axial (left) and coronal (right) images were reconstructed from the sagittal images (center).

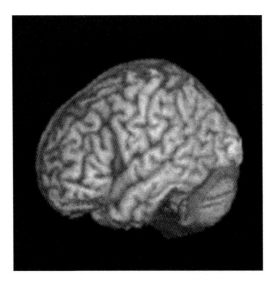

FIGURE 14-4. Real 3D imaging. 3DFT enables breathtaking image representations such as this 3D surface rendering of the brain.

signal only from the slice; signal is limited to that generated by the number of protons residing within the slice. In 3DFT, on the other hand, each RF pulse generates signal from the *entire* slab. That is, signal at each location within each "page" of *k*-space is derived from *all of the protons in the entire volume*. Thus, each time we sample the MR signal during a 3DFT pulse sequence, we measure a much greater signal, and the signal to noise of our image will be greater than that of a comparable 2DFT acquisition. With higher signal to noise, we can generate images with much smaller voxels and still have acceptable image quality.

15
Parallel Imaging: Acceleration with SENSE and SMASH

Why Another Imaging Technique?

We have already seen many ways to image faster and better. Why do we need to develop another class of imaging techniques and another set of MRI acronyms? MR people do seem to be quite fond of those! Parallel imaging, it turns out, is a truly revolutionary development, a quantum leap, that overcomes many of the practical limitations of high-speed imaging techniques like EPI. Looking back at the improvements in gradient performance that we benefit from today, it is easy to imagine even faster imaging by using faster and more powerful gradient magnetic fields and spacing echoes closer together. Other than the practical limitation of achieving such high performance, there are other real issues surrounding such gradient-intensive techniques. Very-high-gradient duty cycles can and do lead to painful peripheral nerve stimulation, and close spacing of RF pulses increases power deposition creating safety concerns (see Chapter 11). Image quality can also suffer, especially in EPI, where magnetic susceptibility artifacts may manifest as severe signal loss and distortion. All of these issues become more problematic at higher field strength. Parallel imaging methods accelerate imaging without any of these nasty effects. Although they have only become available recently, we are likely to see widespread development and dissemination of these methods in the near future.

So What's New?

The parallel imaging techniques accelerate imaging by reducing the number of lines of k-space (phase-encoding steps) that must be acquired but without compromising image resolution. As we know well by now, the number of phase-encoding steps is a direct determinant of imaging time (if this is not clear, refer back to Chapter 6). Using special multielement coils, we can derive unique spatial information from each coil that allows us to fill in the data for those "skipped" phase-encoding steps. Commercial MR scanners are currently available with 16 RF channels, and 32-channel systems will likely be available by the time this book appears in print. Investigational use of even larger RF arrays is under way, but it remains to be seen whether the sky is the limit and more is really always better when it comes to RF channels for parallel imaging.

Basics of Parallel Techniques

As the term implies, *parallel imaging* methods are based on acquiring multiple signals *in parallel*, that is, simultaneously. The techniques differ in the manner in which we process those independent streams of information. Before detailing the major types of parallel imaging, sensitivity encoding (SENSE) and simultaneous acquisition of spatial harmonics (SMASH), we will describe the common ground. These are basic requirements for any parallel imaging acquisition.

Parallel Radiofrequency Systems

In order for parallel imaging to work, we must not only have a multielement coil, but each coil must have its own dedicated receiver and processing stream. This requirement means that any MR scanner cannot be used for parallel imaging by simply adding the right coil and software. Additional hardware is necessary. At least two separate coil elements (typically embedded in a single shell or covering) must be used and the data from each processed through a separate receiver channel. Typical systems in use at the time of this writing employ six to eight channels.

Coil Sensitivity

Parallel imaging methods are based on the fact that a coil will have maximum sensitivity in its immediate vicinity. Thus, though each element in an array of coils will detect all signal, each will be maximally sensitive to signal arising closest to it. It is this pattern of coil sensitivity that is exploited to generate spatial information about the MR signal. In order to use this information, the pattern of coil sensitivities must be known. Because coil sensitivity changes with coil loading and positioning, it must be assessed each time we image a subject. Special images are acquired that determine the spatial sensitivity of each coil element. These images may not look like much (Fig. 15-1C, D), but they provide essential information that will be used in processing the MR signal into a meaningful image.

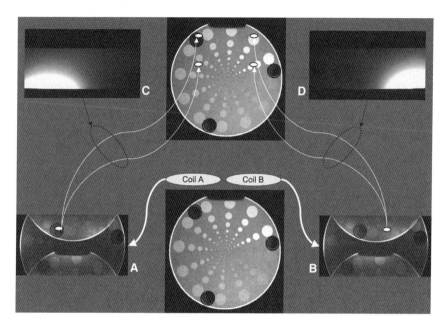

FIGURE 15-1. SENSE reconstruction: two-channel example. Two coil elements are used to acquire two separate images (A and B) of a phantom (center bottom). Neither coil has adequate sensitivity to the entire region encompassed by the phantom. Coil sensitivity is measured by acquiring a coil sensitivity image (C and D). For the actual SENSE acquisition, images (A and B) are acquired simultaneously from each coil, using half the number of phase-encoding steps required in the final image (center top). Signal from each pixel containing aliasing necessarily comes from two locations in the real object (thin white curved arrows). The aliased component images are "unfolded" using knowledge of coil sensitivity and solving the simultaneous equations as shown in the "Unfolding the SENSE Image" text box in this chapter. (Images used to create this figure courtesy of Philips Medical Systems America.)

Acquisition Schemes

Parallel imaging techniques are similar in that they acquire an image with lower resolution in the phase-encoding dimension than will be present in the final image field of view. Imaging is accelerated exactly because we must acquire fewer phase-encoding steps. However, if we separately submit the signal acquired by each coil element directly to the Fourier transform without further processing, each will yield a low-resolution image with aliasing along the phase-encoding dimension. Sensitivity Encoding (SENSE) and simultaneous Acquisition of spatial Harmonics (SMASH) differ in the way in which they combine the acquired signal from each coil element to produce a complete image of the full field of view without aliasing.

Sensitivity Encoding: SENSE, Integrated Parallel Acquisition Techniques–Modified SENSE (iPAT-mSENSE), Array Spatial Sensitivity Encoding Technique (ASSET)

SENSE was the first and is still the most widely used implementation of parallel imaging. As in all parallel imaging techniques, we acquire a smaller number of phase-encoding steps than the resolution we desire in the final image. A multielement coil is used, and the signal received by each coil element is processed independently on a separate RF channel. Data are processed through the Fourier transform, yielding one image for each coil element. Because of the small number of phase-encoding steps, each of these images, while it contains signal from the entire image, will show aliasing (Fig. 15-1a, b). The final steps in SENSE image processing use our knowledge of coil element sensitivity to "unfold" the aliased images.

Consider a case in which we wish to ultimately generate an image with 512 pixels along the phase dimension. We have eight coil elements that are arrayed along the phase-encoding dimension of the image, and, to reduce

Unfolding the SENSE Image

Eight simultaneous linear equations can be solved for signal at each section of the final FOV (S_n):

$$SI_1 = C_1S_1 + C_1S_2 + C_1S_3 + C_1S_4 + C_1S_5 + C_1S_6 + C_1S_7 + C_1S_8$$

$$SI_2 = C_2S_1 + C_2S_2 + C_2S_3 + C_2S_4 + C_2S_5 + C_2S_6 + C_2S_7 + C_2S_8$$

$$SI_3 = C_3S_1 + C_2S_2 + C_3S_3 + C_3S_4 + C_3S_5 + C_3S_6 + C_3S_7 + C_3S_8$$

$$SI_4 = C_4S_1 + C_4S_2 + C_4S_3 + C_4S_4 + C_4S_5 + C_4S_6 + C_4S_7 + C_4S_8$$

$$SI_5 = C_5S_1 + C_5S_2 + C_5S_3 + C_5S_4 + C_5S_5 + C_5S_6 + C_5S_7 + C_5S_8$$

$$SI_6 = C_6S_1 + C_6S_2 + C_6S_3 + C_6S_4 + C_6S_5 + C_6S_6 + C_6S_7 + C_6S_8$$

$$SI_7 = C_7S_1 + C_7S_2 + C_7S_3 + C_7S_4 + C_7S_5 + C_7S_6 + C_7S_7 + C_7S_8$$

$$SI_8 = C_8S_1 + C_8S_2 + C_8S_3 + C_8S_4 + C_8S_5 + C_8S_6 + C_8S_7 + C_8S_8$$

where C_n, coil sensitivity factor. SI_n, composite signal measured at the coil element.

imaging time, we will acquire 64 phase-encoding steps (a factor of 8 reduction), but simultaneously from all eight coil elements. Thus, we have a total of 512 samples, but only 64 unique strengths of the phase-encoding gradient. Subjecting data from each coil to the Fourier transform will produce eight images, each demonstrating aliasing by a factor of 8. That is, eight different sections of the image are superimposed on each other. We can actually consider our complete image as divided into eight sections with each coil element maximally sensitive to the section closest to it and progressively less sensitive to sections that are increasingly farther away. Whereas each coil element will produce the same aliased (times 8) image, the intensity of each component of the aliased image will vary depending on the coil element used. A coil sensitivity factor (C) will tell us the proportion of signal (S) from each section of the image that contributes to the composite signal (SI) in each aliased image. For those of you who *must know* the details, we develop a separate equation describing the components of the signal seen in each coil element's image in terms of the eight subsections of our final image (see the box in this section). Because we end up with eight equations and eight unknowns, we can solve for the signal at each section of the image (S_{1-8}), generating the complete, large FOV image in one eighth the imaging time but with no loss of resolution.

Simultaneous Acquisition of Spatial Harmonics: SMASH, Integrated Parallel Acquisition Techniques–Generalized Autocalibrating Partially Parallel Acquisition (iPAT-GRAPPA)

These techniques differ from SENSE in the way the data acquired from each coil element are handled and processed. In SMASH and related techniques, signal from each coil element is *not* subject to the Fourier transform separately. Rather, the spatial sensitivity of the coil elements is used to recombine signal from the different coil elements to create data for the "missing" lines of k-space. Thus, we develop a complete set of k-space data (in our example, 512 lines) from which we can generate our image. Improvement in the acquisition time obtainable with SMASH is the same as with SENSE. However, data processing for SMASH may be slightly more time efficient.

What Do We Actually Gain and at What Cost?

Speed

Clearly, parallel imaging techniques facilitate dramatic improvement in imaging efficiency. Although imaging time can theoretically be reduced by a factor as high as the number of parallel RF channels used, at this time, acceleration factors of more than 2 or 3 tend to lead to aliasing artifacts. Nonetheless, even this potential degree of acceleration is huge. Aside from the obvious financial potential inherent in being able to slide more patients through your scanner per unit of time, imaging speed has actual importance for image quality as well. Enhanced imaging speed is important for minimizing artifacts due to gross patient motion but also due to physiologic motion. Contrast-enhanced MRA techniques (see Chapter 16) require that we complete imaging during the brief peak concentration of the contrast bolus. Dramatic improvements in imaging time hold promise for time-resolved MRA methods, with temporal resolution matching or exceeding that of conventional x-ray angiography. Functional imaging methods like perfusion, diffusion, and functional MRI benefit from the ability to acquire more data in less time. Finally, decreasing the number of echoes required in a high-speed, fast spin echo acquisition decreases the overall RF power deposition. This safety concern becomes especially problematic as we space echoes closer together and image at higher field strengths. At high field, SENSE or SMASH may allow execution of otherwise unsafe single-shot fast spin echo acquisitions.

Susceptibility

Because we acquire fewer phase-encoding steps, parallel imaging methods are less gradient intensive and are much less affected by signal loss and distortion due to magnetic susceptibility–related effects (see Chapters 10 and 18). This is particularly important at higher field strength where these effects are more problematic. EPI in particular is improved by the reduction in the number of gradient echoes required to complete readout of the signal.

Signal to Noise

The price to pay, not surprisingly, is measured in signal. Because we acquire fewer lines of k-space, we have less signal intensity to contribute to the image. Nonetheless, the imaging methods that benefit most from parallel imaging, such as fast spin echo, generally have enough signal to benefit from parallel acceleration without significant loss of image quality. If we are able to generate the image by sampling fewer echoes, we can complete sampling before relaxation has caused extensive loss of signal. Finally, imaging at increasingly high field strength provides additional signal that offsets losses incurred due to parallel acceleration.

16
Flow and Angiography: Artifacts and Imaging of Coherent Motion

What Is Magnetic Resonance Angiography Anyway?

Magnetic resonance angiography (MRA) uses the same MRI system and methods we have been discussing to make images of blood vessels. Though the MRA images are cross-sectional images just like all other MR images, 3D rendering is commonly used in MRA, and you are probably most used to looking at these 3D images (Fig. 16-1).

MRA has revolutionized the evaluation of patients with vascular disease. In the days before MRA, high-resolution imaging of blood vessels was done only with x-ray angiography. Angiography is an invasive procedure that requires placement of a plastic catheter into the blood vessel of interest and injection of contrast material while radiographs are taken. MRA introduced high-resolution vascular imaging that was entirely noninvasive. However, the nature of the images and the type of information they convey about blood vessels is very different from that provided by x-ray angiography.

X-ray angiography (and by extension CT angiography) is, forgive the analogy, just a barium enema. For a barium study of the gastrointestinal system, we fill a cavity (viscus) with contrast material (barium) and use x-ray images to see the inner surface of that cavity in relief. For an x-ray angiogram, we fill a cavity (an artery or vein) with contrast material (iodine) and use x-ray images to see the inner surface of that cavity in relief. Both procedures provide detailed information about the anatomy of the inner surface of the cavity under study. Acquiring multiple images in sequence at a high frame rate also allows us to observe the "flow" of contrast over time. Nevertheless, x-ray angiography is still an anatomic study of the inner surface of the vessel wall. MRA depicts motion; it is *not*, in almost every case, an anatomic study of the vessel wall. Thus, before we can embark on a discussion of MRA techniques, we must come to a common understanding of the principles of motion and flow that make MRA possible.

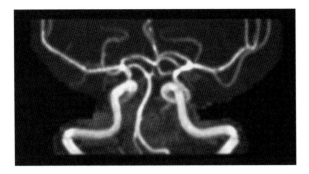

FIGURE 16-1. Maximum intensity projection (MIP). The MRA images are rendered using an algorithm that reports the maximum signal intensity from each of multiple vantage points. The result is a 3D model of the vasculature that can be rotated in any direction.

Basic Principles of Flow for Students of MRI

First, let's be clear about the simple but easily overlooked fact that blood flow is just a special case of motion. There is nothing really different about the flow of blood through an artery, urine through the ureters, or CSF through the cerebral aqueduct. Keep this in mind, because the same principles used to make MRA images of the arterial system can be used to make similar images of, for example, CSF flow.

Flow is depicted as a vector. This vector describes both the direction (vector orientation) and speed (vector length) of flow. Recognize that the fluids whose motion we will be demonstrating with MRA are composed of particles. If we consider the red blood cells that comprise arterial blood, for example, a vector will represent each individual red cell, describing its direction and speed of flow. If we then observe a volume of arterial blood, the net flow detected within that volume would be determined by the individual flow vectors of all red cells within the volume of interest. In MRA, signal depends on the net flow vector present within a voxel of flowing blood.

What then does the net flow vector look like? Let's begin by examining flow within a phantom. To simulate flow through an artery, we will pump blood through an idealized cylinder at a typical velocity found in a medium-sized artery. The cylinder used for our phantom is perfectly straight and has perfectly smooth and parallel walls. Given the straight course of the tube, all red cells will flow in the same direction. Because each cell's individual flow vector has the same orientation as all others, net flow within the tube will be represented by a single vector with its magnitude corresponding with the mean velocity of all cells flowing through the tube.

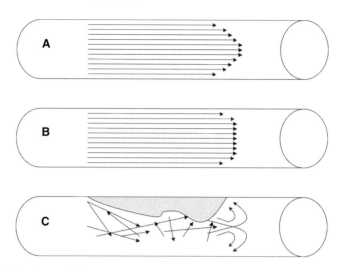

FIGURE 16-2. Types of flow relevant to MRI. (A) Ideal laminar flow shows a parabolic profile with flow velocities declining toward the periphery. (B) A blunted velocity profile occurs in real life and is called plug flow. (C) Turbulent flow results whenever the contour of the vessel deviates from an ideal parallel-walled cylinder. The curved arrows at the right indicate vortex flow that occurs where the vessel widens following an area of narrowing.

Laminar Flow

Because, in our example, we are using a single pump to force blood through the tube, do individual cells in fact flow at different velocities? They do. Velocity will actually be maximal at the center of the tube and will decrease as we examine cells farther from the center. If we plot velocity on a cross section of the tube, we will find concentric rings of decreasing velocity as we move from center to periphery. This is termed *laminar flow*. The velocity profile of laminar flow (Fig. 16-2A) is parabolic. This shape indicates that there is a range of velocities, ranging from maximum at the exact center of the tube to virtual stasis at the extreme periphery. In real life, the velocity profile is truncated, and we have what is termed *plug flow* (Fig. 16-2B). This blunted profile indicates that the flow profile across the center portion of a real blood vessel will be more limited than under the ideal conditions of our model. Nonetheless, velocity does in fact decrease toward the periphery. We will see that this concept of laminar/plug flow has very real impact on the appearance of flowing blood on MR images.

Turbulent Flow

Several features of real blood vessels distinguish them from our flow phantom. The walls of an artery, for example, are not perfectly smooth, straight, and parallel, but they have at least some degree of irregularity, curve, and taper. Perhaps, most importantly, real arteries bifurcate and branch. This branching makes it inevitable that red cells traveling with the idealized straight-line laminar flow we discussed above will meet an obstruction. They will collide with the vessel walls where they turn, taper, or branch. In the presence of narrowing such as that due to atherosclerotic plaque, the red cells will impact the plaque. The end result of these collisions is a disorganization of flow. Cells move in various random directions, and both the net flow vector and the velocity profile are dramatically altered (Fig. 16-2C).

Impact of Flow on the MR Signal

MRA images are just MRI images made particularly sensitive to flow. Before getting to the business of generating such flow-sensitive images, we must understand the way in which the MR signal can be altered by motion. There are three separate mechanisms by which the MR signal is *reduced* by motion such as flow and one process by which *increases* in signal can be induced by flow. Keep in mind that *in the absence of flow*, the signal of blood is not much different from other soft tissues. MRA does not show us the distribution of blood per se but the effects of motion on its signal. As we will see, each effect is characteristic of a unique way in which motion interacts with an aspect of the MR signal or pulse sequence.

High-Velocity Signal Loss

Let's examine an imaging experiment using the flow phantom we employed in the previous sections. As shown in Figure 16-3, we will place the phantom so the direction of flow is parallel to B_0. We will then use a simple spin echo pulse sequence to acquire a single slice perpendicular to the direction of flow. Assuming we are modeling arterial flow, the time required for the

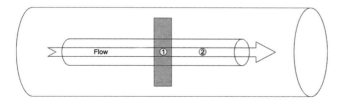

FIGURE 16-3. High-velocity signal loss. Spins are excited by the 90° RF pulse while they reside within the slice (*1*). By the time the 180° pulse is delivered, however, they have moved on (*2*) and do not experience the effects of the slice-selective 180° RF pulse.

volume of blood within the slice to completely traverse the slice is significantly less than the time TE/2 that elapses between the 90° and 180° RF pulses. At the time we generate the MR signal using a slice-selective 90° RF pulse, all spins within the slice including those within the phantom will be excited. During the time TE/2 that elapses, all the excited spins within the phantom will flow downstream and out of the slice. As a result, when we apply the slice-selective 180° refocusing RF pulse at TE/2, the stationary spins will be refocused, but flowing spins that were excited by the 90° RF pulse will not. Refocusing, of course, leads to an increase in signal as T2' effects are recovered (see Chapter 3). The end result is that stationary spins have higher signal than flowing spins (Fig. 16-4). Remember, this phenomenon only affects flow (or the component of flow) that traverses the slice before TE, typically seen in vessels oriented relatively orthogonal to the plane of section.

If the rate of flow is slow enough or the time TE/2 is short enough (as in a very short TE) that spins remain within the slice during application of both the 90° and 180° RF pulses, signal loss will not occur. This is why we call it high-velocity signal loss; the combination of high-velocity flow and a spin echo pulse sequence leads to lower signal from flowing spins. Note that it is in fact not loss of signal from the flowing spins but the fact that their signal *is not augmented by the 180° refocusing RF pulse* as the signal arising from stationary spins is.

What happens if we repeat our experiment using a gradient echo pulse sequence? Both stationary and flowing spins that reside in the slice when the 90° RF pulse is applied are excited. However, because the gradient echo

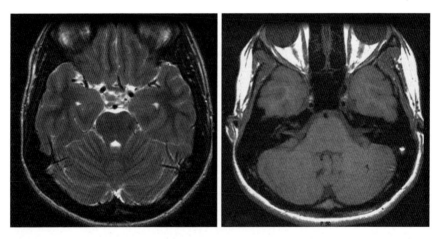

FIGURE 16-4. High-velocity signal loss. Vessels traveling orthogonal to the plane of section (e.g., the basilar artery) show significant signal loss that increases with TE as in the T2-weighted TSE image at left compared with the T1-weighted TSE image at right.

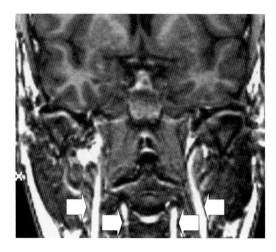

FIGURE 16-5. Lack of flow-related signal loss in gradient echo images. High signal in the internal carotid and vertebral arteries (arrows) is present due to the absence of the 180° RF pulse. No high-velocity signal loss occurs.

pulse sequence does not (by definition; see Chapter 8) contain a 180° refocusing RF pulse, stationary and flowing spins all relax with the time constant T2*. Thus, when we measure the signal at TE, both stationary and flowing spins will induce similar signal in the receiver coil (Fig. 16-5).

You may be wondering at this point: "If the flowing spins no longer reside in the slice, how do we receive their signal and place it correctly in the image?" Remember that the receiver coil detects all signal that is within range of the coil. The only way we localize signal to the slice is by exciting only spins within the slice. The flowing spins in our example are spatially localized to the slice and are flowing exactly perpendicular to the slice. While they move out of the slice (along z), the xy location of the spins does not change between the 90° RF pulse and TE. It is true that the x and y gradient magnetic fields used subsequently to complete spatial localization will be applied after the flowing spins have left the slice. Remember, however, that the gradient magnetic fields are not slice selective and the x and y gradients do not vary along z. Thus, we will accurately place signal arising from flowing spins within the slice at the exact location the spins occupied at the time of the 90° RF pulse.

Dephasing Due to Movement Along a Gradient Magnetic Field

We learned in Chapters 5 and 6 that, in the presence of a gradient magnetic field, adjacent spins will experience different magnetic field strength, precess

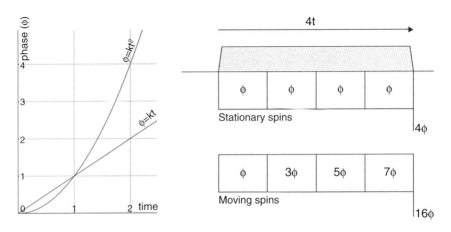

FIGURE 16-6. Gradient-induced dephasing. Spins in motion gain phase (φ) in proportion to the square of time (t) rather than the linear increase exhibited by stationary
spins. The block diagram on the right shows the amount of phase gained during each
unit of time. On the far right, we see the total phase gained over 4 units of time: 4
times greater for the spins in motion compared with the stationary spins.

at different frequencies, and undergo dephasing resulting in signal loss. How
do things change if spins are in motion? It turns out that as spins move
along a gradient magnetic field, they gain phase more rapidly than when
they are constantly exposed to the same field strength. When spins are
exposed to a constant gradient magnetic field strength, dephasing and signal
loss change in a linear fashion as a function of the time they are exposed
to the gradient magnetic field. When spins are in motion along a gradient
magnetic field at a constant velocity, however, phase and signal change in
a quadratic fashion as function of the time they are exposed to the gradient
magnetic field (Fig. 16-6). Thus, as spins move (flow) along a dimension
across which a gradient magnetic field has been applied, the moving spins
gain phase more rapidly than stationary spins. The consequence of this
greater/more rapid accumulation of phase is greater signal loss affecting the
moving spins (Fig. 16-6).

We will see later in this chapter and in Chapter 17 that the concept of
signal loss due to movement along a gradient magnetic field can be exploited
to generate MRA images (phase-contrast MRA), can be corrected by
applying compensatory gradient magnetic fields (gradient-moment nulling),
and is also the basis for diffusion MRI.

Phase Misregistration

When we consider blood vessels oriented so that flow occurs within the
slice, only rarely will flow be exactly parallel to the phase or frequency-

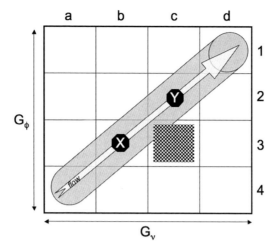

FIGURE 16-7. Phase misregistration. Spins (X) are in row 3 when the phase-encoding gradient is applied. Although they are in column b at this time, they are not encoded along the frequency dimension until they enter column c (Y). Thus, the signal is encoded to a location (cross-hatched region) *adjacent* to the true location of the vessel.

encoding directions. The inevitable occurrence of flow along oblique trajectories within the plane of the slice leads to a unique effect on our image. The basis of the phenomenon of phase misregistration lies in the fact that the two components of in-plane spatial encoding occur at distinct points in time, typically separated in time by at least a few milliseconds and often more. As diagrammed in Figure 16-7, spins are first encoded on the phase dimension. Because the spins have moved through the slice before we sample the signal and encode location on the frequency dimension, we have encoded the "location" of the spins to a point adjacent to the true position of the blood vessel. This misregistered signal sums with signal arising from the stationary tissue at this location adjacent to the vessel. The result is bright signal adjacent to the true location of the vessel. Because no signal is misregistered to the location of the vessel, voxels within the vessel contain no signal and appear very dark. Thus, we see two parallel lines: one dark and one bright (Fig. 16-8). If we know which direction has been used for phase and frequency encoding, the appearance of the phase misregistration artifact actually tells us the direction of flow!

Odd Echo Dephasing and Even Echo Rephasing

In the early years of clinical MRI, William G. Bradley reported an interesting phenomenon demonstrated by dual-echo spin echo imaging. He noticed that when two echoes are acquired in sequence *and TE$_2$ is twice as long as*

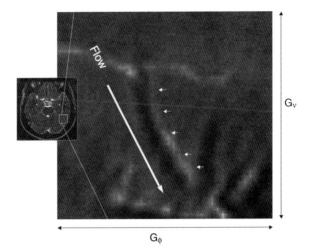

FIGURE 16-8. Phase misregistration. The small white arrows indicate a bright line representing the misregistered signal adjacent to a black line that reflects the true location of the vessel. Based on the location of the misregistered signal and the phase (G_ϕ) and frequency (G_v) encoding direction, we can determine the direction of flow within this cerebellar vein.

TE_1, signal within blood vessels was low on the first echo and high on the second echo. To understand the phenomenon, we need to look at the way phase changes with time. Looking at Figure 16-9, notice that stationary spins gain one unit of phase for each unit of time the gradient magnetic field is on. Thus, for two units of time, two units of phase are gained. Flowing spins, on the other hand, gain phase with the square of time. Thus, over two units of time, moving spins gain four units of phase.

Let's consider the effects of flow only along the frequency-encoding direction. Exposure to the gradient magnetic fields leads to signal loss such that, at TE, flowing spins acquire a net phase shift of –2. This is *odd echo dephasing* and will result in lower signal within the area of flow. If we add a 180° RF pulse, the phase shift becomes 2. After experiencing the effects of the additional frequency encoding gradient application and 180° pulse required to generate the second spin echo of our dual-echo pulse sequence, the flowing spins have completely recovered all phase shifts leading to higher signal. This is *even echo rephasing* and will result in higher signal within the area of flow. Notice that the net phase shift of stationary spins is zero for both TE_1 and TE_2.

Gradient-Moment Nulling (AKA Flow Compensation)

As we have seen (Fig. 16-9), as long as the stationary spins are exposed to an equal number of positive and negative gradient lobes, they will experi-

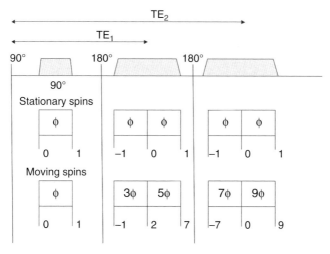

FIGURE 16-9. Even echo rephasing. The symbol ϕ indicates one unit of accumulated phase. In this spin echo pulse sequence, each time a 180° RF pulse is applied, phase of the spins is inverted. For example, if a phase shift of 1 is accumulated, the 180° RF pulse transforms the phase of the spins to −1. Accumulation of phase for stationary and moving spins is otherwise exactly as in Figure 16-6. Numbers within the blocks represent the phase accumulated for each increment of time. Numbers below the blocks indicate the total accumulated phase before or after each block. On the first (odd) echo, moving spins have a nonzero accumulated phase indicating that they are out of phase. This is odd echo dephasing. On the second (even) echo, the net phase for the moving spins is zero. This is even echo rephasing. The same pattern would continue for subsequent odd and even echoes as long as the time between echoes remains the same.

ence a net zero phase shift. The minimum number of gradient lobes required to arrive at a net zero effect is two: one negative and one positive. We can, of course, apply more than two lobes and still end up with a no net effect as long as the total of the negative and positive gradients applied sums to zero. Moving spins, however, will not necessarily end up with net zero phase shift because they gain incrementally more phase with each successive gradient lobe than stationary spins. However, there is a means by which we can deliver a net zero effect on the phase of *both* stationary and moving spins.

In order to compensate the gradient-induced phase shift experienced by stationary spins, we simply have to apply additional gradient lobes in a specific sequence (Fig. 16-10). Remember that moving spins will undergo an increasingly larger phase shift during each successive increment of time. Thus, to correctly compensate the gradient-induced phase shift due to flow, we apply a larger amount of gradient amplitude and induce a larger amount of dephasing *before* the final frequency-encoding gradient is applied. The

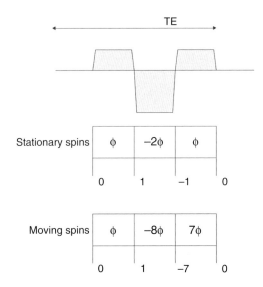

FIGURE 16-10. Gradient-moment nulling (AKA flow compensation). The symbol ϕ indicates one unit of accumulated phase. The pattern of gradient lobes is designed to induce a net zero phase shift on both stationary and moving spins. To this end, the middle (negative) lobe induces "extra" dephasing that is then recovered by the final (positive) lobe.

final gradient application will then correct this large preexisting phase shift. Ultimately, the phase shift for both flowing and stationary spins is zero at TE.

Dephasing Due to Turbulence

Now relax . . . This concept is probably the easiest to understand. Turbulence occurs when straight-line flow hits an obstruction. Whether the obstruction is due to a curve in the vessel, a bifurcation, or a stenosis, the result is the same: disorganization of flow. If the flowing spins have been excited and have signal, the net M_t will decline when the individual magnetization vectors of the flowing spins are sent into disarray because of turbulence. What we have is dephasing due to mechanical disruption of the spins' orientation.

Time-of-Flight Effect

How then can flow manifest as increase in signal intensity? Let's look back at the phantom experiment we used to demonstrate high-velocity signal loss (Fig. 16-3). We saw that because flowing spins "see" only the 90° but not the 180° RF pulse, they generate less signal than stationary spins that are refocused by the 180° RF pulse. Remember that, in a real pulse sequence, we must execute multiple repetitions of the pulse sequence in order to fill all the lines of k-space and generate an image. An unavoidable consequence of the repetitive RF pulses is saturation; spins that are subject to the long series of RF pulses are forced into a steady state where they recover less M_z and thus generate less M_t (signal) than they would after a single RF pulse. Notice that because flowing spins constantly transit the slice during these multiple repetitions of the RF pulses, "new" flowing spins will be found in the slice immediately prior to each subsequent RF pulse. These "new" spins have never "seen" an RF pulse and arrive with their full M_0; they are not saturated. Thus, flowing spins will have higher signal than stationary spins. In fact, even in a spin echo pulse sequence where the flowing spins do not "see" the 180° RF pulse and are not refocused, they will still have higher signal than the stationary spins. This is because the increment in M_z relative to the saturated stationary spins results in more M_t than that recovered by the stationary spins during the 180° RF pulse. This is the *time-of-flight (TOF) effect*, and, yes, it is the basis for time-of-flight MRA (TOF-MRA).

Entry Slice Phenomenon

If we look at a real-life example in which we acquire multiple slices using multislice imaging, it happens that the flowing spins will in fact "see" multiple RF pulses and become partially saturated. This occurs because spins that "see" the 90° RF pulse selective for slice 1 might be, for example, in slice 3 when its 90° RF pulse is applied. Thus, as spins flow farther into the volume, their signal will decline. You can probably see that time-of-flight effects will be most apparent in the initial slices of the volume. This is why the time-of-flight effect is also known as the *entry slice phenomenon* (Fig. 16-11). The most fitting term perhaps is *flow-related-enhancement of signal*.

The phenomenon of laminar flow is nicely demonstrated using the time-of-flight effect, as the degree to which flowing spins will be saturated depends on the velocity of flow. Faster-flowing spins will traverse more slices during the interval between successive RF pulses and thus reach farther into the volume before becoming saturated. The opposite of course is true of slower-flowing spins. Very slow flowing spins in fact will become saturated just like stationary ones. Because the highest velocities of flow are found in the center of the vessel, we will see a progressive narrowing of the area of flow-related enhancement within the center of the vessel (Fig. 16-11). Because high signal can also be characteristic of methemoglobin seen in thrombus (see Chapter 18), it is important to recognize the flow-dependent phenomenon and not misdiagnose normal flow-related enhancement as, for example, a thrombus floating in the basilar artery.

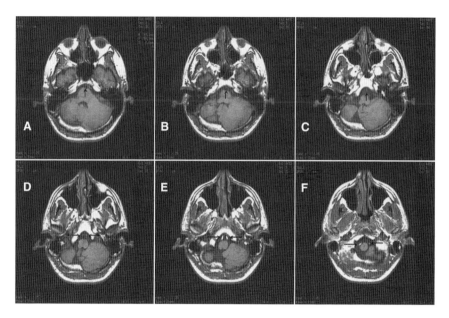

FIGURE 16-11. Time-of-flight effects. High signal is present in the vertebral and basilar arteries toward the bottom of the imaged volume (E, F). The intensity of the intravascular signal declines as we move into the volume (C, D) until it is completely saturated and the vessel displays high-velocity signal loss (A, B). Notice that the diameter of the flow-related enhancement appears to get smaller as saturation progresses, a manifestation of laminar flow.

Time-of-Flight MRA

MRA images are simply MRI images designed to maximize contrast between flow and stationary tissue. This contrast is maximized even at the expense of other tissue contrast. As a result, whereas MRA images are excellent for detection of motion, they otherwise have very poor tissue contrast. The name of the game in MRA is to maximize the difference in signal intensity between flowing spins and stationary spins. To do so, we will use multiple approaches to (1) maximize signal from flow and (2) suppress signal from stationary tissue. The parameters that are adjusted to achieve enhancement of flow-related signal and suppression of stationary tissue signal are summarized in Table 16-1.

Maximizing Signal from Flow

Our approach to maximizing flow-related signal focuses on two concepts: (1) minimize the effects of the three mechanisms of flow-related signal loss discussed at the beginning of this chapter and (2) maximize the MR signal

TABLE 16-1. Maximizing flow-related contrast by parameter optimization.

Parameter	Effect on flow signal?	Effect on background signal?
Gradient echo	Increase	No effect
No multislice	Increase	No effect
Short TE	Increase	Increase
Short TR	No effect	Decrease
Large α	Increase	Decrease
GMN	Increase	No effect
Field strength	Increase	Increase
Gadolinium	May increase	May increase
MTC	No effect	Decrease
Fat suppression	No effect	Decrease
Subtraction	No effect	Decrease

in general. To minimize high-velocity signal loss, we employ a gradient echo pulse sequence. In the absence of a 180° refocusing pulse, this phenomenon does not occur. Gradient-moment nulling (AKA flow compensation) is used to minimize signal loss due to in-plane flow along the gradient magnetic fields. Decreasing voxel size can minimize signal loss due to turbulence. The smaller the number of spins generating signal, the less likely their orientation will become completely random. Bear in mind, however, that decreasing voxel size also reduces the overall signal-to-noise of the image. MRA pulse sequences avoid multislice imaging. This is because if we excite adjacent slices one after the next, signal due to flow will tend to be exposed to multiple successive RF pulses leading to saturation of flow-related signal.

If we maximize the MR signal in general, it follows that we will be maximizing signal due to flow. For this reason, using a very short TE and large (90°) flip angle are advantages. The flip angle ensures we turn all M_z into signal, and the TE ensures that we sample the signal before it has decayed. One of the clearest advantages of higher field strength MR scanners is the increase in flow-related signal. Using gadolinium can provide enhancement of flow-related signal provided the gadolinium is exclusively intravascular. For this reason, only very rapid MRA acquisitions (discussed later in this chapter) benefit from the addition of gadolinium contrast agents.

Suppressing Background Signal

Techniques to minimize signal arising from stationary background tissue include approaches that maximize saturation and tissue suppression techniques. We ideally wish to drive the stationary spins to a steady state where almost no M_z is recovered prior to each successive RF pulse. Remember, because new flowing spins enter the slice before each RF pulse, signal from flow will not become saturated, assuming we image one slice at a time (see earlier discussion). Use of a very short TR (of the order several milliseconds) and a 90° flip angle will achieve maximum saturation of stationary tissue signal. Depending on the body region being imaged, tissue suppression techniques may be useful as well. In abdominal MRA, for example, fat suppression might be used to eliminate signal from the visceral and retroperitoneal fat surrounding the aorta and its major abdominal branches. Intracranial MRA benefits from background suppression achieved using magnetization transfer contrast (MTC). In the past, one more way to suppress background signal was to choose a TE at which fat and water will be out of phase (see Chapter 12). As a result, signal within voxels containing both fat and water will be suppressed. I say "in the past" because it is probably more beneficial to maximize overall signal by using the shortest TE possible.

What Type of Contrast Do MRA Images Have Anyway?

When you look at an MRA image (Fig. 16-12; one of the axial source images, not the maximum intensity projection [MIP] reconstructions), it will have notably low signal-to-noise, with the exception of flow, and tissue contrast will be hard to discern. If you had to identify the relaxation parameters most important for image contrast, however, what would you say? T1? T2? T2*? Looking at the parameters of the MRA pulse sequence, we see a gradient echo acquisition with a short TE. This should minimize contrast

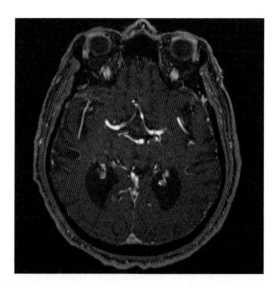

FIGURE 16-12. Axial MRA "source image." Intense flow-related enhancement is present with poor tissue (e.g., gray matter vs. white matter) contrast. Note that tissues with very short T1 such as fat also have relatively high signal.

due to T2 or T2*. The TR of our MRA acquisition is very short, which, as we discussed in Chapter 8, should not impact contrast too much in a gradient echo acquisition. The 90° flip angle, however, brings out contrast due to T1 differences in the tissue (also discussed in Chapter 8). It turns out, then, that MRA images are "T1-weighted." If that is so, it must be that the T1 of flowing blood is much shorter than that of stationary tissue. The only problem with this inference is that it is absolutely *not* true. Blood, flowing or not, has a T1 very similar to soft tissue.

How then do we explain the high signal seen due to flow on these "T1-weighted" images? If we think back to the T1 relaxation curves of Chapter 3 (or look at Fig. 3-1), we will notice that tissues with short T1 are those that recover M_z more rapidly and, as a result, generate a large amount of M_t. What if, perhaps magically, some spins just always happen to have a large M_z, not because they recover more quickly? As we come to the end of each TR and apply the next RF pulse, this very large M_z will be transformed into a very large amount of M_t, which, of course, is detected as a very large amount of signal. When we measure the very large amount of signal at TE, we cannot tell whether it is so large because those spins recovered signal very rapidly (i.e., have a very short T1) or because, *magically*, they always have a very large M_z. If the case is that the spins recovered M_z rapidly, we can say that those spins generating high signal do so because they have a very short T1. In the case of our magical spins, however, T1 may be exactly the same as that of the stationary spins. Nonetheless, it *looks like* those spins have a very short T1. Thus, what matters is not the actual T1 of the spins, but their *apparent T1* (AKA $T1_{app}$). Now let's deal with those magical spins. The magic, of course, is the time-of-flight effect. Because flowing spins enter the slice having never experienced any prior RF pulses, they always have a large amount of M_z; it is the infinitely short $T1_{app}$ of those spins that makes them generate so much signal. Keep this concept in mind because it will be relevant in our future discussions of contrast-enhanced MRA.

Arteries or Veins

Anyone who has looked at a TOF-MRA, say of the carotid arteries, knows that we see only the arteries even though there is certainly plenty of flow through the veins. Similarly, when we examine MR venography (MRV) images, say of the intracranial veins and dural sinuses, we see only veins. How is it that our MRA is selective for arterial or venous flow? Thinking about the time-of-flight effect, after all, it really should make no difference which direction the spins enter the slice from. In fact, TOF-MRA as we have described it to this point will equally show flow from arteries and veins.

In order to make an artery-only or vein-only image, we employ spatial presaturation pulses (Fig. 16-13). To image the carotid arteries, an RF

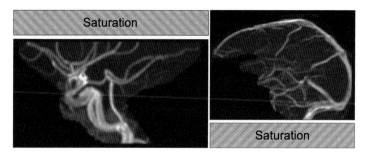

FIGURE 16-13. Use of saturation to selectively sample flow direction. Placing a spatial presaturation pulse (shading) suppresses flow entering the imaged volume from the side on which the presaturation pulse is placed.

saturation pulse selective for the region cranial to the slice of interest is applied immediately before the MRA pulse sequence begins. As a result, spins flowing in the head-to-foot direction are saturated and, when they flow into the MRA slice, have no M_z to be turned into signal. One caveat: if this saturation pulse is applied far from the level of the MRA slice (say, over the head in an MRA of the cervical segments of the carotid arteries), the flowing spins exposed to the presaturation pulse will recover some M_z as they flow from the region of the presaturation to the location of the slice. For this reason, we employ a "walking" saturation band; the presaturation is not applied in the same location for every slice but is moved to just above the slice that will be sampled next. This process is repeated for each and every slice in the stack of 2D images that will make up our MRA study.

Two-dimensional or Three-dimensional

What Do We Mean by 2D TOF-MRA?

Everything we have discussed so far describes what we call 2D TOF-MRA. "2D," of course, indicates the fact that we acquire a series of 2D slices. In practice, we actually acquire overlapping slices; 2-mm-thick slices might be spaced at only 1-mm increments, giving us 50% overlap of the slices. This overlapping scheme provides for cleaner 3D reconstructions. Nonetheless, because each slice is acquired *independently* (remember, MRA acquisitions do *not* employ multislice imaging, so that we do not saturate signal from flowing spins), if the patient moves, there will be obvious misregistration between the slices (Fig. 16-14).

There Is Another Way: 3D TOF-MRA

An alternative approach to 2D MRA is the use of a 3D Fourier transform approach. Remember (see Chapter 14) that this means we excite the entire

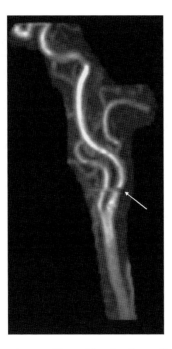

FIGURE 16-14. Misregistration artifact: The horizontally oriented discontinuity (arrow) in the internal and external carotid arteries on this MIP image is due to patient motion between acquisition of two adjacent axial "source images." Note that the remainder of the reconstruction is unaffected.

volume of tissue, not just one slice, at once. The 3D data are then separated into slices using a third iteration of the Fourier transform, hence 3DFT. This is beneficial for two principle reasons. First, as we saw in Chapter 14, 3DFT images have higher signal-to-noise than 2DFT images. Second, with the 3DFT approach, we can achieve much higher spatial resolution in the slice direction; instead of slices of several millimeters thick in 2D MRA, 3D MRA is routinely performed with slice (AKA partition) thickness of 1 mm or less. Improved signal-to-noise supports our ability to image at very high spatial resolution, which confers the following specific benefits in MRA:

- **Dealing with tiny vessels:** The smaller the blood vessel is relative to the voxel size, the less signal due to flow will be apparent as it is averaged with signal from stationary (saturated) spins residing in the voxel.
- **Dealing with in-plane flow:** The model case of MRA we have been discussing, where flow is perpendicular to the plane of the slice, is obviously contrived and not consonant with reality. In real life, blood vessels are also oriented so that flow runs parallel to the plane of the slice. Due to in-plane flow, flowing spins will experience many RF pulses before they

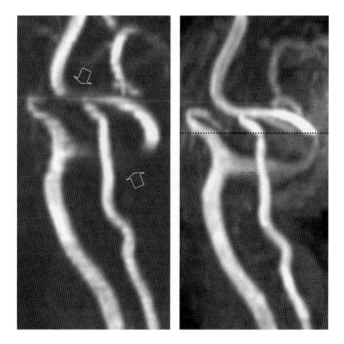

FIGURE 16-15. Saturation of in-plane flow. In the 2D TOF MIP image of the cervical carotid bifurcation (left), flow within the plane of the "source images" results in saturation of flow-related enhancement (open arrows). Because of higher spatial resolution (smaller voxels/thinner partitions) and optimized RF excitation (TONE pulse), flow-related enhancement is much more uniform, saturation is minimized, and the appearance of "stenosis" resolved in the 3D acquisition (right).

exit the slice. As a result, signal from flow becomes saturated. If we make the slice (partition) thinner, the course of in-plane flow will be shorter and saturation will be less of a problem (Fig. 16-15).

- **Dealing with turbulence:** As we discussed at the beginning of this chapter, turbulence leads to signal loss because the random orientation of many spins that results from turbulence sums to a lower amount of M_t than in the absence of turbulence. It follows that if we can reduce the number of spins per voxel, we will have a lesser range of orientations and see less loss of signal. This effect is extremely important in MRA examinations of the cervical segment of the carotid arteries where turbulence in the region of a stenosis may lead to substantial signal loss and the appearance of complete occlusion (Fig. 16-16).

Limitations of 3D MRA and Their Solutions

Despite the advantages of the 3D MRA technique, there is an important limitation of 3D MRA. Remember that in 2D MRA we image one slice at

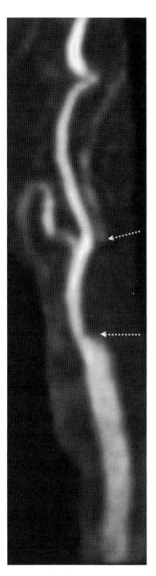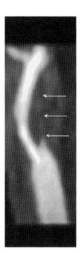

FIGURE 16-16. 2D TOF versus 3D TOF. The 2D TOF image (left) provides much more extensive coverage without saturation of flow-related enhancement. However, the area of high-grade stenosis is seen as absent flow-related enhancement (dotted arrows) indistinguishable from occlusion. This is due to signal loss resulting from turbulence at and beyond the stenosis. 3D TOF (right) is less affected by turbulence and shows a thin extension of flow-related enhancement (solid arrows) indicating patency of the carotid lumen.

a time. If we would employ multislice imaging, signal from flow would become saturated as it experienced the successive RF pulses used to excite the individual slices. In 3DFT imaging, we excite a thick slab of tissue with each RF pulse. Because spins do not fully traverse the thick slab within one TR, they experience multiple RF pulses, and signal from flow becomes saturated. Two options exist to address this issue:

- **Slab thickness:** Quite simply, using a thinner slab minimizes the amount of saturation that will occur because, for a given velocity of flow, spins will transit a thinner slab faster and thus see fewer RF pulses and suffer less saturation.
- **RF pulse optimization:** Because of saturation, the M_z of flowing spins will be progressively smaller as the spins move deeper into the slab. If we apply a relatively narrow flip angle to the portion of the slab the spins enter first, we will generate less M_t, but also less saturation. If we then apply a larger flip angle to the portion of the slab the spins exit from, we can actually generate a similar amount of M_t as we did at the entry portion of the slab. The end result is a relatively even amount of M_t generated at all points through the thickness of the slab and little evidence of saturation. This approach, which depends on no small feat of engineering, employs a TONE (tilted optimize nonsaturating excitation) RF pulse.

Which Way Do You Go? Two-dimensional Versus Three-dimensional

What then is the best method for MRA, 2D or 3D? Strictly speaking, 2D MRA is the most sensitive technique and provides the greatest anatomic coverage in the slice direction. We say most sensitive because small amounts of flow or slow flow will be detected without concern for the saturation effects inherent in 3D MRA that could render such small amounts of flow undetectable. We say "strictly speaking" because this statement, though printed without qualification in some texts, is really only true if the voxel size in the 2D and 3D acquisitions are the same. In reality, flow-related signal will be attenuated somewhat in 2D MRA due to the partial volume effect of the larger voxel size (larger due to the thicker slice dimension): flow-related signal is averaged with signal from stationary tissue. Because voxels are much smaller in 3D MRA, partial volume effects are much less of an issue. Signal loss due to saturation, however, is an important issue. In the end, the partial volume effect seen in 2D MRA and saturation effect seen in 3D MRA tend to balance out so that sensitivity is equivalent. As a result, if the only difference between 2D MRA and 3D MRA were sensitivity to flow, we could write the epitaph for 2D MRA.

There is another important difference between 2D MRA and 3D MRA: anatomic coverage in the slice direction. Because 2D MRA is performed one slice at a time, increasing the extent of coverage (number of slices) will not cause any additional saturation of flow-related signal. In 3D MRA, however, as we make our slab thicker, more saturation of flow-related signal will occur. Thus, for areas where extensive coverage is essential, 2D MRA may be the better option. Our practice for some time was to perform both 2D MRA and 3D MRA of the carotids (Fig. 16-16). The 2D images were useful because we could survey the entire neck and localize the carotid bifurcation. Next, a much smaller area centered on the carotid bifurcation was imaged using 3D MRA. This latter acquisition would delineate the carotid bulb and any stenosis much better than the 2D technique because of decreased susceptibility to turbulence-induced signal loss and saturation of in-plane flow.

It Really Is Better if You Go Both Ways: Multiple Overlapping
Thin-Slab Acquisition

We described the combined use of 2D MRA and 3D MRA in the past tense for a good reason: We do not do it any more. The best way to solve the sensitivity versus coverage dilemma is with a hybrid approach called multiple overlapping thin slab acquisition (MOTSA). Although MOTSA is not edible, its ability to give us the best of both worlds is truly "delicious." The thin slabs are 3D MRA acquisitions made thin enough to avoid saturation. We then acquire a whole series of them, stacked one atop the other. To improve the quality of the 3D reconstructions, we position the slabs so that they overlap each other.

The number of slabs (also called stacks or chunks) depends on the coverage required. As an example, the cervical carotids might be imaged with five to seven slabs and the head with two to three. The balance between slab thickness and number of slabs really depends on the velocity of flow and field strength. In children, for example, fewer slabs can be used because flow is so fast. At high field strength, fewer slabs may be required; as so much signal is available, saturation is less problematic.

In the best case, when looking at 3D MIP images from a MOTSA acquisition, you cannot even tell that multiple acquisitions were used. More likely, a faint line will be evident at the interface of adjacent slabs (dotted line in Fig. 16-15). This occurs because saturation of signal is maximal at the "far end" of each slab whereas it is minimal in the adjacent "near end" of the next slab. Thus, we tend to see an abrupt transition to higher flow–related signal when moving from one slab to the next. Some tapering of the vessels may also occur at the "far end" of individual slabs. If the patient moves between acquisition of neighboring slabs, misregistration, reminiscent of 2D TOF, can show up in the MIP images at the interface of adjacent slabs.

Something Different: Contrast-Enhanced MRA

Table 16-1 tells us that using gadolinium contrast *might* improve flow-related signal but also *might* increase signal from background tissue. What determines which *might* is right? It ultimately depends on where the

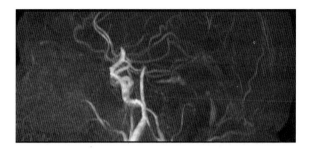

FIGURE 16-17. Effects of gadolinium contrast on TOF-MRA. In this patient, a large dose of contrast material was infused for an abdominal MRI examination performed *before* this MRA of the head. Notice the extensive background signal, reducing the contrast-to-noise of flow versus background.

gadolinium is. If it is *only* intravascular, the T1 of blood will be shortened, leading to increased flow-related signal. Perhaps this could compensate for saturation effects in 3D MRA? The problem is that the contrast agents currently available in the United States all leave the circulation and enter tissue to some degree after the first pass. The obvious problem, then, is that extravascular contrast will increase extravascular signal, worsening the contrast between flow and stationary tissue (Fig. 16-17). If we could, however, image rapidly enough that the entire MRA pulse sequence was executed during the first pass of a contrast bolus, administering contrast agents could, in fact, improve MRA quality (Fig. 16-18). We could do this and call the new technique contrast-enhanced MRA (CE-MRA). The catch is that it takes several minutes to acquire a 3D MRA while the first pass of the contrast agent occurs over a few seconds.

Notice that the concept of CE-MRA is of a true T1 contrast technique. In CE-MRA, we do not rely on inflow of unsaturated spins. Rather, we rely on dramatic shortening of intravascular T1 compared with extravascular tissue. This is unlike TOF-MRA where the very short $T1_{app}$ of flowing blood is due to the fact that flowing spins never experience saturation. In CE-MRA, we look at T1, not $T1_{app}$.

The key to CE-MRA, then, is imaging fast enough to "catch" the contrast bolus. There are several important factors to consider when setting up the CE-MRA acquisition:

- **Imaging speed:** At this point, it should be clear that speed is the name of the game when it comes to CE-MRA. The foundation of the CE-MRA acquisition, however, is really the same as in noncontrast MRA. We use a fast gradient echo pulse sequence with an extremely short TR (a few seconds at most). In order to image as fast as possible, we will not use gradient-moment nulling (flow compensation) because it adds

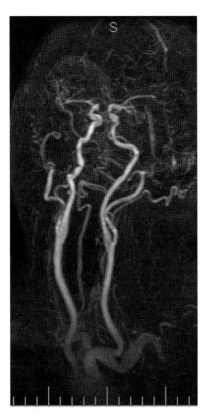

FIGURE 16-18. CE-MRA. This MIP reconstruction shows the extensive coverage and high contrast-to-noise achievable with dynamic CE-MRA. In this case, the cerebrovascular system is shown from the origin of vessels at the aortic arch through the circle of Willis.

additional imaging time, which is required to apply the extra gradient lobes.

- **Orientation:** As we learned in Chapter 8, the number of slices is one of the major determinants of imaging time. Though we do not want to limit coverage, we can orient the slab we are imaging so that the slice select dimension runs perpendicular to the longest dimension of the body region we are imaging. With this orientation, we will require the smallest number of slices and minimize imaging time.

- **Exploiting our knowledge of k-space:** Even if we use a superfast gradient echo pulse sequence and optimize our slice position, we still may not be able to complete imaging during the peak of the intravascular phase of the contrast injection. A newer approach to tackling this problem exploits the nature of k-space, discussed in Chapter 6. As we learned, it is the central lines of k-space that governs image contrast, whereas the periphery of k-space determines spatial information in the image. What matters most, then, is that we acquire the entire *central portion* of k-space during the peak of the contrast bolus. Because acquisition of those central lines of k-space requires less time, it suddenly becomes possible to complete imaging (or at least the portion of imaging that governs contrast) within the time that intravascular contrast is maximal.

If it seems to you that we are now acquiring our k-space data out of order, you are exactly right! It makes no difference what temporal sequence we acquire the data in as long as we enter the data in k-space in the correct order. That order, of course, is the order of phase-encoding gradient strength. There are two options for collecting the central k-space data in this manner. First, we can simply collect the central lines and immediately afterward collect the peripheral lines of k-space. Note that in this manner we collect the complete central lines of k-space (including the right and left edges that do not contribute to image contrast) during the time of the bolus peak. Alternatively, we can use what has been termed *centric data acquisition*. This process fills k-space in a somewhat spiral fashion; not only the top and bottom lines of k-space, but also the right and left edges are not filled at the beginning of the acquisition. Centric filling makes more efficient use of the precious seconds that the bolus is at its peak; only the essential central data points of k-space are filled.

- **Bolus timing:** Once we can image fast enough to capture the bolus peak, we must make sure that we in fact image during this peak. Three approaches are available to achieve proper timing. First, we can just use a fixed delay from the time of the injection until we begin imaging. We estimate, based on experience, how long a delay will be optimal for a certain portion of the vascular system. Second, a "timing run" (AKA "test bolus") can be used. In this approach, we set up a single-slice MRA pulse sequence so that we acquire a series of images, perhaps one image every second or every other second. A small dose of contrast material is injected and imaging begun *before* we expect the contrast to arrive. After the images have been acquired, we measure the intravascular signal and plot it against time. The resulting curve allows us to determine the moment at which the bolus will peak and to determine the optimal delay between injection and imaging. Finally, MR scanners often have the ability to perform bolus tracking and triggering. A pulse sequence is employed to acquire signal from a single voxel within the artery of interest. The scanner measures signal intensity in this voxel every second or so, and, when signal amplitude surpasses a threshold intensity, the MRA scan is triggered. The threshold is generally set as a relative change from the baseline precontrast signal intensity. In the event that the bolus-tracking algorithm fails to trigger the scan after a fixed delay has elapsed, the MRA scan proceeds anyway. This is done in order to avoid, in the event the bolus tracking algorithm fails, missing the opportunity to scan during the bolus altogether.

Don't Forget This Pitfall!

As the MRA techniques discussed above all detect flow based on its short T1 (or $T1_{app}$), we must be prepared to deal with the effects of anything that has a very short T1 for reasons other than flow. This *T1 shine-through* artifact is most commonly seen in the presence of fat or hemorrhage (methemoglobin), both of which have very short T1. In the case of hemorrhage, for example, even though signal may be within stationary tissue, the very short T1 conferred by methemoglobin prevents saturation from occurring (Fig. 16-19). One particular case in which confusion can occur is in the case of arterial dissection. Because dissection is essentially a mural hematoma, we may have difficulty distinguishing thrombus in the dissection from normal flow (Fig. 16-20).

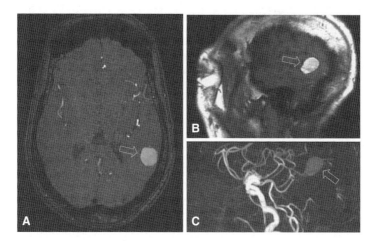

FIGURE 16-19. T1 shine-through artifact. The cortical hematoma (open arrows) in this patient has signal intensity indistinguishable from flow on the 3D TOF-MRA. Whereas it appears connected to the vasculature on the source image (A) and on the MIP MRA (C) images and might be mistaken for an aneurysm, review of other images (B) demonstrates that it is not.

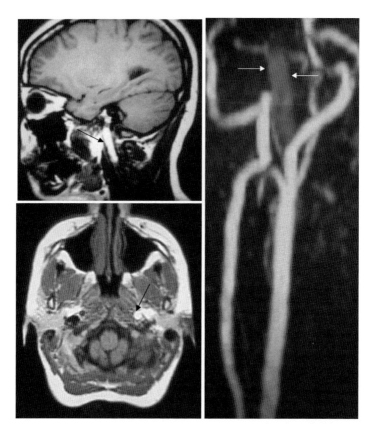

FIGURE 16-20. T1 shine-through artifact. In this case of carotid dissection, mural hematoma (white arrows) appears similar to flow on the MIP image (right). Its somewhat lower signal on the MIP image and inspection of structural images (black arrows, left) lead to the correct diagnosis of thrombus in the wall of the carotid.

Phase-Contrast MRA

The Concept

Phase-contrast MRA (PC-MRA) tends to be used much less in clinical practice compared with TOF-MRA and CE-MRA. Nonetheless, it has unique and important characteristics that make it worthwhile to understand. A simple, but not inaccurate, way to conceptualize PC-MRA is as a variation on gradient moment nulling (GMN). In GMN, we apply additional gradient lobes to compensate for phase changes due to flow along a gradient magnetic field. We apply these additional gradient lobes in a manner that imposes no net phase shift on stationary spins. In PC-MRA, we first acquire such a flow-compensated image (i.e., with GMN). Next, we acquire

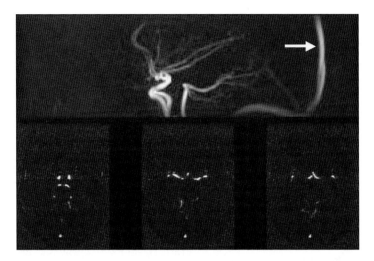

FIGURE 16-21. PC-MRA. The "source images" (bottom row) and MIP reconstruction (top) exhibit two hallmarks of PC-MRA: (1) excellent background suppression and (2) lack of directional selectivity. Notice flow in the venous sinuses (arrow).

an image where we compensate phase shifts of stationary spins in a manner that *does not* rephase flowing spins. Because stationary spins exhibit the same signal in both images, when we subtract the flow-compensated and non–flow-compensated images, the result shows *only* flow. Notice then that PC-MRA is truly a flow-sensitive technique. Only if spins are in motion will they have a different appearance on the two images. As a result, PC-MRA generally has better background suppression (Fig. 16-21) than TOF techniques and is not susceptible to T1 shine-through artifacts.

Direction Sensitivity in PC-MRA?

The answer is yes *and* no. PC-MRA is direction-selective in the sense that we can *only* detect flow parallel to the direction of the flow-encoding gradient. Because B_{net} does not change along the directions perpendicular to a gradient magnetic field, any component of flow perpendicular to the gradient will not result in a phase shift and will not be detected. For this reason, we must apply flow-encoding gradients along each of three orthogonal directions if we are to accurately depict three-dimensional flow.

On the other hand, PC-MRA is just like TOF-MRA where we saw that the technique is not intrinsically direction sensitive: whichever direction flow enters the slab from, flow-related signal will be detected. Flow-related signal in PC-MRA, of course, is not due to inflow effects. As long as flow is parallel to the flow-encoding gradient, phase shifts will occur. In the neck, for example, both arterial (foot-to-head) and venous (head-to-foot) flow will generate phase shifts, and the MRA image will show both arteries and veins. The saturation pulses used to suppress arterial or venous flow in order to make time-of-flight MR arteriograms or venograms will have *no* effect in PC-MRA where phase shifts occur within the imaging volume regardless of initial M_z (Fig. 16-21).

Velocity Encoding and Another Type of Aliasing

As we learned at the beginning of this chapter, the total accumulated phase due to flow is a function of velocity (speed *and* direction). How so? For a given strength of the flow-encoding gradient, increasing velocity will result in an increasing phase shift according to the quadratic formula we detailed earlier. The formula is $\theta = \kappa t^2$, but you do *not* need to memorize it. It is sufficient to recall that spins moving along the gradient magnetic field gain more phase than stationary spins. It follows that if we examine the phase of spins (by generating a phase image as in Chapter 5),

Speed Versus Velocity

Remember that the term *velocity* describes both direction and speed of motion. PC-MRA images are generally designed to show the presence of flow in any direction but not to distinguish the absolute direction of flow at any given location. For this reason, it is actually more accurate to say that PC-MRA images represent speed, not velocity. Of course, this is a fine semantic point, mentioned for those perfectionists who might otherwise take issue with the description in the text.

we should be able to deduce speed of flow from the phase shift imparted on the flowing spins by the flow-encoding gradient. In practice, this will only be accurate if the phase shift is exactly 180°. If flow is faster, a greater phase shift, perhaps 270^0, will result. As shown in Figure 16-22, however, higher-velocity flow will be indistinguishable from the phase shift produced by lower-velocity flow *in the opposite direction* that could yield a phase shift of –90°. This phenomenon is called *velocity aliasing* and is worth being aware of. The good news, however, is that unless we are trying to quantify flow velocity, aliasing does not matter too much. When all we are trying to do is make pictures of blood vessels, flow is flow. . . .

How do we maximize the contrast between flow and background in PC-MRA? Because the PC-MRA image is a subtraction of the flow-encoded image and the flow-compensated image, flow will be most obvious when the phase shift imparted on the flowing spins is the most different from the flow-compensated image. This occurs when flowing spins undergo a phase shift of 180°. As we discussed above, an 180° phase shift will only occur when the flow-encoding gradient amplitude is appropriately selected for the velocity of flow. At this gradient setting, our images are most

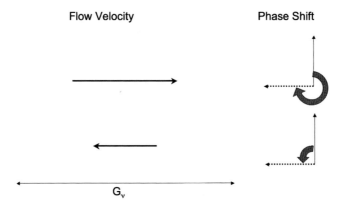

FIGURE 16-22. Velocity aliasing in PC-MRA. The velocity diagram at left shows flow at two different velocities, both parallel to the flow-encoding gradient magnetic field. The phase shift (right) is proportional to velocity, but the sign of the phase shift changes with flow direction. Ultimately, the phase shift in both cases yields indistinguishable phase of the signal.

sensitive to a specific flow velocity. The scanner operator must specify the VENC (velocity ENCoding), which is the velocity to which our images will be maximally sensitive. The value specified for VENC will determine if we generate images that show arterial, venous, or perhaps CSF flow (Fig. 16-23).

Making the PC-MRA Image

At this point, we have generated a flow-compensated image and a flow-encoded image, optimized to detect a specific flow velocity by choosing the appropriate VENC. Actually, we must acquire three separate flow-encoded images, one sensitized to flow along each of three orthogonal directions. Remember that if we would apply all three gradients at once, our images would only be sensitized to flow along one compound oblique direction. Hence, a major limitation of PC-MRA: it takes a long time.

To generate our PC-MRA image, we first combine velocity information from the three flow-sensitized images. Because we are combining all of the directional information to generate a single value for each pixel in the final PC-MRA image, the actual directional information is lost and we have signal amplitude that reflects speed (S). For those who must know, we do this by taking the square root of the sum of squares at each voxel:

$$S = \sqrt{(v_x)^2 + (v_y)^2 + (v_z)^2}$$

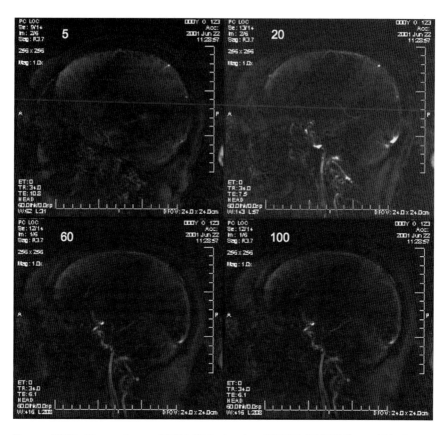

FIGURE 16-23. Dependence of PC-MRA signal on VENC. VENC (in cm/s) is shown in white numerals. At lower VENC, slower-velocity flow, such as due to CSF or venous flow, will achieve a 180° phase shift and show up as the greatest intensity. Higher VENC generates images depicting arterial flow and high-velocity venous flow.

Direction and Quantification of Flow Derived from PC-MRA Images

Actual directional information can be displayed by reconstructing each directionally sensitive image separately. These images are somewhat noisy, and flow direction is displayed as black or white corresponding with the direction of the phase shift (Fig. 16-24). Do not forget, however, that the direction can be misleading if our VENC was not chosen appropriately and aliasing is present (Fig. 16-22).

Velocity of flow can be quantified from the PC-MRA data. To do so, phase images must be reconstructed from each directionally sensitized

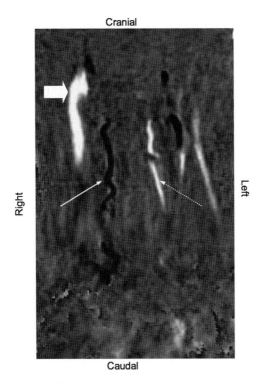

Cranial

Right

Left

Caudal

FIGURE 16-24. Directional PC-MRA. In this coronal image (a single "source image" slice, not a MIP image), flow has been encoded based on the absolute direction of flow along the craniocaudal dimension. The large white arrow shows flow in the internal jugular vein telling us that white encodes flow in the head-to-toe direction. Black encodes flow in the toe-to-head direction as seen in the right vertebral artery (solid white arrow). White within the left vertebral artery (dotted white arrow) indicates abnormal toe-to-head flow in this patient due to subclavian steal syndrome.

image (see Chapter 5). The phase image provides a quantitative measure of phase at each pixel. The phase shift results from the combination of motion (flow) and gradient amplitude. Because we know both the phase shift and gradient parameters, we can solve for the quantitative velocity.

Note that direction and phase information are encoded within the basic PC-MRA image data. No additional acquisition and, therefore, no additional imaging time are required to derive this quantitative information. However, commercial scanners do not always provide direction and velocity images by default.

Where Do We Go from Here?

There are so many different MRA options that it can be overwhelming. What is the "right" or "best" choice for your patient? Although it is dangerous to make generalizations and each situation must be judged on its unique circumstances, we can suggest a few overall principles. First, in any case in which motion is an issue, high-speed CE-MRA has a clear advantage. This makes it the method of choice for almost all body MRA applications. Second, cases that demand resolution of very small vessels, such as spinal and extremity MRA, especially of the foot, benefit from CE-MRA. This is not because of motion suppression but because of improved contrast between vessels and other tissue. Third, there is a role for noncontrast TOF-MRA. Typical head and neck MRA is accomplished quite nicely using MOTSA. Single-slab 3D TOF and 2D TOF, however, probably no longer have much of a role to play. The role of CE-MRA in the head is unclear, with the exception of time-resolved studies. CE-MRA of the neck allows coverage to extend from the aortic arch through the circle of Willis but with a penalty in spatial resolution. As a result, studies of the neck will benefit from inclusion of noncontrast MOTSA, even when CE-MRA is performed. Finally, there is a limited role for PC-MRA. Studies requiring quantification of flow, including cardiac applications, require this technique. Fast, low-resolution PC-MRA acquisitions are useful to create "scout" images for planning the position of a subsequent 3D MRA volume. MR venography, particularly of the head, is best performed using PC-MRA. This is especially so because it avoids the T1 shine-through pitfall in cases of venous thrombosis that so commonly are the indication for these MRA studies. Although the array of choices can indeed be bewildering, keep in mind that it is our ability to apply knowledge of these techniques that allows us to tap their diagnostic power.

17
Diffusion: Detection of Microscopic Motion

Introduction

Mention *diffusion* to most MR users and they will most likely think of the techniques for diffusion-weighted MRI that came into routine clinical use during the 1990s after FDA approval for use of these methods in the diagnosis of stroke. Indeed, that is the largest application of diffusion in clinical MRI. We will see, however, that effects of diffusion are always present in all MRI images. "Diffusion imaging" results when we structure MR images to make them especially sensitive to the effects of diffusion.

What Is Diffusion?

Water molecules in the samples we image are not stationary; they are in constant motion. Absent any barriers to movement, the direction of motion will be completely random. This random molecular movement is an example of Brownian motion. Those who study diffusion describe the path of Brownian motion as a case of the mathematical *random walk*. The random walk, however, only results when water molecules can move in any direction without impediment; that is, if we are dealing with a freely diffusible solvent (one with no structure that might impede movement in any direction, say a bottle of distilled water), and our sample is at a temperature above absolute zero. This uninhibited pattern of diffusion will be present within "pure" body fluids like urine, bile, and cerebrospinal fluid (CSF).

Diffusion also occurs in tissue. However, cellular, subcellular, and extracellular structure (such as cell and organelle membranes) and large molecules (such as collagen) impede movement of water molecules through tissue to some degree. As a result, the "velocity" of diffusion is lower in tissue than, for example, in CSF. The velocity of diffusion is referred to simply as diffusion (D). Because of the effects of tissue structure as well as limitations on the accuracy at which we can measure D, we will speak of the apparent diffusion coefficient (ADC), which we can measure.

As we discussed in Chapter 16, velocity implies not just a rate (speed) but also direction. Similarly, diffusion through tissue can be described by its rate (ADC) and also by its direction. In a "pure" fluid like CSF, the direction of diffusion will be entirely random. In most other tissues, the nature of tissue structure does not tend to confer a preferred direction of diffusion. However, certain tissues, such as brain white matter, have a highly organized tissue structure that leads to predominance of a single direction of diffusion. This directionality will be addressed in more detail in the section of this chapter on diffusion tensor imaging (DTI).

Effect of Diffusion on the MR Signal

Recall that in Chapter 16 we described the effects of flow on the MR signal. When spins flow along a gradient magnetic field, accumulation of phase by moving spins exceeds that incurred by stationary spins. Accumulation of phase, of course, leads to a decline in net M_t and, therefore, signal. The amplitude of the gradient magnetic field and the velocity at which the spins are moving will determine the amount of signal loss incurred. Because diffusion is just movement of spins, we expect diffusion along a gradient magnetic field to result in signal loss as well. This signal loss is the signature of diffusion in an MRI image. Notice, by the way, that, because *all* MRI images require the application of gradient magnetic fields, all will demonstrate some degree of signal loss due to diffusion. Because the magnitude of the gradient magnetic fields used for imaging and the velocity at which spins move due to diffusion are both relatively low, only minimal signal loss due to diffusion will actually manifest in a typical MR image.

Making the MR Image Sensitive to Diffusion

Signal loss due to diffusion is proportional to the net amount of gradient strength applied to the diffusing spins. This net effect is a function of the strength of the gradient magnetic field and the time spins are subject to it. To maximize signal loss due to diffusion then, we should apply the strongest gradient magnetic field for a very long time. As we will shortly see, it is also important to accomplish imaging very quickly if we wish to observe the effects of diffusion and not have the small-scale motion due to diffusion overwhelmed by larger-scale physiologic or gross patient motion. Because the duration of the gradient magnetic field applications must be brief, gradient amplitude is the parameter that will govern the degree of signal loss due to diffusion.

To sensitize our image to diffusion, we apply additional gradient magnetic fields in a manner reminiscent of phase-contrast MRA (PC-MRA). Typically, a pair of gradient pulses is applied at high gradient amplitude

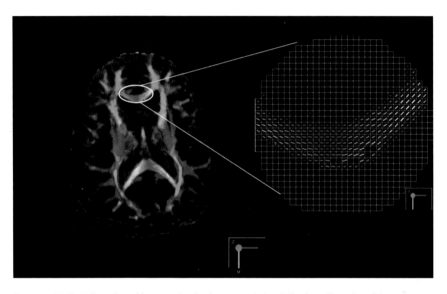

FIGURE 17-5. Directional image. In the image at left, diffusion direction (the orientation of the principle eigenvector) is color-coded to represent orientation along the three principle directions (cranial-to-caudal = blue; right-to-left = red; anterior-to-posterior = green). The enlarged view (right) shows the principle eigenvectors for each voxel in a region of interest in the genu of the corpus callosum. Notice that hue of each vector changes based on fiber orientation.

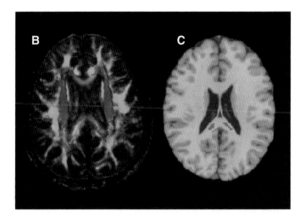

FIGURE 17-6. Fractional anisotropy. Visual inspection of grayscale (A) and color-encoded (B) FA images of a patient with traumatic brain injury do not demonstrate low FA. Yet, statistical analysis of this subject's FA images with reference to a group of age-matched control subjects' images identifies very significant (p = 0.0001) decrease in FA within the splenium of the corpus callosum in this patient (C).

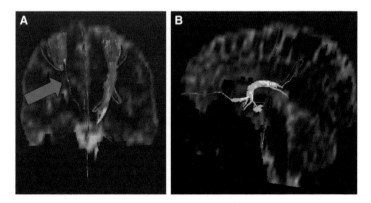

FIGURE 17-7. DTI fiber tracking. The corticospinal tracts (A) and fornix (B) have been delineated using DTI. Notice marked attenuation of the right corticospinal tract (magenta arrow) due to prior brain hemorrhage.

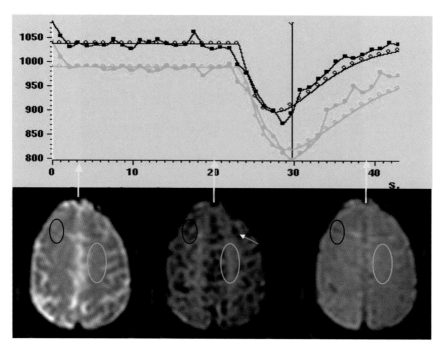

FIGURE 18-5. Time series for perfusion imaging. Signal loss occurs with wash-in of the contrast bolus and resolves with washout. Colored circles (bottom) indicate the regions of interest from which the time versus signal curves (top) were extracted.

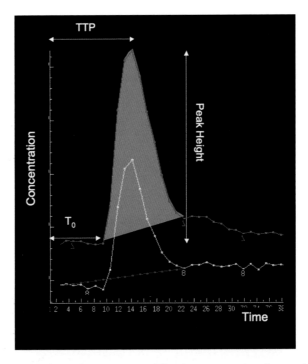

FIGURE 18-6. Hemodynamic parameters. The time versus signal curve is essentially the inverse of the time versus concentration curve (shown here after gamma variate fitting). Timing is easily measured as indicated by T_0 and TTP. Area under the curve (shaded in green) is proportional to CBV, and peak height has been used as a very rough estimate of relative CBF.

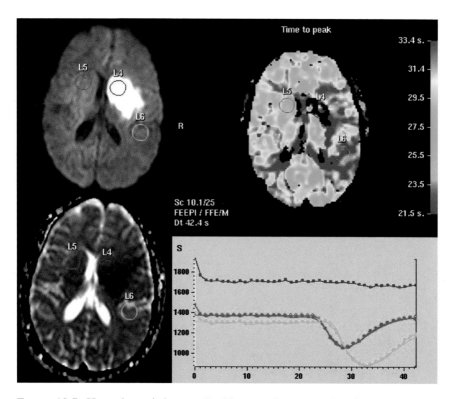

FIGURE 18-7. Hemodynamic images. In this case of acute stroke, diffusion imaging (DWI at upper left and ADC at lower left) confirm a region of infarction. The TTP map (upper right) shows delayed arrival of the contrast bolus in an area much larger than indicated by the DWI images. Time versus signal curves extracted from regions of interest in the core (dark blue) and periphery (turquoise) of the infarct as well as the unaffected contralateral cerebral hemisphere (magenta) confirm the presence of an ischemic penumbra surrounding the infarct core.

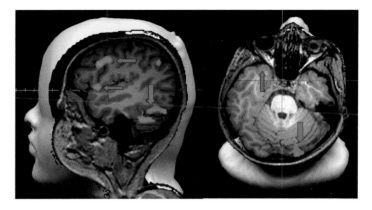

FIGURE 18-10. Three-dimensional display of fMRI results. Colored regions indicate areas where signal increased in sync with the onset of the stimulus. The subject viewed and was required to name pictures of common objects shown on a video screen. Responses are thus detected in visual (magenta arrows) and language (blue arrows) areas.

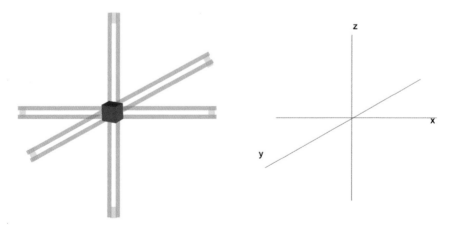

FIGURE 19-5. Spatial localization. Three orthogonal slices intersect so that the only spins that receive all three RF pulses are those within the voxel defined by the intersection of the slices.

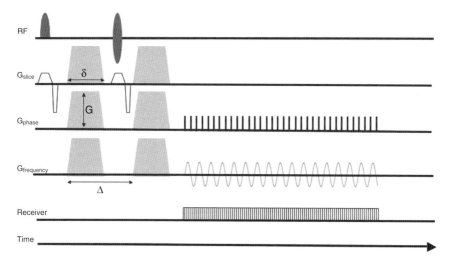

FIGURE 17-1. Diffusion-weighted MRI pulse sequence. This is a standard spin echo EPI pulse sequence (see Chapter 13) with the addition of gradient magnetic field pulses before and after the 180° RF pulse (gray trapezoids) to sensitize to diffusion. The b-value is determined from gradient amplitude (G), gradient duration (often referred to as mixing time) (δ), and the interval between gradients (Δ). (For an explanation of the striped and solid symbols, see Figure 8-1.)

straddling a 180° RF pulse (Fig. 17-1). Although diffusion sensitization can be applied to many different types of pulse sequences, ultrafast EPI acquisitions are most commonly employed. Spins in motion along the gradient magnetic field accumulate phase leading to signal loss.

The net amount of gradient strength applied is determined by the gradient amplitude (G) and the time the gradient is kept on (δ). The term *b-value* (in units of s/mm^2) is used to express the net gradient effect, and, therefore, amount of diffusion sensitization, concisely. Increasing the b-value will make the image more sensitive to small amounts of diffusion. Keep in mind, however, that increasing the b-value also leads to a decrease in the overall amount of signal in the diffusion-sensitive image and, as a result, its signal-to-noise ratio. Typically, a b-value of 700 to 1000 is used in clinical diffusion-weighted imaging.

Which gradient direction is used for diffusion sensitization? If we apply the diffusion-sensitizing gradient along the frequency-encoding dimension only, signal loss due to diffusion will only occur along this dimension; our image will only be sensitive to diffusion in one linear direction. The clinical question addressed by diffusion-weighted imaging, however, is whether the magnitude of diffusion is decreased (perhaps due to stroke) regardless of its direction. To generate an image that is sensitive to diffusion in all directions, we apply the diffusion-sensitizing gradients along all three orthogonal dimensions *simultaneously* (Fig. 17-1). It is true, as we discussed in Chapters

5 and 6, that simultaneous application of multiple gradient magnetic fields is equivalent to applying a single obliquely oriented gradient magnetic field described by the vector sum of the three component gradient magnetic fields. This does not mean, however, that our image is sensitive to diffusion only along this dimension. For this oblique gradient magnetic field to exist, gradient strength must change in all directions. The change in gradient strength is what matters. To be sensitive to diffusion in all directions, spins must experience a change in B_{net} no matter in which direction they move.

What Do Diffusion-Sensitized Images Look Like?

Using the method described above, any MR image can be sensitized to diffusion. In practice, however, we employ high-speed EPI pulse sequences for diffusion imaging. Because imaging is so fast that it essentially "freezes" gross patient motion and physiologic motion, we are left with motion due to diffusion as the only cause of signal loss in the diffusion-sensitive image. As we discussed in Chapter 13, because of the nature of single-shot imaging techniques like EPI, T1 contrast is generally not present. Thus, diffusion imaging generally employs a T2-weighted EPI image; inversion recovery EPI such as FLAIR can also be used. The diffusion-sensitizing gradient pulses induce signal loss in proportion to the rate of diffusion.

In CSF, for example, diffusion is very fast due to the complete lack of tissue structure. As a result, a very large degree of signal loss occurs in voxels containing CSF. Although CSF has very high signal on the T2-weighted EPI image, it demonstrates almost no signal on the diffusion-weighted version of the same image (Fig. 17-2). Brain tissue undergoes a

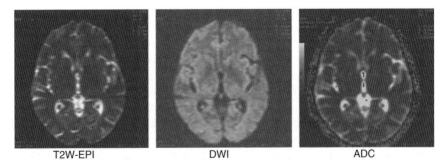

| T2W-EPI | DWI | ADC |

FIGURE 17-2. Diffusion images. When diffusion-sensitizing gradients are added to the T2-weighted EPI image (left), a diffusion-sensitized or diffusion-weighted image (DWI) (center) results. The magnitude of diffusion can be quantified and displayed as an ADC image, often called an ADC map (right).

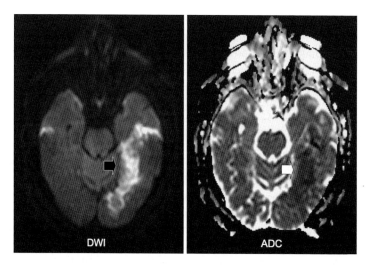

FIGURE 17-3. Acute stroke shown by diffusion imaging. High signal in the diffusion-weighted image (DWI) (black arrow) is due to diminished diffusion and manifests as low ADC in the quantitative ADC image (white arrow).

decline in signal as well, but not to the same degree as CSF, because tissue structure impedes the movement of water molecules and "slows down" the rate of diffusion.

In disease states that alter the magnitude of diffusion, signal on the diffusion-weighted image will be affected accordingly. Acute brain infarction leads to a dramatic decrease in diffusion and, as a result, relatively little attenuation of signal on the diffusion-sensitive image. For this reason, acute infarction manifests as very high signal on the diffusion-weighted image (Fig. 17-3). Conversely, vasogenic edema, such as that surrounding a brain tumor, represents an increase in extracellular water and an increase in the magnitude of diffusion. Thus, vasogenic edema leads to greater signal loss and lower signal on the diffusion-weighted image in comparison with normal white matter.

In certain cases, a large area of demyelination, for example, a lesion, may have very high signal on the T2-weighted image while its diffusion is not very different from that of normal tissue. Because the magnitude of diffusion is similar to normal brain, the signal intensity of the lesion will be attenuated by the diffusion-sensitizing gradients to a degree similar to normal brain. Nonetheless, the lesion will demonstrate very high signal on the diffusion-weighted image. Whereas it might *look* similar to infarction, the high signal does not represent a decline in diffusion; even with the reduction in signal due to diffusion, signal on the diffusion-weighted image is still high because the initial signal on the T2-weighted image is so high. This pitfall is called *T2 shine-through* because it is the very long T2 of the lesion that leads to its high signal. From this example, it should be clear that we cannot be sure that every high-signal lesion seen on a diffusion-weighted image will actually be due to a decline in diffusion. Making the distinction requires that we actually *measure* diffusion, not just look at its effects on signal intensity.

Quantitative Diffusion Imaging: The ADC

For a given b-value (net applied diffusion-sensitizing gradient), signal loss due to dephasing is a function of the rate at which spins move along the diffusion-sensitizing gradient magnetic field; greater diffusion results in more signal loss. If we plot signal intensity from an image without diffusion sensitization (referred to as a b = 0 image because the strength of the diffusion-sensitizing gradient is 0) and that from a diffusion-sensitized image, the slope of the resultant line will approximate the apparent diffusion coefficient (ADC). We thus have a quantitative measure of diffusion. Because this approach actually measures the degree of signal loss due to the diffusion-sensitizing gradient, it may solve the problem of T2 shine-through. Whereas a lesion with very high signal on the b = 0 image might show high signal on the diffusion-weighted image, measuring the ADC will show a value similar to normal tissue. In the case of infarction, the ADC will be very low (Fig. 17-3).

The ADC "Map"

In practice, a routine diffusion imaging study will consist of the acquisition of two sets of T2-weighted EPI images: one with addition of diffusion-sensitizing gradients (the diffusion-weighted image) and one without these additional gradients (the b = 0 image). Because the spatial dimensions of the two image sets are identical, we can calculate the ADC, as described above, for each and every voxel. These ADC data are commonly displayed as a third set of "images" where the pixel values are the actual ADC measurements from corresponding voxels in the diffusion imaging data. The ADC values can be displayed as a grayscale or color image and compared with the diffusion-weighted images (Fig. 17-2).

Regions containing abnormally decreased magnitude (sometimes called restricted) diffusion will have relatively low "signal" on the ADC image (sometimes referred to as an ADC "map"). Remember, however, that it is wrong to describe the pixel intensity on an ADC image as signal; the ADC image is a calculated image, and the pixel values are actual measurements of ADC. Rather than just memorize them, we can now actually understand the patterns of signal seen on diffusion-weighted and ADC images. Areas with large magni-

Quantitative images do not lie.

tude diffusion such as CSF exhibit a large degree of signal loss due to dephasing. Thus, low signal on the diffusion-weighted image corresponds with high "signal" on the ADC image. Conversely, an area with decreased diffusion will exhibit little signal loss. Because spins move less, they accumulate less phase and do not lose very much signal. As a result, these areas will exhibit high signal on the diffusion-weighted image. Low "signal" on the ADC image will reflect the low-magnitude diffusion (Fig. 17-2).

In summary then, the finding of high signal on a diffusion-weighted image has high sensitivity for detection of abnormally decreased diffusion. The images are not as specific, however. Very high signal on the $b = 0$ image can also lead to the same signal intensity. We use the quantitative ADC image to solve the problem of T2 shine-through. Quantitative images do not lie, and diffusion imaging should never be interpreted without them.

Accuracy in Measurement of the ADC

In describing measurement of the ADC using the $b = 0$ and one diffusion sensitive image, we said:

> If we plot signal intensity from an image without diffusion sensitization (referred to as a $b = 0$ image because the strength of the diffusion-sensitizing gradient is 0) and that from a diffusion-sensitive image, the slope of the resultant line will *approximate* the ADC.

The reason we used the modifier *approximate* is that two points do not suffice for accurate measurement of the ADC. If we acquire multiple diffusion-sensitive images, each using a different b-value, the resultant plot will be much more accurate. Our two-point method is only a very gross approximation of the actual ADC. This approach is, nonetheless, sufficiently accurate for clinical applications where detection of large changes in ADC is the goal. An important caveat emerges from this seemingly technical detail: ADC images are relatively insensitive to very small alterations in diffusion. A slight decrease in diffusion might lead to increased signal on the diffusion-weighted image but no alteration of "signal" on the ADC image. In this setting, again, the diffusion-weighted images are maximally sensitive, but not specific. In the setting of mildly restricted diffusion, the ADC image is increasingly likely to yield a false-negative result and is not reliable for exclusion of subtle acute ischemia.

Directional Information: DTI

Until now, we have discussed the measurement of the magnitude of diffusion. Because diffusion is a vector quantity, we can also discuss its direction. Measurements of directional information are on the cutting edge of MRI and include powerful ways to detect disease and display anatomy. We will discuss two types of directional information: (1) absolute direction of diffusion and (2) homogeneity of direction within a voxel.

Real Life: Anisotropy

Whereas the human body might be largely composed of water, tissue does not behave like a glass of water, at least not as far as water diffusion is concerned. As we discussed at the beginning of this chapter, diffusion approaches a *random walk* in pure fluids. Because such motion is equally likely to occur in any direction, its spatial pattern is termed *isotropic diffusion*. In tissue, structure restricts the directions along which water molecules can move. The resultant diffusion occurs along selected directions and is termed *anisotropic diffusion*. Certain tissues, most notably white matter, possess a highly ordered structure that facilitates diffusion along a single direction and restricts diffusion in all other directions. White matter thus has very high anisotropy. Keep in mind that anisotropy describes the degree to which diffusion occurs along a single direction but does *not* describe the absolute direction of diffusion.

Encoding the Direction of Diffusion

Sensitizing our image to diffusion along all three major directions simultaneously will not suffice to generate an image that can provide information about the direction of diffusion. We will require a series of images, each sensitized in a unique direction. The more images acquired, each sensitized along a unique direction, the better we will be able to accurately determine the absolute direction of diffusion. Each additional direction along which we sensitize, however, requires an additional set of images and requires additional imaging time.

The optimal number of diffusion-sensitizing directions is a subject of debate, with some investigators suggesting the more the better. What is clear is that a minimum of six noncollinear directions is required. High-resolution DTI is commonly performed with 25 to 30 directions, but it can be done with less. Most commonly, the number of directions is a limitation of the scanner system.

Describing Diffusion Direction: The Diffusion Tensor

Signal intensity under each diffusion-sensitizing direction at each voxel is used to compute a representation of diffusion orientation for each and every voxel in the data set (usually a series of contiguous slices covering the entire brain). The mathematical construct is called a tensor, but we will not delve into its computation. For our purposes, the tensor represents a three-dimensional ellipsoid (Fig. 17-4). I would just call it fat cigar, but that

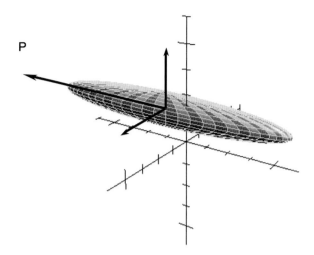

FIGURE 17-4. The diffusion tensor: This graphical representation of the diffusion ellipsoid (tensor) describes the magnitude and direction of diffusion at a single voxel. The principle eigenvector (P) indicates the main diffusion direction at this location.

might require that this book carry a parental advisory. The preferred direction of diffusion at a given voxel is the orientation of the long axis of the ellipsoid. This is referred to as the *principle eigenvector*. By determining the principle eigenvector for each voxel in our data set, we can describe the preferred direction of diffusion at each voxel, commonly displayed as a color-coded image (Fig. 17-5, see color plate).

The girth of the ellipsoid tells us how much diffusion is occurring in other directions, each represented by an additional vector. Most commonly (and most simply), we can describe the ellipsoid using three vectors, one along its length (the primary eigenvector described earlier) and two orthogonal to it and to each other. In an idealized case where diffusion is present *only* along one dimension, the ellipsoid will become a line. Conversely, if diffusion is entirely random, perhaps as in CSF, the ellipsoid will become a sphere. Thus, the girth-to-length ratio provides a means for describing the homogeneity of diffusion direction within a voxel, that is, its anisotropy.

Measuring Anisotropy

The degree of anisotropy at each voxel in our data set is described by the unitless parameter *fractional anisotropy* (FA). FA ranges from 0, where the tensor ellipsoid is a sphere, to 1, where the tensor ellipsoid is a line. It is common, however, for the FA values to be scaled by some factor—perhaps 10,000—in order to optimize the display of FA images. The FA image (Fig. 17-6A, B, see color plate for part B only) is, like the ADC image, a calculated

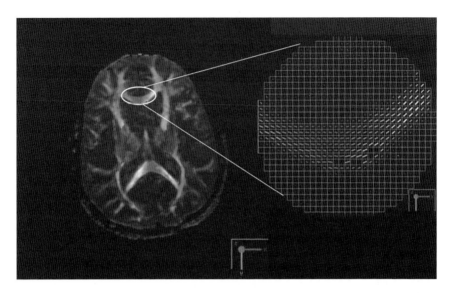

FIGURE 17-5. Directional image. In the image at left, diffusion direction (the orientation of the principle eigenvector) is color-coded to represent orientation along the three principle directions (cranial-to-caudal = blue; right-to-left = red; anterior-to-posterior = green). The enlarged view (right) shows the principle eigenvectors for each voxel in a region of interest in the genu of the corpus callosum. Notice that hue of each vector changes based on fiber orientation. (See color plate.)

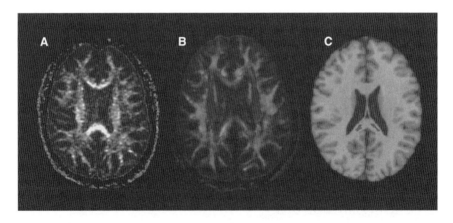

FIGURE 17-6. Fractional anisotropy. Visual inspection of grayscale (A) and color-encoded (B) FA images of a patient with traumatic brain injury do not demonstrate low FA. Yet, statistical analysis of this subject's FA images with reference to a group of age-matched control subjects' images identifies very significant (p = 0.0001) decrease in FA within the splenium of the corpus callosum in this patient (C). (See color plate, for parts B and C only.)

image. Thus, it is incorrect to speak of the signal intensity of an FA image. High pixel values, such as within normal white matter structures like the corpus callosum, reflect high degrees of anisotropy, and lower pixel intensities in gray matter and CSF correspond with lower FA. FA images may be presented using a grayscale display or color-coding. When color-coded, color indicates the direction of the principle eigenvector (as discussed earlier), and intensity represents the magnitude of FA. Additionally, the absolute degree of decrease in FA that might indicate a white matter lesion is not known and may be too small to be detected by simple observation. Quantitative analysis of FA images, however, has been used to detect white matter abnormalities in several disorders and may become a clinically relevant tool in the near future (Fig. 17-6C, see color plate).

Tractography

Arguably the most dramatic visual display of diffusion imaging has been achieved using relatively new techniques for white matter fiber tracking. Many approaches have been described for delineating white matter anatomy using DTI data, and it is still unclear which approach is best. Full treatment of these various approaches is well beyond the scope of our discussion. The essential concept of fiber tracking is that, if we begin at a single voxel—called the seed voxel—and identify the principle eigenvector (the dominant diffusion direction), we can next examine all surrounding contiguous voxels in an attempt to identify a continuous path of end-to-end alignment of principle eigenvectors as we traverse the data set. For example, choosing a seed voxel in the white matter of the centrum semiovale might result in depiction of a "fiber tract" following the corticospinal tract along its full length (Fig. 17-7A, see color plate). The resultant fiber tracts can be

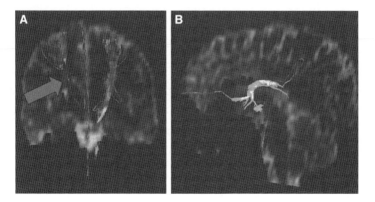

FIGURE 17-7. DTI fiber tracking. The corticospinal tracts (A) and fornix (B) have been delineated using DTI. Notice marked attenuation of the right corticospinal tract (magenta arrow) due to prior brain hemorrhage. (See color plate.)

used to assess the integrity of a white-matter pathway or show displacement of a tract by a mass lesion. Tractography may also be performed using two seed voxels (usually called a seed voxel and a target voxel, respectively) at points that might be connected by a white-matter pathway. The fiber-tracking algorithm will then determine if in fact a continuous diffusion path connects these two locations. This approach can be used to determine if connectivity exists between two brain regions (Fig. 17-7B, see color plate).

18
Understanding and Exploiting Magnetic Susceptibility

What Is Magnetic Susceptibility (χ) Anyway?

The term *susceptibility* often comes up in conversations about MRI images. Yet, in an admittedly nonscientific poll of MRI users, I found it rare that anyone really had a good idea what the term actually means. Coming to an understanding of magnetic susceptibility is worthwhile (really!) because it drives home the nature of what we will call susceptibility-related effects that we can observe in images. Those effects can be both informative and annoying, sometimes simultaneously. And, they are very common. Fortunately, the concept of magnetic susceptibility is pretty straightforward, even encoded, as a permanent reminder, in the term itself:

Magnetic susceptibility is the degree to which a substance becomes magnetized when exposed to a magnetic field.

Susceptibility-related effects result from spatial variability in the static magnetic field strength.

Effects on Magnetic Field Strength (B_{net})

Magnetic susceptibility is simply the degree to which a substance or tissue becomes magnetized on exposure to a magnetic field. We can think of magnetization as the generation of a local magnetic field B_χ by the substance when we apply a magnetic field B_0. Yes, that is the same B_0 used for imaging. B_χ is induced when the applied magnetic field, B_0, induces motion of electrons in the outer orbitals of a paramagnetic substance. That electron motion, in turn, induces a new magnetic field B_χ.

B_χ is a vector quantity just like any other magnetic field, and, therefore, it sums with the applied magnetic field B_0 that induced it in the first place! B_χ is small in proportion to B_0. Thus, in proximity to the paramagnetic substance, B_{net} will be the sum of $B_0 + B_\chi$. B_χ declines with distance from its source, and, far from it, $B_{net} = B_0$.

Whereas magnetic susceptibility always modulates field strength, B_χ will assume different orientation with respect to B_0 depending on the substance, and, as a result, different substances will cause a decrease or increase in field strength when B_χ sums with B_0. Diamagnetic substances lead to a decrease in field strength because B_χ is oriented opposite B_0, whereas paramagnetic substances cause a net increase in field strength because they induce B_χ oriented the same as B_0. It turns out that the effects of diamagnetism are quite small and generally do not lead to a meaningful alteration in B_0. Paramagnetic substances, on the other hand, may have very profound effects on field strength. Such paramagnetic substances are the cause of the susceptibility-related effects mentioned earlier.

Déjà Vu (See Chapter 1): Nuclear Paramagnetism

Just as the interaction of an applied magnetic field with orbital electrons in the sample will generate new magnetic fields in proportion to the magnetic susceptibility of the sample, interactions with nuclear charged particles can also result in such paramagnetic effects. This *nuclear paramagnetism* is in fact the very phenomenon we discussed in Chapter 1 that makes certain atoms produce the NMR effect. So what's the difference between electrons and protons? The difference is not absolute, but one of scale. Both electrons and protons can undergo NMR (called electron spin resonance or ESR when we are dealing with electrons) *and* produce paramagnetic effects. Nuclear paramagnetism is much stronger for protons (NMR) than for electrons (ESR) due to the much greater mass of the protons. Paramagnetism, the generation of bulk magnetization that perturbs the surrounding magnetic field B_0, is much greater for electrons. Both particles, however, exhibit both classes of effects to at least a small degree, so small that it may be virtually irrelevant and undetectable in MRI.

Those are the effects on static field strength. But who cares? We do not measure static field strength to make an MRI image.

Where It Really Counts: Effects on B_0 Homogeneity

What if we introduce a paramagnetic substance so that it is present at an absolutely uniform concentration and modulates field strength to exactly the same degree throughout the sample? All spins in the sample will precess at the same frequency, but that frequency will differ from ω_0 by a very small degree. Such small variation in the absolute frequency commonly occurs from day to day simply due variations in patient size and density or ambient temperature. We will ultimately see no effect on the signal we record or the appearance of the image we generate!

Principle Magnetic Susceptibility–Related Effects: Signal Loss and Distortion

Magnetic susceptibility–related effects occur only when B_0 is modulated in a manner that produces spatial variation in field strength. When B_{net} varies from point to point, neighboring spins precess at slightly different frequencies depending on the B_{net} they experience. This produces the susceptibility-related effects we see in an MRI image: signal loss due to dephasing and geometric distortion due to frequency shifts. We cannot emphasize enough that it is the induction of *variability* in the static magnetic field that produces the susceptibility-related effects we see in MR images. The paramagnetic substances do not produce any MR signal themselves. We only know that they are there as a result of their effect on the homogeneity of the static magnetic field.

A gradient of magnetic susceptibility will be present when adjacent tissues have different magnetic susceptibilities. The result is that a different B_χ is induced for each tissue's magnetic susceptibility, and we have a gradient of magnetic field strength. The consequence for our MRI image is the same as the consequence of an applied gradient magnetic field, such as those we have been dealing with since we introduced them in Chapter 5. When adjacent spins experience different B_{net}, they will precess at different ω_{net}. Each of two consequences of this spatial variation of ω_{net} will lead to one of the two principle susceptibility-related effects.

First, because the magnetic susceptibility gradients are continuous across the sample, they result in gradients across very small distances, even within a voxel. Thus, spins within a given voxel experience different B_{net}, precess with different ω_{net}, and, over time, lose phase coherence. The end result is lower M_t (AKA signal intensity) due to the magnetic-susceptibility gradient. This susceptibility-related signal loss is the first of our two principle susceptibility-related effects (Fig. 18-1).

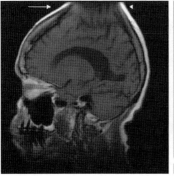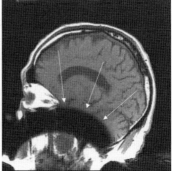

FIGURE 18-1. Magnetic susceptibility effects. A hairpin (left) causes gross distortion of the image (arrows) in the absence of signal loss. A necklace (right), though causing dramatic signal loss (arrows), leads to little distortion.

Second, we have been making extensive use of gradient magnetic fields to perform spatial localization in a variety of MR pulse sequences. The fundamental role of these linear gradient magnetic fields is to create an orderly and predictable gradient of B_{net} with a resultant orderly and predictable gradient of ω_{net}. If the spatial variability of ω_{net} is not predictable or even knowable, we cannot place signal in its appropriate spatial location. This is exactly what happens in the presence of a gradient of magnetic susceptibility. When we set up our pulse sequence and transform the signal into an image, we assume that ω_{net} is determined by the sum of the effects of the static and gradient magnetic fields ($B_0 + G$). In reality, due to magnetic susceptibility effects, ω_{net} is the sum of $B_0 + B_{net} + B_\chi$ (Fig. 18-1).

Proton-Electron Dipole Interactions: The Other Face of Paramagnetism

The paramagnetic phenomena we have discussed result from spatial gradients induced in the static magnetic field. An additional effect of paramagnetism occurs when unpaired electrons of the paramagnetic element interact on a one-to-one basis with the water protons that provide the MR signal. These effects are referred to as proton-electron dipole interactions (PEDIs), and they principally result in acceleration of the T1 and T2 relaxation processes. That is, paramagnetic substances shorten T1 and T2. As a result, we will see increased signal on a T1-weighted image and decreased signal on a T2-weighted image in the presence of paramagnetic substance. However, these are one-to-one interactions between a proton and an unpaired electron and will only occur if the distance between the proton and electron is less than 3 Å. Note that this requirement does not apply to the paramagnetic phenomena that result from magnetic field variability.

Examples of the PEDI in clinical MRI include the detection of hemorrhage and the effects of gadolinium-based contrast agents. Whereas PEDI does result in shortening of both T1 and T2, the effect on T2 is modest in comparison with the potentially profound shortening of T1. Thus, small amounts of a paramagnetic substance (such as the typical intravenous dose of gadolinium-containing contrast agents) will not noticeably alter signal due to T2 shortening.

Susceptibility-Related Effects I: Artifacts

The manifestations of the magnetic susceptibility artifact are discussed in Chapter 10 and demonstrated in Figure 18-1. Note that any paramagnetic material such as blood or stainless steel can produce these artifacts (Fig. 18-2). The severity of the artifact (signal loss or distortion) will scale with

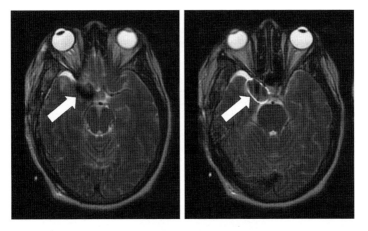

FIGURE 18-2. Nonferromagnetic metal causing magnetic susceptibility artifact. This patient's MRI-safe, nonferromagnetic Elgiloy aneurysm clip (Sugita Elgiloy, Mizuho Medical, Tokyo) causes modest signal loss and distortion (arrow). A ferromagnetic clip (that should, of course, *never* be imaged with MRI) would create a dramatically larger artifact.

the magnitude of the magnetic susceptibility gradient conferred by the paramagnetic material. The artifacts can be troublesome, as in dramatic image distortion due to orthodontic hardware (see Fig. 10-5), but can also provide diagnostic information as in the detection of blood products.

Susceptibility-Related Effects II: Hemorrhage

The exquisite ability of MR images to distinguish different blood breakdown products and, as a result, to accurately determine the age of a hematoma is well-known and of great clinical value. Diagnostic information derives from the paramagnetic nature of hemoglobin and its effect on the MR image. The hemoglobin molecule is made of four subunits, each containing a single atom of iron (Fe). The oxidation state of hemoglobin as well as the shape of the hemoglobin molecule governs the effect of hemoglobin on the MRI signal; hemoglobin does not itself produce any MRI signal. We detect its effect on signal arising from tissue water protons.

An overview of hemoglobin breakdown and the effects of each stage on relaxation parameters and signal intensity are shown in Table 18-1. Images showing the different stages are shown side-by-side in Figure 18-3. Note that the evolution of hemoglobin breakdown is a *continuum*. It is likely that you will see evidence of more than one stage in a single image. Because a hematoma evolves from the outside in, changes will occur first in the

TABLE 18-1. Evolution of hemorrhage: timing, physiology, and MRI.

Time frame	Blood product	Location	Susceptibility	T1	T2	T2′	T1 weighted	T2 weighted	T2* weighted
Hours	Oxyhemoglobin	Intracellular	Diamagnetic	—	—	—	—	—	—
Days	Deoxyhemoglobin	Intracellular	Paramagnetic	—	—	⇓	—	⇓	⇓⇓
Weeks	Methemoglobin	Intracellular	Paramagnetic	⇓	⇓	⇓	⇑	⇓	⇓⇓
Months	Methemoglobin	Extracellular	Paramagnetic	⇓	⇓	—	⇑	—	—
Months	Hemosiderin	Intracellular	Super-paramagnetic	—	—	⇓⇓	⇓	⇓⇓	⇓⇓⇓⇓
Months	Ferritin	Extracellular	Ferromagnetic	—	—	⇓⇓	⇓	⇓⇓	⇓⇓⇓⇓

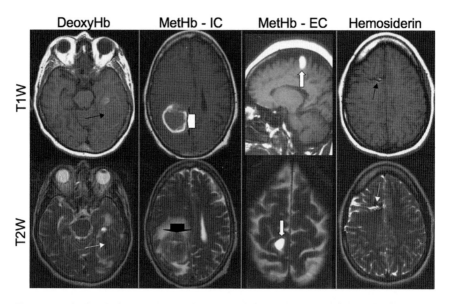

FIGURE 18-3. Evolution of hemorrhage on MRI images. The top row shows spin echo images acquired with short TE and short TR to confer T1 contrast. The bottom row shows TSE images acquired with long TE and long TR to confer T2 contrast (second from right is a spin echo image, rather than TSE). The hemorrhagic tumor (far left) shows intermediate signal on the T1-weighted image (black arrow) and low signal on the T2-weighted image (white arrow), reflecting deoxyhemoglobin (DeoxyHb). A different hemorrhagic tumor (second from left) shows a slightly later stage. Only the periphery of the hematoma shows high signal on the T1-weighted image (large white arrow) due to methemoglobin. The entire hematoma exhibits low signal on the T2-weighted image (large black arrow), as intracellular methemoglobin (MetHb-IC) and deoxyhemoglobin both induce signal loss. The primary cortical hemorrhage (second from right) exhibits high signal on both images (thick arrows) due to extracellular methemoglobin (MetHb-EC). The chronic primary hematoma (far right) shows a dark rim (white arrow) at the periphery of an area of volume loss. The appearance of high signal on the T1-weighted image (black arrow) is due to distortion and displacement of signal caused by the superparamagnetic hemosiderin and ferromagnetic ferritin.

periphery of a hematoma, with earlier stages of hemoglobin breakdown persisting the longest within the center of the hematoma.

Oxyhemoglobin: The "Hyperacute" Phase

In normal arterial blood, more than 90% of hemoglobin will be present as oxyhemoglobin. Although the iron in each subunit of the oxyhemoglobin molecule is paramagnetic (Fe^{+2}), because of the complementary effects of bound oxygen, oxyhemoglobin is diamagnetic. As a diamagnetic substance, oxyhemoglobin will not modify the relaxation parameters of tissue. As a result, we will not detect it, per se, using MRI. "Hyperacute" hematoma can alter the signal on the MR image very slightly. This, however, is due to the serum component of blood (water and protein) and *not* oxyhemoglobin. Most importantly, oxyhemoglobin vanishes so quickly that patients are almost never imaged soon enough to detect it.

Deoxyhemoglobin: The "Acute" Phase

Once hemorrhage occurs and blood has left the circulation, oxygen is rapidly depleted and deoxyhemoglobin becomes the predominant species within the hematoma during the first days. Whereas the state of iron in the deoxyhemoglobin molecule (Fe^{+2}) is unchanged, the absence of bound oxygen leaves the hemoglobin paramagnetic. As a result, we would expect two effects to result: magnetic susceptibility gradients and PEDI.

Gradients of magnetic susceptibility are a prominent characteristic of deoxyhemoglobin. It is actually the gradient of magnetic susceptibility between the intracellular space containing deoxyhemoglobin and the extracellular space where it is absent that leads to prominent signal loss on T2*-weighted images such as GRE.

Despite the fact that deoxyhemoglobin is quite paramagnetic, it does not demonstrate signal enhancement due to the PEDI. This is because the conformation

Can't a spin echo recover signal lost due to magnetic susceptibility effects?

Although we expect that a spin echo pulse sequence should compensate for signal loss due to magnetic susceptibility gradients, the reality is otherwise. Signal loss will also be quite evident on a T2-weighted spin echo image. This is thought to be due to the fact that protons are constantly diffusing both within and across the red cell membranes during the imaging process. As a result, the distribution of protons and hemoglobin and, as a result, the gradient of magnetic susceptibility is constantly changing. Recall that in Chapter 3 we learned that the spin echo is only able to compensate for variability in the static magnetic field if the spatial distribution of spins with respect to the variability of the magnetic field is invariant.

of the deoxyhemoglobin molecule shields the Fe^{+2} from water protons. Because water protons and iron electrons cannot come within 3 Å of each other, PEDIs will not occur. Thus, deoxyhemoglobin will cause neither signal loss nor augmentation on a T1-weighted image.

Methemoglobin: The "Subacute" Phase

After two days or so, deoxyhemoglobin will be oxidized to methemoglobin (pronounce it met-hemoglobin), with the iron moving to the Fe^{+3} state. The additional unpaired electron (five total) makes methemoglobin more strongly paramagnetic than deoxyhemoglobin. Perhaps most importantly, methemoglobin undergoes a significant conformational change that exposes the Fe electrons. They can now interact with water protons. As a result, the PEDI becomes a prominent feature of methemoglobin. In fact, methemoglobin is the *only* blood product to exhibit signal enhancement due to the PEDI. That's a little pearl that can make it much easier to keep the appearances of hemorrhage straight: if you see high signal on a T1-weighted image, the *only* blood product it can be due to is methemoglobin.

Methemoglobin manifests as low signal on T2- and T2*-weighted images for the same reason as deoxyhemoglobin. However, this characteristic of methemoglobin lasts only as long as the red cells themselves.

Location, Location, Location!

During the weeks that methemoglobin is present, another important change occurs. As the red cells degrade and die, they will swell and ultimately lyse. As a result, methemoglobin held within the cells will be released into the extracellular space. The importance of this event for MRI is that the concentration of paramagnetic methemoglobin becomes much more uniform throughout the now liquefying clot. When methemoglobin resides within the red cells, large gradients of magnetic susceptibility exist between the intracellular compartment containing paramagnetic methemoglobin and the extracellular space where no paramagnetic material is present. After the red cells lyse, we have paramagnetic methemoglobin dispersed at a relatively uniform concentration throughout the hematoma. Remember that, without a *gradient* of magnetic susceptibility, we will not have spatial variation in the magnetic field and will not see signal loss due to that variability.

In the absence of magnetic susceptibility gradients, signal is dominated by the serum components of the hematoma. The T2 of serum, longer than that of tissue, confers higher signal on T2-weighted images. High signal on T1-weighted images due to the PEDI persists unchanged because it depends only on the proximity of Fe in the hemoglobin and water protons. This high signal intensity remains *the* hallmark of methemoglobin whether it is intra- or extracellular.

Hemosiderin and Ferritin: The "Chronic" Phase

In the months and years after hemorrhage, the hematoma is completely liquefied, leaving a cavity filled with fluid and perhaps heme pigments. Iron is scavenged by macrophages that infiltrate the margins of the cavity to remain there forever. These cells are laden with hemosiderin and, to a lesser extent, ferritin. Both are composites of numerous hemoglobin molecules with a core containing thousands of Fe^{3+} atoms embedded in a relatively thick jacket of protein. These highly paramagnetic molecules are described as superparamagnetic and ferromagnetic, respectively. They have much more profound effects on magnetic field variability and thus lead to profound signal loss. The signal loss is typically distributed in a ring surrounding the hematoma cavity. Signal loss is increasingly noticeable on T1-weighted, T2-weighted, and T2*-weighted images, respectively. The dramatic increase in the intensity and extent of signal loss seen on T2*-weighted images compared with T2-weighted (i.e., spin echo) images is termed *blooming* (Fig. 18-4). The degree of magnetic field gradient induced by both hemosiderin and ferritin may in fact cause distortion of the MR image (Fig. 18-4).

Analogous to the case of deoxyhemoglobin, the Fe atoms in both hemosiderin and ferritin are shielded from close interaction with water protons because of the thickness of the protein portion of the molecule surrounding the iron core. As a result, PEDI cannot occur. Because the electrons of the iron core and water protons cannot get closer than 3 Å, we will not see

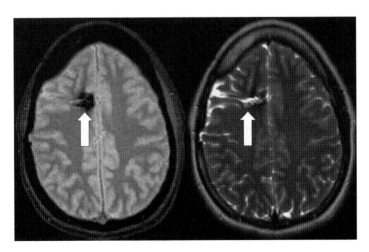

FIGURE 18-4. Blooming. The area of hemosiderin deposition (arrow) demonstrates much greater signal loss on the gradient echo image (left) than on the TSE image (right).

increase in signal on T1-weighted images despite the strong paramagnetism of the iron-containing molecules.

Susceptibility-Related Effects III: Contrast Agents

Several contrast agents are available for use in MRI, each falling into one of several classes. It is important to recognize that these agents are drugs. Although they have been extensively tested and shown to be effective and safe, they do have toxicity and should be used with prudence. The detailed study of contrast agents, particularly their chemistry and pharmacology, is well beyond the scope of our discussion and will not be addressed here. We will, however, take a brief look at two classes of agents based on their physical effects during MRI.

Exploiting the PEDI Effect

The most commonly used MRI contrast agents are based on the gadolinium (Gd) ion, which is strongly paramagnetic, possessing nine unpaired electrons. We will not consider the various Gd-based agents, as they all function in essentially the same manner from the point of view of the image. The most widely used effect of these paramagnetic contrast agents is their ability to profoundly shorten T1, even at low concentration. This effect was demonstrated in Chapter 4 (see Figs. 4-5 and 4-6). Whereas T2 is also shortened due to the PEDI effect, the magnitude of that effect is small and of little consequence in imaging.

Creating Spatial Variability in the Magnetic Field

If a paramagnetic substance accumulates in the region we are trying to enhance, it will generate variability in field strength that can be detected as signal loss. Several agents have been developed that exploit this effect. Very small ferromagnetic particles (superparamagnetic iron oxides, or SPIOs) have been injected intravenously, after which they are taken up by the reticuloendothelial system, including liver Kupffer cells. As a result, signal within normal liver is dramatically attenuated, causing pathologic tissue such as metastases to stand out. Similar particles or even smaller ones have been used to create an intravascular contrast agent and to bind to bioactive molecules for service as functional contrast agents. These agents are not, however, currently approved for clinical use in humans. Intravascular contrast can also be achieved by delivering a rapid bolus of a Gd-based contrast agent. In sufficient concentration, large local magnetic susceptibility gradients will develop in the bloodstream. Delivery of a compact bolus, requiring high volume and rate as well as rapid imaging, is essential if a substantial effect is to be detected.

Susceptibility-Related Effects IV: Perfusion Imaging

This type of perfusion imaging is generally referred to as *dynamic suscep-tibility perfusion MRI*. This is because we detect the movement of blood as signal loss caused by temporal change in magnetic susceptibility gradients induced by changes in the concentration of the contrast agent over time. Using a large, rapid bolus injection of a Gd-based contrast agent during rapid imaging, we can observe the transit of a bolus through the cerebro-vascular circulation and use our observations to generate information about and images of cerebral hemodynamics. Although we will discuss the appli-cation of this technique to brain perfusion imaging, the same techniques are relevant to perfusion measurements in other organs.

Time Series

To understand perfusion MRI, we must first clarify the concept of a time series. Quite simply, we image the brain over and over again at a fixed interval. Let's say we require 30 axial slices to cover the whole brain. We would then, using a high-speed EPI pulse sequence, acquire the same 30 slices in exactly the same way every 1.5 seconds until we have a total of 40 sets of images (1200 slices). We now have 40 sequential samples of signal from each and every voxel in our 30-slice set of brain images, acquired in about a minute.

Let's make things a bit more complex. Ten seconds after the beginning of the time series, we will inject a bolus of Gd-based contrast material. Typi-cally, this will be 0.1 mmol/kg in 20 mL of contrast followed by a chaser of an equal volume of saline, all delivered at 5 mL/s using a power injector. Imaging and the injection occur in parallel with no interruption in the imaging time series.

After we have completed the time series, a computer is used to interro-gate the data. We can extract signal intensity from a region of interest (ROI) in cortex, for example, and plot the signal from that ROI in *each and every* image on a graph where signal intensity is on the y axis and time (i.e., image number) is on the x axis (Fig. 18-5, see color plate). Ultimately, the computer will plot this curve for each and every voxel in each of our 30 slices of the brain, and we will compute hemodynamic parameters for each voxel in order to generate images displaying the hemodynamic parameters.

The time versus signal intensity curve shows the change in signal intensity that occurs with transit of the contrast bolus. An initial sharp decline in signal is followed by recovery as the first pass of contrast washes out of the tissue. Signal does not, however, return quite to baseline. There is a second shallow dip followed by a return closer, but still not all the way, to the pre-injection baseline. Signal does not return all the way to baseline because a small fraction of the contrast agent crosses the capillary membrane into

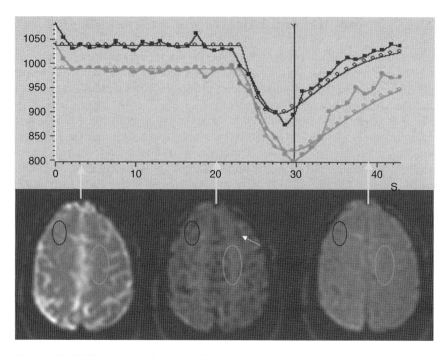

FIGURE 18-5. Time series for perfusion imaging. Signal loss occurs with wash-in of the contrast bolus and resolves with washout. Colored circles (bottom) indicate the regions of interest from which the time versus signal curves (top) were extracted. (See color plate.)

tissue. Subsequent release of this absorbed contrast agent leads to a second smaller dip. Yes, this does occur even in the presence of the intact blood-brain barrier. Newer agents have been developed that bind Gd to larger molecules that remain completely intravascular. These agents, which are not yet available in the United States, may be important if they truly facilitate measurement of purely intravascular blood flow.

Hemodynamic Measures

It turns out that the time versus signal intensity curve is essentially the inverse of the time versus concentration curve for the contrast agent. That is, signal declines in proportion to the change in concentration of Gd at a given voxel. We can thus use the time versus concentration curve to compute the hemodynamic parameters that describe transit of the bolus. Figure 18-6, see color plate, details the computation of several commonly measured parameters. Arrival time (T_0) and time to peak (TTP) are simply the time interval from injection to the initial deflection and peak height of the time versus concentration curve, respectively. The mean transit time (MTT)

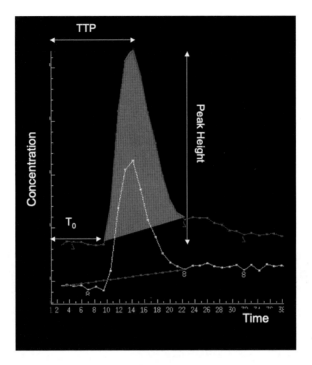

FIGURE 18-6. Hemodynamic parameters. The time versus signal curve is essentially the inverse of the time versus concentration curve (shown here after gamma variate fitting). Timing is easily measured as indicated by T_0 and TTP. Area under the curve (shaded in green) is proportional to CBV, and peak height has been used as a very rough estimate of relative CBF. (See color plate.)

represents the time required for the contrast agent to traverse the vascular bed. It can be estimated as the full-width at half-maximum (FWHM) of the time versus concentration curve. Cerebral blood volume (CBV) is a measure of microvascular volume and is derived from the area under the time versus concentration curve. Cerebral blood flow (CBF) cannot be measured directly, but it can be computed by using the central volume theorem:

$$CBF = \frac{CBV}{MTT}$$

Peak height is also used as a *gross* estimate of CBF. The results of these calculations will not be quite accurate, however, because the equations assume that the contrast agent arrives at a single instant in time. The equation can be made more complex to account for the actual delivery of the contrast agent, but it is generally simpler to treat dynamic susceptibility MRI as a relative measurement. Thus, it is useful to compare parameters across brain regions. Making comparisons of absolute measurements across scans and subjects is more likely to be fraught with error.

Hemodynamic Parameter Images

Each hemodynamic measurement is generally displayed as an image. Values of CBV, for example, will be assigned to a color or a gray scale, and the color or the shade of gray corresponding with the CBV measured at a given voxel will be entered into the appropriate pixel in the image. Such hemodynamic images permit the visual assessment and display of spatial variations in a given parameter, such as those due to ischemic penumbra surrounding an infarct (Fig. 18-7, see color plate). It is also important to

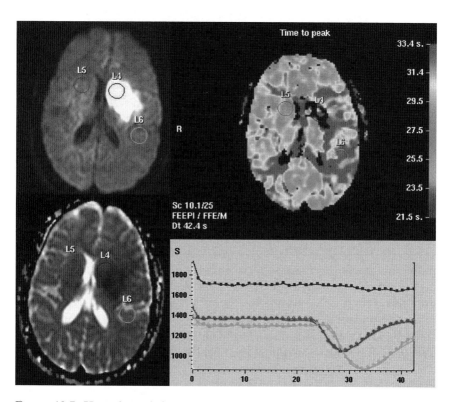

FIGURE 18-7. Hemodynamic images. In this case of acute stroke, diffusion imaging (DWI at upper left and ADC at lower left) confirm a region of infarction. The TTP map (upper right) shows delayed arrival of the contrast bolus in an area much larger than indicated by the DWI images. Time versus signal curves extracted from regions of interest in the core (dark blue) and periphery (turquoise) of the infarct as well as the unaffected contralateral cerebral hemisphere (magenta) confirm the presence of an ischemic penumbra surrounding the infarct core. (See color plate.)

examine the time versus intensity curves, comparing curves from several ROIs side by side to confirm that a significant difference is present.

Susceptibility-Related Effects V: Functional MRI

Many of the MRI techniques we have discussed, diffusion and perfusion for example, evaluate physiology rather than structure. Although we might consider these functional imaging techniques, the term *functional MRI* (fMRI) specifically connotes the imaging of brain activity. At this time, however, MRI is not capable of directly measuring electrical neural activity in a useful way. What we can measure is the hemodynamic phenomenon that goes hand-in-hand with such electrical activity. In 1990, Seiji Ogawa described the principles that ultimately led to the current explosion of interest in and application of fMRI. The science and practice of fMRI has become so sophisticated that even a basic discussion is beyond our scope. What we will do is introduce the basic physiologic principles of fMRI, describe a simple acquisition scheme, and take a basic look at the results we can expect. Several excellent resources for further study are provided in Appendix 4.

Consider a clinical example. A patient with intractable epilepsy is referred for presurgical fMRI. The proposed surgical procedure may put brain regions that govern language at risk of damage, and the surgical team wishes to determine the location of the patient's language areas prior to surgery. The fMRI team has designed a test to stimulate activity in the brain regions involved in language processing. The patient will be shown pictures of common objects and asked to think of the name of each object as it pops up on a video screen.

Physiology of fMRI

The principal effect in fMRI is termed *blood oxygen level–dependent* (BOLD) contrast. This refers to a change in the ratio of deoxyhemoglobin to oxyhemoglobin detected as a change in signal intensity due to the variation in local magnetic susceptibility. Local is key: these effects occur in the immediate vicinity of brain activity while other uninvolved brain regions maintain normal baseline hemodynamics.

When, as in the example above, a brain region becomes active, neurons in that region will exhibit more electrical activity than in the resting state. Such neural activity requires metabolism, which in turn requires the basic substrates of metabolism: oxygen, and glucose. Initially, extraction of oxygen from the blood tips the balance toward deoxyhemoglobin. Subsequently, a local hemodynamic response develops whereby both CBV and CBF increase in the immediate vicinity of the active brain region. As a result, supply of oxygen exceeds prior demand, and the hemoglobin ratio favors oxyhemoglobin. Other brain regions that remain in the resting state do not receive the same hemodynamic response and show no change in signal intensity.

The hemodynamic response, diagrammed in Figure 18-8, requires about 6 to 9 seconds to fully evolve in response to a single stimulus. Initially, signal intensity drops with the increase in oxygen extraction. This event occurs very early and is of very small magnitude. As a result, it is only detected under special conditions and is not relevant to typical fMRI applications. Subsequently, a progressive increase in signal intensity occurs until a plateau. This increase in signal is the BOLD contrast we detect with fMRI. If the stimulus is repeated or maintained (in our example, we will continue the task for a total of 30 seconds), the plateau will persist. After stimulation ceases, signal will return to baseline over several seconds.

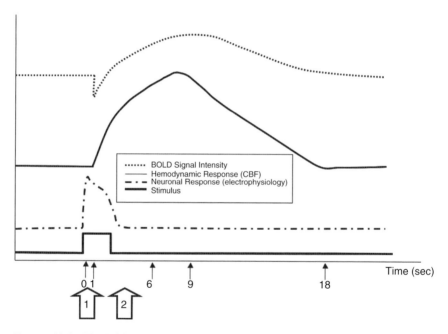

FIGURE 18-8. The BOLD effect. Shortly after onset of the neural response, increase in neuronal metabolism elicits, at first, an increase in oxygen extraction that causes a brief and small increase in the local concentration of deoxyhemoglobin and decrease in the MRI signal (open arrow 1). The onset of the hemodynamic response to neuronal activity results in an increase in the local concentration of oxygenated hemoglobin and in the MRI signal (open arrow 2). (Reprinted with permission from Yarmish G, Lipton ML. Functional MRI: from acquisition to application. *Einstein Journal of Biology and Medicine* 2003;20(1):2–9.)

The fMRI Acquisition

Like perfusion imaging, fMRI employs a time series. During the acquisition of a series of brain volumes at some set interval (typically 2 to 3 seconds), the subject will perform the task for periods of time interspersed with periods of a control task or simply rest periods. Many different stimulus paradigms have been described for use in fMRI. We will use a simple block design for our example. In this scheme, blocks of task performance (naming the pictures that show up on the screen) alternate with equal time periods where the subject simply stares at a small X in the middle of the screen.

fMRI Data Processing

A plot of signal intensity versus time, for our time series, is shown in Figure 18-9, in parallel with a plot of the stimulus paradigm. These data were extracted from a single voxel in a brain region that responded to the stimulus paradigm. As we can see, the MRI signal increases in sync with the stimulus paradigm, lagging behind by about 2 seconds. This response identifies the language region we were looking for. The full data analysis involves a computer examining the correlation between the time-course of signal change and the stimulus paradigm independently for each and every voxel. Voxels showing a good correlation are considered active; those not showing a good correlation are not considered active. We choose a statistical threshold to classify correlations as significant or not.

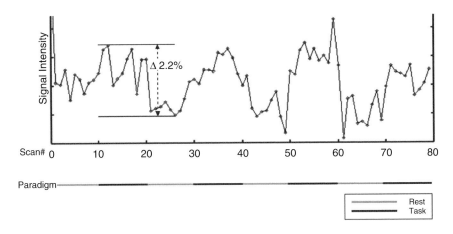

FIGURE 18-9. fMRI signal time course. Increases in signal intensity shortly follow the onset of the task. The delay represents the time required for evolution of the hemodynamic response. (Reprinted with permission from Yarmish G, Lipton ML. Functional MRI: from acquisition to application. *Einstein Journal of Biology and Medicine* 2003;20(1):2–9.)

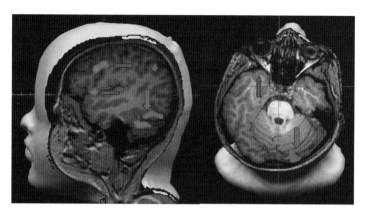

FIGURE 18-10. Three-dimensional display of fMRI results. Colored regions indicate areas where signal increased in sync with the onset of the stimulus. The subject viewed and was required to name pictures of common objects shown on a video screen. Responses are thus detected in visual (magenta arrows) and language (blue arrows) areas. (See color plate.)

The example described highlights essential components of fMRI data processing. In practice, many more steps including correction for head motion, filtering and normalization of signal across the time series, and more sophisticated statistical approaches are used. Once the active regions have been determined, they are shown as colored blobs superimposed on a high-resolution structural image, sometimes in three dimensions (Fig. 18-10, see color plate).

19
Spectroscopy and Spectroscopic Imaging: *In Vivo* Chemical Assays by Exploiting the Chemical Shift

Introduction

Spectroscopy (magnetic resonance spectroscopy; MRS) is often viewed (and marketed) as an advanced application of MRI. It is usually an add-on module that must be purchased from the manufacturer. This viewpoint is a strange one, as NMR was originally used for spectroscopy, and it was only after several "add-ons" that NMR spectrometers came to be used for imaging. Very-high-field research instruments designed for spectroscopy of homogeneous solutions held in test tubes are in fact sold with options to upgrade them for imaging of very small animals such as mice.

The Chemical Basis of MRS

In the early chapters of this book, we considered the signal arising from the sample to precess at one single frequency, ω_0. This is absolutely not true, however, unless we are imaging a completely homogeneous sample such as distilled water. As developed in our discussions of chemical shift in Chapter 12, our sample is composed of a vast array of unique chemical environments, each imposing small, but specific, variations on local magnetic field strength and, consequently, on the precessional frequency of spins in that neighborhood. Thus, spins in our sample or patient precess not at a single frequency but at a spectrum of frequencies. The components of that spectrum and which populations of spins precess at which frequencies on that spectrum are determined by the chemical composition of the sample.

MRS allows us to determine what frequencies are present in the sample and how much of the total signal is produced by spins precessing at each of those component frequencies. If we know the specific chemical environments that confer these frequencies (this has been determined by experiment), we will have, in essence, a chemical assay of living tissue.

What Then Is Spectroscopy (MRS) and How Is It Different from MRI?

Put most simply, spectroscopy results when we take the Fourier transform of the NMR signal *in the absence of applied magnetic field gradients*. Things are not entirely that simple, of course, but the description does encapsulate the basics. Remember, as we learned in Chapter 6, the Fourier transform of the MR signal yields a list of frequencies, each with a corresponding signal amplitude. In the presence of a gradient magnetic field, those frequencies correspond with locations in space along the dimension of the gradient magnetic field. In the absence of gradient magnetic fields, the frequencies are the actual precessional frequencies of spins in the sample. That we detect different frequencies reflects the fact that different populations

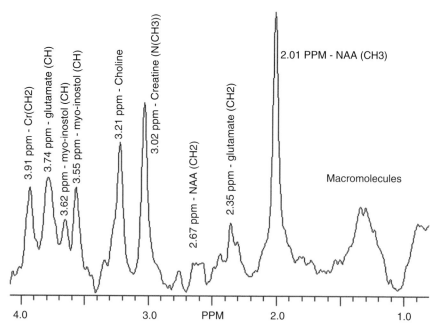

FIGURE 19-1. Normal proton spectrum from human brain. This spectrum acquired using STEAM at 3.0 Tesla demonstrates many resonances as indicated by the labels. Note that the NAA resonance occurs at 2 ppm. (Reproduced with permission from Baslow MH, Guilfoyle DN. Using proton MRI and spectroscopy to understand brain "activation." Brain Language 2007;102(2):153–164.)

of spins are subject to slight variations in static magnetic field strength due to their chemical environment. This is the chemical shift phenomenon described in Chapter 12. Each frequency corresponds with a unique chemical environment, and the magnitude of the signal detected for each frequency tells us the abundance of that chemical species in our sample. When we plot signal intensity on the y axis and frequency on the x axis of a simple line graph, we have the frequency spectrum (Fig. 19-1). The peaks, called *resonances* in the jargon of MRS, on the frequency spectrum represent unique populations of spins associated with one or more chemical shifts.

We speak of a proton spectrum when we are imaging in the proton frequency range. Spectra for other nuclei (e.g., ^{31}P, ^{19}F, ^{13}C) can be obtained by sampling in the range of ω_0 for these nuclei. However, this requires special RF, receiver, and coil hardware optimized for the correct frequency range.

Abundance, Resolution, and Detection

When looking at the proton spectrum, you may not realize that it has been, in a sense, edited. The actual proton spectrum is so dominated by signal from water that, were the water signal not suppressed, we would be unable to see any of the metabolites that we are looking for. The water signal is removed by applying a low-amplitude spectral presaturation pulse (CHESS, see Chapter 12) narrowly tuned to the precessional frequency of water. If tuned properly, water saturation will minimize signal from "pure water" leaving the signal from spins associated with other substances unchanged.

Whereas there are many different resonances of interest in biological samples, each causing a unique chemical shift, we cannot necessarily detect them all. Two main phenomena may impede detection of a given resonance. First, if the abundance of a substance is very low, it may not produce enough signal to be distinguished as a peak. That is, its signal amplitude may not exceed the baseline variability of our signal (the noise). This problem is also a function of the signal to noise of the measurement and may be alleviated by altering the acquisition pulse sequence, shortening the TE, acquiring additional signal averages, or performing the examination at higher field strength. Spectral resolution is the other limiting factor. If we are trying to distinguish two resonances that are very close together (i.e., have very similar chemical shift), we may not be able to identify them as separate resonances as their peaks may merge together. This difficulty is a function of the difference in the chemical shift between the two species. As we learned in Chapter 12, chemical shift is a function of field strength. Imaging at higher field strength yields a greater absolute chemical shift and may resolve closely spaced resonances (Fig. 19-2).

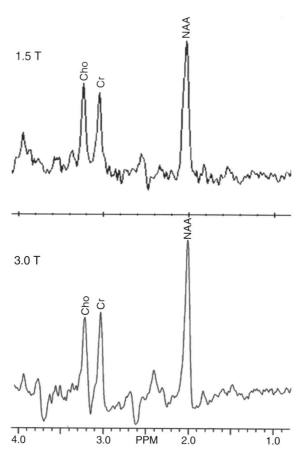

FIGURE 19-2. Field strength effects on spectral resolution. The spectrum acquired at 1.5 Tesla (top) shows a more irregular baseline due to lower SNR. Additionally, peaks are incompletely separated. At 3.0 Tesla, peaks are much better separated with return to baseline between the Cho and Cr peaks.

The Importance of Field Homogeneity

Gradients are the bane of the spectroscopist. In addition to the issue of spectral resolution described above, the ability to distinguish closely spaced resonances is a function of their spectral linewidth. In the presence of a magnetic field gradient, a single resonance that should be represented by, say, a range of 0.1 ppm, will appear to span a greater range of frequencies. As a result of this spectral broadening, adjacent resonances may overlap, limiting our ability to resolve adjacent peaks.

Toward maximizing spectral resolution (and of course, as with imaging, signal to noise), it is essential to ensure that the magnetic field, B_0, is as homogeneous as possible. To start with, the scanner should have good base-line homogeneity. Next, shimming (see Chapter 5) must be optimized over the region from which we will derive our spectrum. This is generally accomplished using a localized shimming routine where shim optimization is restricted to the immediate location we wish to interrogate. Optimally, high-order shims should be used, if available.

It is important to recognize that the advantage in signal to noise and spectral resolution available at higher field strength can be lost if shimming is not optimized. Because shimming becomes increasingly difficult as field strength increases, this concern is not trivial. Neither, however, is it insurmountable. Using appropriate and widely available methods, effective automated shimming can be achieved at high field strengths such as 3.0 Tesla.

Localization: Single-Voxel Methods

If we implement everything we have discussed to this point, the result will be a spectrum derived from all tissue that is excited by our RF pulse. If the RF is applied in the absence of gradient magnetic fields, the spectrum will arise from all signal within the coil. Using a slice selection gradient will cause our spectrum to derive from a known slice, but we will not be able to localize the source of signal to a particular location in that slice. To be useful for detection and characterization of disease, however, it is important to know where in the subject the spectrum arises. For this reason, several techniques have been developed that allow us to generate spectra localized in three dimensions. These techniques are called *single-voxel spectroscopy* (SVS) because we localize the signal to a single prism-shaped voxel. Note that though we may use gradient magnetic fields to select the voxel for excitation, it is essential that *no gradient magnetic field be present within the voxel* at the time we record the signal. If gradients are present, we effectively have a poor shim. Resultant spectral broadening may prevent us from generating a meaningful spectrum.

Two general approaches have been described for localizing a single voxel for *in vivo* spectroscopy. The first, less commonly used, employs gradient magnetic fields that disrupt homogeneity of the magnetic field only *outside* the voxel of interest (Fig. 19-3). As a result, severe spectral broadening occurs in the regions we do not wish to detect, and we will not detect signal from these regions. The second and more commonly applied technique uses slice selection gradients along three orthogonal dimensions in one of several implementations discussed below.

Stimulated Echo Acquisition Mode

In Chapter 3, we discussed the stimulated echo (STE) that results from any series of three (or more) RF pulses (see Fig. 3-7). Stimulated echo

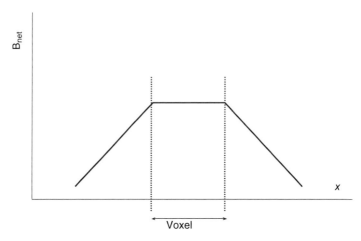

FIGURE 19-3. No gradient is present across the voxel of interest allowing acquisition of high spectral resolution. Gradient slope outside the voxel of interest causes so much broadening of spectral linewidth that signal from these regions does not contribute to the spectrum.

acquisition mode (STEAM) is a spectroscopy pulse sequence (Fig. 19-4) that employs a series of three $90°$ RF pulses, each applied in the presence of a unique slice selection gradient magnetic field. The three slice selection gradient magnetic fields must be orthogonal to each other. Thus, the only spins that experience all three RF pulses are those that lie within the prism-shaped volume of tissue at the intersection of the three slice selection gradients (Fig. 19-5, see color plate). We then space the RF pulses so that our chosen TE coincides with the peak of the resultant STE. Only signal from spins within our voxel generate the STE yielding maximal signal. Signal from spins outside the voxel will be so low that we will not even detect it.

An important advantage of STEAM is its ability to acquire spectra at quite short echo times (30 milliseconds). Using a short TE, of course, is a virtual necessity with STEAM because of the low-amplitude signal of the STE it produces. PRESS (see the next section), on the other hand, was previously limited by a longer minimum TE (144 milliseconds). The major disadvantage of STEAM, and the reason it has lost considerable popularity, is its relatively low signal to noise. It is more difficult to obtain high-quality spectra and to resolve lower-amplitude resonances using STEAM. This is, of course, especially so at lower field strength.

Point-Resolved Spectroscopy

The point-resolved spectroscopy (PRESS) pulse sequence (Fig. 19-6) uses a series of three RF pulses, each slice selective in one of three orthogonal dimensions. We generate signal with the first $90°$ pulse and then refocus that

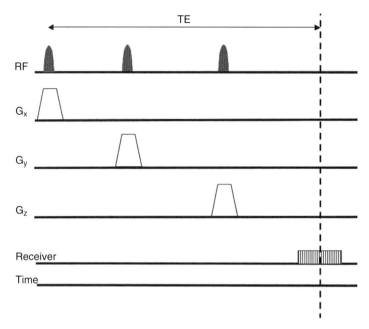

FIGURE 19-4. STEAM pulse sequence. A series of three $90°$ RF pulses, each slice selective in one of three orthogonal planes. Notice that all three gradients are being employed as slice selection gradients, each selecting a slice orthogonal to the other two, and no gradients are applied during signal readout. (For an explanation of the striped and solid symbols, see Figure 8-1.)

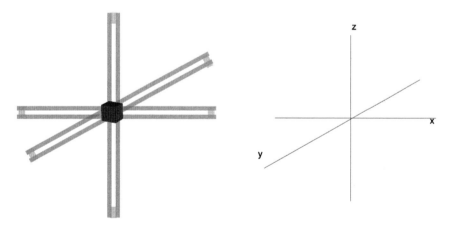

FIGURE 19-5. Spatial localization. Three orthogonal slices intersect so that the only spins that receive all three RF pulses are those within the voxel defined by the intersection of the slices. (See color plate.)

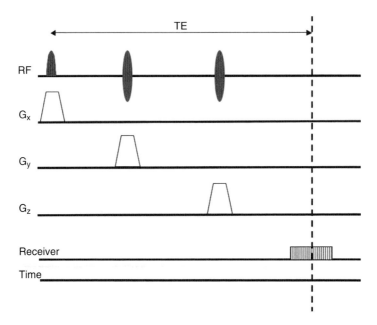

FIGURE 19-6. PRESS pulse sequence. By changing the last two RF pulses of the STEAM pulse sequence to 180°, we sample spin echoes rather than stimulated echoes with consequent improvement in SNR. (For an explanation of the striped and solid symbols, see Figure 8-1.)

signal twice using 180° RF pulses. Only spins at the intersection of the three slice selection slabs will be fully refocused and yield a spin echo at TE. All other spins will be out of phase to the extent that we will not detect their signal. PRESS is essentially a modification of STEAM that improves signal to noise by using 180° rather than 90° RF pulses. This allows us to sample a higher-amplitude spin echo rather than the lower-amplitude stimulated echo sampled using STEAM. Because newer implementations of PRESS allow for acquisition of spectra at short TE, some consider it to have effectively replaced STEAM, and at least one major vendor only provides PRESS as a clinical MRS acquisition tool.

Localization: Chemical Shift Imaging

Chemical shift imaging (CSI), sometimes called multivoxel spectroscopy, provides means for acquiring multiple spectra from a slice of tissue or even from a volume of tissue, all during a single acquisition. The approach is reminiscent of 3DFT imaging as we use multiple gradient magnetic fields, switched to a different strength during each TR, to "phase encode" along more than one direction (Fig. 19-7). These gradients each generate phase

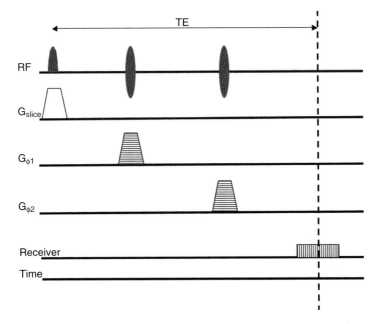

FIGURE 19-7. Chemical shift imaging pulse sequence. In this example of 2D-CSI, a single slice will be acquired using a single setting of G_{slice} but changinh $G_{\phi 1}$ and $G_{\phi 2}$ for each TR. For each setting of $G_{\phi 1}$, we must read-out a signal using each value of $G_{\phi 2}$. This fills one line of k-space. We repeat the entire process, during each repetition employing a unique strength of $G_{\phi 1}$ for each additional line of k-space (and each additional row of voxels) we wish to obtain. A 1D Fourier transform is applied to the group of samples acquired under each unique combination of $G_{\phi 1}$ and $G_{\phi 2}$, yielding a frequency spectrum derived from the entire slice and modulated by the strength of $G_{\phi 1}$ and $G_{\phi 2}$. The 2D Fourier transform is then applied separately to each point on each spectrum, yielding a spectrum for each location in the 2D grid. (For an explanation of the striped and solid symbols, see Figure 8-1.)

changes that reflect spatial information across one dimension of the image at a time. Essentially, we employ phase encoding along two dimensions. This approach is really the only choice, because frequency encoding cannot be used in CSI: the frequency-encoding gradient will create spectral broadening at the time we sample the signal, destroying chemical shift information. The phase-encoding approach utilizes gradient applications *only* during the time period preceding sampling of the signal. *no* gradient magnetic fields are present during readout of the signal.

If we perform this "phase encoding" along two orthogonal directions, we will have localized signal in two dimensions. That is, we will be able to extract spectra from individual locations within the slice that was excited. If we phase encode in all three dimensions, we will have a set of slices representing the 3D slab of tissue originally excited by the RF pulse. Spectra will be produced for each of multiple locations in *each* slice. Note that in

CSI, additional resolution is costly in terms of time, *no matter what dimension we increase resolution on*. For example, a 32 × 16 2D-CSI acquisition with a TR of 1500 milliseconds will cost 12.8 minutes. Increasing the resolution to 32 × 32 will take 25.6 minutes, and a 3D-CSI acquisition of four 32 × 32 slices will require 102.4 minutes of patient cooperation! For this reason, 3D-CSI is not commonly used in clinical practice. Nonetheless, high-resolution volumetric CSI may yet become part of routine practice as many groups are at work on techniques to dramatically accelerate CSI, including the application of parallel imaging techniques (see Chapter 15).

Although we can and do look at the individual spectra from each location in the CSI data set, results are also displayed as images (often called maps) representing the distribution of individual metabolites. The peak heights or areas of the choline resonance, for example, might be assigned specific hues on a color scale and displayed as a color-coded image superimposed on a structural brain image to indicate the distribution of choline. Similar images can be generated for other resonances as well as ratios of metabolites.

Brain Chemistry: Brief Overview of the Proton Spectrum

The major (and currently the only reimbursable) application of MRS is in the evaluation of brain disease. MRS has been applied to many different brain diseases, but it currently has the widest clinical application in the evaluation of brain tumors.

The normal proton spectrum may contain many resonances, but three are quite constant at 1.5 Tesla and above: choline, creatine, and *N*-acetylaspartate (NAA). My suggestion for remembering their locations is that they show up in alphabetical order from left to right, just like we read English (Fig. 19-1).

Neuronal Marker: N-Acetylaspartate

NAA occurs only in neurons, not nonneuronal cells such as glia. Its abundance correlates with neuronal health. Declines in the NAA resonance are seen in disease as well as in neuronal loss due to replacement by nonneuronal cells (e.g., glial tumors as in Fig. 19-8), necrosis, or apoptosis. NAA has a very consistent chemical shift of 2 ppm. This makes it the reference standard for determining scale on the brain spectrum.

Membrane Marker: Choline

The choline (Cho) resonance occurs at 3.2 ppm and generally has a peak height similar to creatine or perhaps a bit lower. This ratio, however, varies

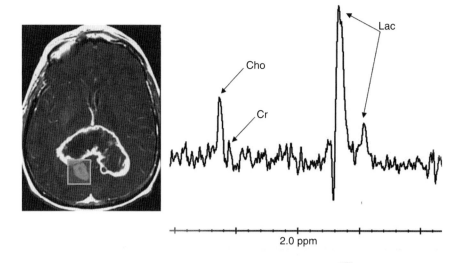

2.0 ppm

FIGURE 19-8. MRS of brain neoplasm. The proton spectrum was acquired from the shaded region using a single-voxel PRESS acquisition at TE = 144 milliseconds. NAA (2 ppm) is undetectable, as this glial tumor (glioblastoma multiforme) contains no neurons. The choline-to-creatine ratio is markedly elevated, indicating a very high degree of cellular proliferation. To the right, a large lactate doublet is present, a consequence of tumor necrosis and indicative of a very-high-grade tumor.

with brain region (e.g., gray vs. white matter). The choline resonance provides information about membrane turnover and destruction. Remember that phosphatidylcholine is an important component of cell membranes. In the presence of a proliferative process such as malignant tumor (Fig. 19-8), the choline level will rise in proportion to the degree of membrane formation. Conversely, in cases of tissue destruction such as infection, choline may decline.

The Reference Standard: Creatine

The creatine (Cr) resonance at 3.0 ppm has been thought to be generally unaffected by brain disease, at least at the precision required for clinical MRS. It represents both creatine and phosphocreatines. Because of its stability, creatine is used as a point of reference for gauging the abundance of the other metabolites. Because the absolute peak heights vary with field strength, scanner, and signal to noise of the individual measurement, referencing the peak height against creatine to create a ratio is very useful. For example, the NAA:Cr ratio is normally about 2:1. The elevations of choline seen in malignancy are judged by observing the Cho:Cr ratio. In fact, the magnitude of elevation of this ratio correlates not only with the presence of malignancy but also with tumor grade (Fig. 19-8). Be advised, however, that recent evidence suggests that Cr does in fact vary in different disease states.

Necrosis: Lactate

A lactate (Lac) resonance is not observed in normal brain. In the presence of necrosis, due to ischemia or tumor for example, a doublet (twin peaks) will manifest at 1.7 ppm (Fig. 19-8). It is important to distinguish the lactate resonance from fat, which, though wider, also occurs at about 1.3 ppm. Fortunately, there is a neat spectroscopy trick for differentiating lactate and lipid/fat. Recall that in our discussions of chemical shift (see Chapter 7) we learned that because fat and water precess at different frequencies, they will alternately come into and out of phase with each other. As a result, depending on the time we choose as TE, fat and water will be either in or out of phase with respect to each other. So, too, for lactate. At a TE of 144 milliseconds, lactate is completely out of phase with respect to the other metabolites. As a result, its resonance will be inverted on the proton spectrum. In addition, at this relatively long TE, signal from fat will be minimal, if present at all. The "take home message" is if you see a resonance to the right of NAA, double check (this might require acquiring a spectrum at TE = 144) whether it is lipid or lactate.

Tissue Loss: Myo-Inositol

This relatively small resonance occurs at 3.6 ppm and is thought to rise when the metabolite is released due to tissue damage such as in neurodegenerative disease. The normal myo-inositol resonance is not consistently seen, particularly at 1.5 Tesla. At higher field strength, it may be easier to detect, but it is most commonly seen when elevated due to disease. Incomplete water suppression may completely mask the small myo-inositol (mI) peak.

Neurotransmitters: Glutamate

A relatively broad peak at the left of the NAA peak (2.1 to 2.5 ppm) is seen due to the resonances of several neurotransmitters, principally glutamate (Glx). This group resonance may be obscured due to low signal to noise or, particularly at lower field strengths, merge with the NAA peak. The individual components cannot be differentiated except using specialized techniques at very high field strength.

Appendices

Appendix 1
Understanding and Manipulating Vectors

What Are They?

Simply put, a vector is a mathematical representation of two features using a single notation. Vectors have both magnitude and direction, making them ideal for representation of motion. For example, a speeding car can be described as traveling at 135 miles per hour. This is the *speed* of the automobile. Speed is a *scalar* quantity. That means that it tells us one thing and one thing only: magnitude. A vector, on the other hand, can be used to describe the *velocity* of the car, a quantity that implies both speed and direction of travel.

Vectors are shown on illustrations using an arrow notation. The orientation of the arrow and the position of the arrowhead indicate the orientation of the vector. The length of the arrow indicates the magnitude of the vector.

What Do We Do with Them?

The essential vector operation needed to understand the explanations used in this book is vector addition. As shown in Figure A1-1,when we plot two vectors that are each parallel to one of the axes of the coordinate system and have one end at the origin (0, 0), we can generate the vector sum or resultant of the two by simply plotting a line between the origin and the point indicated by the magnitude of each vector along the axis it is parallel to.

If we take the resultant vector just created, we can perform the reverse of our vector addition to generate the components of that single vector. This is referred to as vector decomposition.

What happens if the vectors we wish to add are not parallel to the axes? The first step is to decompose each vector into components parallel to the two (or three) axes of our coordinate system. Next, we add the component vectors parallel to each axis to determine a single vector parallel to each axis. Finally, we plot the resultant vector based on these final components (Fig. A1-2).

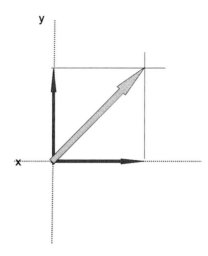

Figure A1-1. Vector addition. In this simple case, the position of the end of each vector (gray arrow) on the axis it parallels is used to plot the ending point of the resultant vector (dotted arrow).

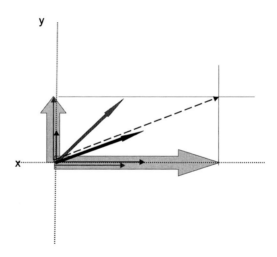

Figure A1-2. A slightly more complex case. In this case, the vectors we are adding (medium gray and black arrows) are not parallel to the axes. We decompose each into two components (thin gray and black arrows) parallel to one of the axes. Adding the components along each axis yields the components of the resultant vector (largest gray arrows). These are added as in Figure A1-1 to yield the resultant (dashed arrow).

Appendix 2
Glossary of Terms

The following list provides brief definitions for many of the terms and the jargon used in this book, with references to the chapters that define and explain the terms and concepts in more detail. Some terms that refer to general MRI terms do not have specific chapter references.

aliasing Misplacement of signal in an image due to undersampling. Other names: wraparound; foldover.

analog-to-digital converter (A2D) Device that periodically samples the analog signal to yield a series of measures of signal amplitude that can then be subject to digital processing. Other names: receiver.

anisotropic Motion *not* equal in all directions.

anisotropy A descriptor of the degree to which motion is anisotropic.

apparent diffusion coefficient (ADC) The measure of diffusion obtained using MRI. Note that ADC is used to describe both speed (no direction information) or velocity (includes direction of diffusion).

artifact Signal not reflecting the expected anatomic or physiologic appearance of the subject being imaged.

ASSET A parallel imaging technique. See Chapter 15.

b value Measure of the magnitude of diffusion sensitization.

b = 0 image An image acquired using the same pulse sequence as that used to acquire diffusion-weighted images but without applying diffusion-sensitizing gradients.

back projection A mathematical algorithm used to reconstruct a tomographic image (slice) from many unique projections through the slice. This approach is used routinely in CT but no longer is used in MRI.

bandwidth A range of frequencies.

blip Very brief application of the phase-encoding gradient during EPI.

bolus tracking A means for automatically detecting peak intravascular contrast concentration to initiate a CE-MRA acquisition. See Chapter 16.

Brownian motion The random movement of water molecules through a freely diffusible solute.

center frequency The frequency at which the dominant MR signal precesses. Although this can theoretically be calculated from the Larmor equation, due to subtle changes in field strength, center frequency must be determined during the prescan process. See Chapter 5.

chemical shift The degree to which the precessional frequency of spins in a given chemical environment differs from some reference frequency. The common reference standard is tetramethylsilane, and the chemical shift is expressed in ppm. See Chapter 7.

chemical shift imaging A form of localized spectroscopy in which unique spectra are obtained from a 2D or 3D array of locations and displayed as metabolic images. See Chapter 19.

coil The device in which the MR signal (M_t) induces voltage that can then be sampled by the receiver.

conjugate symmetry A characteristic of k-space in which diagonally homologous locations have the same value, and, as a result, one value can be used to predict the other.

conservation of energy Energy can only be transferred or transformed to a different state but never irrevocably lost. This is the first law of thermodynamics.

console The computer system that runs the MRI scanner and where the operator specifies the parameters to be used during imaging.

contrast A difference in signal amplitude between two tissues. See Chapter 9.

contrast agent A drug that is injected/instilled in order to enhance the contrast between tissues based on its preferential accumulation in one tissues or location.

contrast-enhanced MRA A high-speed MRA technique that relies on the intravascular concentration of a contrast agent, rather than inflow of non–steady-state spins, to generate high contrast.

contrast to noise A measure of contrast in an image. The difference in signal between two images is compared with the random variability of signal (noise) within the image. See Chapter 9.

cross talk See slice interaction.

cryogen Coolant, such as liquid helium and nitrogen, used to maintain the superconducting magnet coils close to absolute zero. See Chapter 5.

dewar The container containing the magnet coils and cryogens. See Chapter 5.

diamagnetic Substances with a magnetic susceptibility less than zero that interact weakly with a magnetic field causing repulsion of magnetic field lines. See Chapter 18.

diffusion For the purposes of MRI: the movement of water molecules through tissue. See Chapter 17.

diffusion tensor imaging An MRI technique that can determine both speed and direction of diffusion. See Chapter 17.

diffusion tractography An analytical approach to DTI that delineates the anatomy of white matter fiber tracts based on the direction of diffusion along that tract. See Chapter 17.

diffusion-weighted image An MRI image designed to show signal loss in proportion to the speed of diffusion within a voxel. See Chapter 17.

duty cycle The rate at which a circuit is cycled. See Chapter 5.

echo An increase in signal intensity due to RF or gradient pulses. See Chapter 3.

echo spacing The time between successive echoes in a fast spin echo pulse sequence. See Chapter 13.

echo time The time between the RF excitation and the midpoint of signal sampling. See Chapter 3.

echo train The number of echoes acquired during a single TR of a fast spin echo pulse sequence. See Chapter 13.

echoplanar imaging An ultrahigh-speed imaging technique. See Chapter 13.

eddy current Magnetic field gradients induced by the interaction of the gradient magnetic fields with hardware in the scanner bore. (Remember Faraday's law of induction.) See Chapter 5.

energy configuration The distribution across available energy levels. See Chapter 1.

entropy An index of the energy configuration of the system; at high entropy, the system is at a low energy configuration.

entry slice phenomenon Flow-related enhancement due to the entry of unsaturated spins into the slice(s) at the edge of the imaged volume. See Chapter 16.

Ernst angle The flip angle that yields maximum M_t for a given TR and a sample with a given T1. See Chapter 8.

even echo rephasing Signal due to flow that results at the even echoes of a multiecho spin echo acquisition where all TEs are multiples of the first TE. See Chapter 16.

excitation Application of an RF pulse to generate M_t. See Chapter 2. Other names: flip, nutation.

Faraday cage The shield that prevents RF noise from entering the scanner room. See Chapter 5.

Faraday's law of induction A moving magnetic field induces voltage in a nearby conductor. (The reverse is also true!) See Chapter 1.

fat saturation The suppression of signal intensity arising from fat. See Chapter 12.

ferromagnetic Substances with extremely high magnetic susceptibility that retain magnetization even after being removed from an externally applied magnetic field. See Chapter 16.

field of view (FOV) The dimensions of the sample that are represented in the image, *as long as receiver bandwidth (sampling rate) is sufficient to accurately measure all frequencies in the sample.* See Chapter 7.

Flip See excitation.

flow compensation Recovery of signal loss due to flow along gradient magnetic fields used during imaging. See Chapter 16.

flow-related enhancement High signal arising from moving spins that are less saturated than stationary spins. See Chapter 16.

Fourier transform Determines the component frequencies and their associated amplitudes contained within a single composite frequency. A mathematical algorithm used to reconstruct MR images. See Chapter 6.

fractional anisotropy (FA) A measure of the homogeneity of diffusion direction within a voxel. See Chapter 17.

frequency domain *k*-space data *after* the first Fourier transform. See Chapter 6.

frequency encoding Spatial localization by applying a gradient magnetic field *during* signal sampling. See Chapter 6.

functional MRI An MRI technique for detecting localized brain activation in response to a stimulus by measuring changes in blood flow, volume, or oxygenation. See Chapter 18.

gating Timing of the MRI acquisition to begin at a specific time during, for example, the cardiac or respiratory cycle.

gradient echo An echo produced by application of a gradient magnetic field that reverses the dephasing effect of a previously applied gradient magnetic field. See Chapter 8.

gradient-induced dephasing Signal loss due to motion (e.g., flow) along the direction of a gradient magnetic field, leading to phase accumulation and dephasing. See Chapter 16.

gradient magnetic field A magnetic field that changes strength along a linear dimension in space. (In MRI, gradients are *only* linear.) See Chapter 5.

gradient-moment nulling See flow compensation.

gradient speed The time required for a gradient magnetic field to reach full strength. See Chapter 5.

gradient strength The maximum slope of a gradient magnetic field. See Chapter 5.

gyromagnetic ratio A constant that describes the behavior of a specific nucleus when exposed to a magnetic field. See Chapter 1.

Heisenberg uncertainty principle At a fixed moment in time, we cannot—in the world of quantum mechanics—know the precise location and velocity of a particle. See Chapter 1.

hemodynamic response The increased in blood flow and blood volume that follows cerebral activation and is detected using fMRI. See Chapter 18.

high-velocity signal loss Low signal seen within blood vessels on spin echo images due to the fact that spins travel so fast that they are not refocused by the slice-selective 180° refocusing pulse and thus have low signal relative to refocused stationary spins. See Chapter 16.

interleaving The acquisition (excitation) of slices out of order to minimize cross talk. See Chapters 5 and 8.

inversion-recovery imaging A pulse sequence employing a 180° RF pulse prior to the RF excitation in order to impart a unique contrast due to differences in tissue T1 and/or to cause suppression of signal from tissues with a specific T1. See Chapter 12.

inversion time The time between the initial 180° RF pulse and the excitation (90°) RF pulse of an inversion-recovery pulse sequence. See Chapter 12.

isocenter The most homogeneous region of the B_0 field and the center of all gradient magnetic fields within the MRI scanner. See Chapter 5.

isotropic Equal in all dimensions. Generally referring to a cubic voxel or diffusion sensitization that is applied equally along all dimensions.

k-**space** The time-domain MRI data prior to application of the Fourier transform. See Chapter 6.

k-**space trajectory** The order in which data are written to *k*-space.

laboratory frame of reference Viewing precessing spins from an external stationary vantage point. See Chapter 2.

laminar flow Flow through a straight cylinder such that higher-velocity flow is present in the center and lower-velocity flow at the periphery adjacent to the walls of the cylinder. See Chapter 16.

Larmor frequency The frequency of precession at a given magnetic field strength. See Chapter 1.

longitudinal magnetization The component of magnetization whose vector is parallel to the vector describing B_0.

magnetic moment A measure of the strength of nuclear paramagnetism. Other terms: magnetic dipole moment. See Chapter 1.

magnetic susceptibility The degree to which a substance becomes magnetized when exposed to a magnetic field, generating its own magnetic field and thereby causing variation in the strength of the applied magnetic field. See Chapter 18.

magnetization transfer contrast Alteration in signal intensity that occurs after application of an off-resonance RF pulse, in proportion to the concentration of macromolecules. See Chapter 12.

maximum intensity projection A technique used to generate 3D images of the vasculature from MRA images. See Chapter 16.

MR angiography An MR pulse sequence sensitive to motion that is used to generate images of blood vessels. See Chapter 16.

MR hydrography Modification to a fast spin echo pulse sequence with filling of the periphery of *k*-space before the center to create images showing contrast between fluid and all other tissue but having poor soft tissue contrast. The technique is used for urography, myelography, and so forth. See Chapter 13.

multiecho imaging Acquisition of two separate lines of data after a single RF excitation. Each signal is acquired after an 180° RF pulse and is written to a separate *k*-space to generate two images, each with a unique TE. See Chapter 8.

multislice imaging Excitation of multiple slices during the TR of the first slice to improve time efficiency. See Chapter 8.

multivoxel spectroscopy Acquisition of spectra from a grid of multiple adjacent locations during a single acquisition. See Chapter 19.

net magnetization vector The vector sum of the magnetization of all spins in a sample. See Chapter 1.

noise Signal that we are not interested in. See Chapter 9.

nuclear magnetic resonance The basic phenomenon describing the behavior of nuclei in an applied magnetic field and their response to application of RF energy. See Chapters 1 through 3.

nuclear magnetism The magnetic field generated by protons in the nucleus of an atom. See Chapter 1.

nutation See excitation.

Nyquist rule To accurately sample a continuous function, samples must be acquired at least at one-half the period of the function. See Chapter 7.

odd echo dephasing Signal loss due to flow that results at the odd echoes of a multiecho spin echo acquisition where all TEs are multiples of the first TE. See Chapter 16.

opposed phase imaging Images acquired at a TE chosen so that fat and tissue (water) spins are 180° out of phase at the time the signal is sampled, leading to signal loss in voxels containing both fat and tissue. See Chapter 12.

oversampling Acquiring more samples than the desired resolution in order to avoid aliasing. See Chapter 7.

parallel imaging Accelerating imaging by simultaneously acquiring signal from more than one receiver coil and deriving spatial information from the location and sensitivity of the coil. See Chapter 15.

paramagnetic Substances with a magnetic susceptibility greater than zero that interact with a magnetic field causing attraction of magnetic field lines. See Chapter 18.

perfusion The transfer of molecules from the intravascular space to tissue, across the capillary membrane. See Chapter 18.

permanent magnet A magnet composed of ferromagnetic material that maintains its magnetic field without input of energy. See Chapter 5.

phase The orientation of two vectors, precessing around an axis, to each other.

phase coherence When two or more vectors have the same orientation.

phase-contrast MRA An MRA technique that exploits the predictable phase shifts that will occur with movement along a gradient magnetic field at a given velocity. See Chapter 16.

phase encoding The process for localizing signal in space based on the phase shift that occurs with multiple unique applications of a gradient magnetic field. See Chapter 6.

phase misregistration A flow-related artifact that occurs when spins are in different locations during phase and frequency encoding. See Chapter 16.

phased array coil Coordinated use of multiple surface coils to cover a large sample. See Chapter 5.

pixel The smallest element in a digital image.

precession Movement about a magnetic field in a trajectory describing a cone. See Chapter 1.

prescan A series of calibration and optimization procedures that are performed prior to the actual MRI pulse sequence. See Chapter 5.

proton density The number of protons per unit volume. A determinant of the MR signal intensity. See Chapter 4.

pulse Brief application of an RF or gradient magnetic field.

pulse sequence The series of RF and gradient pulses as well as signal sampling used to generate an MR image. See Chapter 8.

pulse sequence diagram A graphical representation of the series of events comprising the pulse sequence. See Chapter 8.

quadrature coil Two coils oriented at 90° to each other and used to simultaneously record two signals that are 90° out of phase, yielding improved SNR and sensitivity to tissue deep within the sample. See Chapter 5.

quantum mechanics A field of physics used to understand and explain the behavior of very small particles. See Chapter 1.

quench The sudden loss of magnetic field strength and boil off of cryogens that occurs when a superconducting magnet loses its superconduction. See Chapter 5.

radiofrequency field The rotating magnetic field used to cause excitation of the sample. See Chapters 3 and 5.

readout Sampling of the signal. See Chapter 6.

receiver See analog-to-digital converter.

receiver bandwidth The range of frequencies the receiver is capable of sampling accurately.

region of interest (ROI) A group of pixels from which a measure of, for example, signal intensity is made.

relaxation The return of spins to the resting state after excitation. See Chapter 3.

repetition time The time interval between successive RF excitation pulses. See Chapter 2.

resistive electromagnet A magnet composed of coils of wire at room temperature through which electric current is run to generate a magnetic field. When the electric current is discontinued, the magnetic field ceases to exist. See Chapter 5.

resonance Energy transfer between two objects will be most efficient when both possess the same natural frequency. See Chapter 2.

right-hand rule When curling the fingers of the right hand in the direction of current flow, the orientation of the thumb describes the orientation of the induced magnetic field.

rise time See gradient speed.

rotating frame of reference Viewing precessing spins from a vantage point rotating at the same rate as the frequency of precession. See Chapter 2.

rotating magnetic field See radiofrequency field. See Chapter 2.

sampling time (T_s) The time over which a single sample of signal is acquired. See Chapter 6.

saturation Reduction in the magnitude of M_z due to the application of successive RF pulses.

second law of thermodynamics Any system will move toward a state of maximum entropy. See Chapter 1.

selective excitation An RF excitation pulse tuned to selectively excite only a subgroup of spins in the sample, most commonly tissue, water, but not fat. Used as an alternative to fat saturation. See Chapter 12.

SENSE A parallel imaging technique. See Chapter 15.

shielding Hardware used to limit the spread of magnetic fields and RF signal. See Chapter 5.

shimming A means for optimizing homogeneity of the magnetic field. See Chapter 5.

signal Magnitude of transverse magnetization.

signal averaging Combining signal from multiple identical images to improve SNR. See Chapter 9.

signal to noise A measure of image quality. See Chapter 9.

single-shot imaging Complete acquisition of signal for an entire image after a single RF excitation. See Chapter 13.

single-voxel spectroscopy Acquisition of a spectrum from a single volume of tissue. See Chapter 19.

slab The volume of tissue excited during a 3DFT acquisition. See Chapter 14.

slew rate A measure of gradient performance. See Chapter 5.

slice The volume of tissue excited during a 2DFT acquisition. See Chapter 2.

slice interaction Saturation occurring when adjacent slices are excited in sequence. See Chapters 5 and 10.

SMASH A parallel imaging technique. See Chapter 15.

spatial presaturation An RF excitation used to eliminate M_z from tissue at a specific location so that it will not contribute signal to the image. See Chapter 12.

spatial resolution Voxel size, which determines the smallest increment that can be delineated by the image. See Chapter 1.

specific absorption rate A measure of RF power deposition. See Chapter 11.

spectral presaturation An RF excitation used to eliminate M_z from tissue with a specific frequency of precession so that it will not contribute signal to the image. Commonly used to suppress signal from fat. See Chapter 12.

spectroscopic imaging Multivoxel spectroscopy.

spectroscopy An NMR/MR technique designed to measure the signal strength of specific subpopulations of spins based on their unique precessional frequencies (chemical shift). See Chapter 19.

speed Rate of movement without specification of direction.

spin The smallest unit from which the NMR signal can be derived. Other terms: proton, nucleus. See Chapter 1.

spin angular momentum A phenomenon causing the spin to precess about B_0 rather than simply rotate. See Chapter 1.

spin echo An increase in signal that occurs after a 180° RF pulse. See Chapter 4.

Spin-lattice (longitudinal) relaxation The process of regrowth on longitudinal magnetization after an RF excitation. See Chapter 3.

Spin-spin (transverse) relaxation The process of decay of transverse magnetization after an RF excitation. See Chapter 3.

spoiling Destruction of residual phase coherent transverse magnetization. See Chapter 10.

steady state The magnitude of M_z that returns after a series of RF pulses. See Chapter 8.

stimulated echo An increase in signal after three or more RF pulses. See Chapter 3.

superconducting magnet A type of electromagnet that requires no ongoing input of electric current because the material used to make the magnet coils, if kept at a temperature close to absolute zero, conducts electricity without resistance. See Chapter 5.

surface coil A single loop of conductive material placed adjacent to the sample and used to record the MR signal. See Chapter 5.

T1 shine-through High signal due to very short T1, but not due to flow, that appears in a TOF-MRA image. See Chapter 16.

T2 shine-through High signal due to very long T2, but not due to low ADC, that appears in a diffusion-weighted image. See Chapter 17.

time domain The raw MR data prior to the Fourier transform. See Chapter 6.

time series Acquisition of multiple images or sets of images (e.g., brain volumes) in sequence. Commonly used for perfusion imaging and fMRI. See Chapter 18.

transverse magnetization Signal intensity. See Chapter 2.

truncation A limitation that becomes apparent when too few samples are input to the Fourier transform, which can lead to an MRI artifact. See Chapter 10.

turbulence Chaotic flow, as in the presence of luminal irregularity or stenosis. See Chapter 16.

undersampling Collecting of too few samples of the MR signal to correctly resolve all frequency components of the sample, leading to aliasing. See Chapter 7.

velocity Description of speed *and* direction of movement.

velocity encoding Setting of the flow-sensitizing gradient magnetic fields used in PC-MRA to be sensitive to a specific range of flow velocity. See Chapter 16.

voxel The volume of tissue from which signal is measured for each pixel in an MR image. See Chapter 6.

water suppression A form of spectral presaturation used to eliminate signal from tissue water. Essential for spectroscopy. See Chapters 12 and 19.

zeugmatomography An early form of MR image reconstruction. See Chapter 5.

Appendix 3
Glossary of Common MRI Acronyms, Abbreviations, and Notations

The following list contains many acronyms, abbreviations, and symbols that are in more or less common use in MRI. Not all of the items on this list are necessarily used in the book. I include them here for reference when you need to know what your local physicist is talking about when he insists on running MOSES or B0-PEEP on your next patient. MRI people have a real penchant for cute and unique acronyms, so there is no way this list could ever be considered complete. It is highly likely that many, many more such acronyms will be coined as this book goes to press!

α	Flip angle
γ	Gyromagnetic ratio
ϕ	Phase
ν	Frequency
ω	Precessional frequency
χ	Magnetic susceptibility
δ	Diffusion-sensitizing gradient duration
Δ	Diffusion-sensitizing gradient amplitude
ω_0	Larmor frequency
ω_{net}	ω due to B_{net}
2DFT	Two-dimensional Fourier transform
3DFT	Three-dimensional Fourier transform
ACR	American College of Radiology
ADC	Analog-to-digital converter
ASL	Arterial spin labeling
ASSET	Array spatial sensitivity encoding technique
B	Magnetic field strength
b	Diffusion sensitization
B_χ	Magnetic field strength due to magnetic susceptibility effects
B_0	Static magnetic field strength of the MR scanner
B_{net}	Net static magnetic field strength (=B_0 + G)
BOLD	Blood oxygen level–dependent

BTFE	Balanced turbo field echo
CASL	Continuous arterial spin labeling
CBF	Cerebral blood flow
CBV	Cerebral blood volume
CE-MRA	Contrast-enhanced magnetic resonance angiography
CHESS	Chemical shift selective
CNR	Contrast-to-noise ratio
CPMG	Carr Purcell Meibloom Gill
CSF	Cerebrospinal fluid
CSI	Chemical shift imaging
D	Diffusion
DAC	Digital-to-analog converter
DE	Dual echo or driven equilibrium
DFT	Digital Fourier transform
DICOM	Digital Imaging and Communications in Medicine
DRIVE	Driven equilibrium
DTI	Diffusion tensor imaging
DWI	Diffusion-weighted imaging
EFGRE	Enhanced fast gradient recalled echo
EPI	Echoplanar imaging
EPISTAR	Echoplanar imaging and signal targeting with alternating radiofrequency
EPR	Electron paramagnetic resonance
ESR	Electron spin resonance
ETL	Echo train length
EVI	Echo volume imaging
FA	Flip angle
FAIR	Flow-sensitive alternating inversion recovery
FAME	Fast acquisition with multiphase EFGRE
FC	Flow compensation
FE	Field echo
FFE	Fast field echo
FFT	Fast Fourier transform
FGR	Fast gradient recalled echo
FGRE	Fast gradient recalled echo
FID	Free induction decay
FIESTA	Fast imaging employing steady-state acquisition
FIRM	Fast inversion recovery for myelin
FISP	Fast imaging with steady-state precession
FLAIR	Fluid attenuated inversion recovery
FLASH	Fast low angle shot
fMRI	Functional magnetic resonance imaging
FOV	Field of view
FRFSE	Fast recovery fast spin echo

FSE	Fast spin echo
FSPGR	Fast spoiled gradient recalled echo
FT	Fourier transform
FWHM	Full-width at half-maximum
G_ϕ	Phase-encoding gradient magnetic field
G_v	Frequency-encoding gradient magnetic field
Gd	Gadolinium
G_{sl}	Slice select gradient magnetic field
rGE	Gradient echo
GHz	Gigahertz
GMN	Gradient moment nulling
GMR	Gradient moment rephasing
GRA	Gradient recalled acquisition
GRAPPA	Generalized autocalibrating partially parallel acquisition
GRASE	Gradient and spin echo
GRASS	Gradient recalled acquisition in the steady state
GRE	Gradient recalled echo
GSE	Gradient and spin echo
H	Magnetic field inductance
HASTE	Half Fourier acquisition single-shot turbo spin echo
Hz	Hertz
iPAT	Integrated parallel acquisition techniques
IR	Inversion recovery
ISIS	Image selected *in vivo* spectroscopy
kHz	Kilohertz
KT-BLAST	k-space time broad-use linear acquisition speed-up technique
LAVA	Liver acquisition with volume acceleration
M_0	Proton density
MAST	Motion artifact suppression technique
MDEFT	Modified driven equilibrium Fourier transform
MHz	Megahertz
MinIP	Minimum intensity projection
MION	Monocrystalline iron oxide nanocompounds
MIP	Maximum intensity projection
MOSES	Multiple oversampled slabs EPI sequence
MOTSA	Multiple overlapping thin-slab acquisition
MPR	Multiplanar reformat
MP-RAGE	Magnetization-prepared rapid gradient echo
MRA	Magnetic resonance angiography
MRCP	Magnetic resonance cholangiopancreatography
MRI	Magnetic resonance imaging
MRS	Magnetic resonance spectroscopy
MRSI	Magnetic resonance spectroscopic imaging

MRV	Magnetic resonance venography
mSENSE	Modified sensitivity encoding
M_t	Transverse magnetization (=signal intensity)
MTC	Magnetization transfer contrast
MTT	Mean transit time
M_z	Longitudinal magnetization
NAA	N-Acetylaspartate
NEX	Number of excitations
NMR	Nuclear magnetic resonance
NMV	Net magnetization vector
N_p	Number of phase-encoding steps
NPW	No phase wrap
NSA	Number of signal averages
N_{sl}	Number of slices
OVS	Outer volume suppression
PACS	Picture archiving and communication system
PASL	Pulsed arterial spin labeling
PCA	Phase contrast angiography
PEDI	Proton electron dipole interaction
PEEP	Phase-encoded echoplanar
PEPSI	Proton echoplanar spectroscopic imaging
POMP	Phase ordered (offset) multiplanar
PPG	Peripheral pulse gating
PPM	Parts per million
PPU	Peripheral pulse unit
PRESS	Point resolved spectroscopy
PRESTO	Principles of echo shifting using a train of observations
PROPELLER	Periodically rotated overlapping parallel lines with enhanced reconstruction
PWI	Perfusion-weighted imaging
Q-Flow	Flow quantification
QUIPPS	Quantitative imaging of perfusion using a single subtraction
RARE	Rapid acquisition with relaxation enhancement
REST	Regional saturation technique
RF	Radiofrequency
ROAST	Resonant offset averaging in the steady state
RSSARGE	Radiofrequency spoiled steady-state acquisition rewound gradient echo
RT	Respiratory triggered
RUFIS	Rotating ultrafast imaging sequence
SAR	Specific absorption rate
SARGE	Spoiled steady-state Acquisition Rewinded Gradient Echo
SE	Spin echo

SENSE	Sensitivity encoding
SI	Signal intensity
SMASH	Simultaneous acquisition of spatial harmonics
SNR	Signal-to-noise ratio
SPGR	Spoiled gradient recalled echo
SPIO	Superparamagnetic iron oxide
SPIR	Spectral presaturation with inversion recovery
SPOILED GRASS	Spoiled gradient recalled acquisition in the steady state
SSFP	Steady-state free precession
SSFSE	Single-shot fast spin echo
STE	Stimulated echo
STEAM	Stimulated echo acquisition mode
STIR	Short tau inversion recovery
SVS	Single voxel spectroscopy
T_0	Arrival time
T1	Longitudinal relaxation time
$T1_{app}$	Apparent T1
T2	Transverse relaxation time constant due to energy exchange between spins
T2*	Transverse relaxation time constant due to all effects
T2′	Transverse relaxation time constant due to B_0 variability
TE	Echo time
TE_{eff}	Effective TE
TFE	Turbo field echo
THRIVE	T1-weighted high-resolution isotropic volume examination
TI	Inversion time
TOF	Time of flight
TONE	Tilt optimized nonsaturated excitation
TR	Repetition time
TRICKS	Time resolved imaging of contrast kinetics
T_s	Sampling time
TSE	Turbo spin echo
TSI	Turbo spectroscopic imaging
TTP	Time to peak
Turbo-FLASH	Turbo fast low angle shot
UFSE	Ultrafast spin echo
UNFAIR	Uninverted flow-sensitive alternating inversion recovery
USPIO	Ultrasmall superparamagnetic iron oxide
VCG	Vector cardiogram
VENC	Velocity encoding
VEST	Volume excitation stimulated echoes

VIBE	Volumetric interpolated breath-hold examination
VIBRANT	Volume imaging for breast assessment
VINNIE	Velocity encode cine imaging
VOSY	Volume selective spectroscopy
WATS	Water selective excitation
ZIP	Zero fill interpolation processing

Appendix 4
Resources for Reference and Further Study

The following print and electronic sources are provided for those who wish to delve into one or more areas in more depth or just to see a topic from another vantage point.

American College of Radiology (2007). MRI Accreditation Program. Available at http://www.acr.org/accreditation/mri/mri.html. Retrieved January 10, 2007.
This site is an excellent resource on MRI QA as well as a source for the now famous ACR QA phantom.

Elster, A. D. and J. H. Burdette (2000). *Questions and Answers in Magnetic Resonance Imaging*, Second ed. Philadelphia, Mosby.
This outstanding book takes MR topics in small bites and, in a question-and-answer format, addresses them in great, yet understandable, depth. Even MR physicists find this a useful reference.

Haacke, E. M., R. M. Brown, et al. (1999). *Magnetic Resonance Imaging: Physical Principles and Sequence Design.* New York, John Wiley & Sons.
Not for the faint of heart, but an outstanding resource for a full mathematical treatment of MRI basics and extensive detail on the building of a pulse sequence.

Hornak, J. P. (2007). The basics of MRI. Available at http://www.cis.rit.edu/htbooks/mri/. Retrieved January 10, 2007.
This popular Web site provides concise explanations, often with animated illustrations, for the full range of MRI topics.

Jezzard, P., P. M. Matthews, et al. (2003). *Functional MRI: An Introduction to Methods.* New York, Oxford University Press.
An excellent introduction (in some detail) to fMRI from leaders in the field and authors of one of the preeminent fMRI software packages.

Kanal, E., J. P. Borgstede, et al. (2004). American College of Radiology White Paper on MR Safety: 2004 update and revisions. *American Journal of Roentgenology* 182(5):1111–1114.

Kanal, E., J. P. Borgstede, et al. (2002). American College of Radiology White Paper on MR Safety. *American Journal of Roentgenology* 178(6):1335–1347.
These two papers have become the standard for safe MRI practice.

Lipton, M. L. (2004). Keeping it safe: MRI site design, operations, and surveillance at an extended university health system. *Journal of the American College of Radiology* 1(10):749–754.

Practical implementation of an MRI safety plan with emphasis on site security and surveillance.

Mori, S., J. Zhang (2006). Principles of diffusion tensor imaging and its applications to basic neuroscience research. *Neuron* 51(5):527–539.

Although pitched for a basic neuroscience audience, this excellent review provides a lucid overview of DTI in significant detail.

Index

NSA. *See* Number of signal averages
Nuclear magnetic resonance (NMR),
    4–10, 37, 246, 285
  measurement of, 37
  prerequisites for, 6, 7–9
  quantum mechanics and, 12
Nuclear paramagnetism, 246
Nuclear spin, 6, 10
Nucleus, 6
  nuclear magnetism in, 9
Null point, 167
Number of signal averages (NSA), 106
Nyquist, Harry, 103
Nyquist rule, 103, 285
Nyquist-Shannon theorem, 103

O

Oblique gradient magnetic field, 60
Observer offset, 72
Odd echo dephasing, 207–208, 209, 285
Ogawa, S., 259
1DFT. *See* One-dimensional Fourier
    transform
One-dimensional Fourier transform
    (1DFT), 89–90, 96
Open-design permanent magnet, 48
Opposed phase shifting
  chemical shift and, 285
  TE and, 285
Orientation
  in CE-MRA, 223
  of magnetism, 17
  of NMV, 24–25
  of slice, 288
    location of, 81
Oscillating magnetic field, 22–23
Oscilloscope, 65
Outer volume suppression, 171
Oversampling, 106–107, 285
  aliasing and, 105–106
Oxyhemoglobin, 250–251

P

Parallel imaging, 194–199, 285
  acquisition schemes in, 196
  coil sensitivity in, 195
  contrast resolution in, 194–195
  imaging time in, 198–199
  k-space in, 194–195

phase encoding in, 194–195
  SNR in, 199
  susceptibility effects in, 199
Paramagnetic contrast agents. *See*
    Contrast agents
Partial flip angle, 124–127
Partial volume artifact. *See* Partial
    volume effect
Partial volume effect, 76
Partition. *See* Slice thickness
Passive shims, 54
PC-MRA. *See* Phase-contrast MRA
PEDI. *See* Proton-electron dipole
    interaction
Penetration panel, 70
Perfusion imaging, 285
  susceptibility and, 255–259
Period, 91
Permanent magnets, 49, 285
  SNR of, 50–51
  vertical fields and, 50–51
Phantoms, 130, 136, 137
  in MRA, 201
Phase, 285
  detection of, 92–93
  measurement of, 93
  rate of change to, 93–94
Phase coherence, 17, 92, 285
  of M_t, 24
  spin echo and, 32–33, 34
Phase encoding, 90–97, 286
  in 3DFT, 188–191
  with CSI, 271–272
  in parallel imaging, 194–195
Phase images, 64
Phase misregistration, 286
  in MRA, 206–207
Phase shift, by gradient magnetic field,
    92
Phase-contrast MRA (PC-MRA), 206,
    226–232, 285
  direction sensitivity in, 227–228
  VENC in, 228–230
Phased array coils, 64–65, 286
Phase-encoding direction, 106
Phase-encoding gradient, 97
Pixels, 76, 82, 286
  DFT and, 87
Plug flow, 202

Printed in the United States of America